Physiology and Pathophysiology of Iron in Humans

Physiology and Pathophysiology of Iron in Humans

Editor: Rosalia Kripke

AMERICAN
MEDICAL PUBLISHERS
www.americanmedicalpublishers.com

AMERICAN
MEDICAL PUBLISHERS
www.americanmedicalpublishers.com

Cataloging-in-Publication Data

Physiology and pathophysiology of iron in humans / edited by Rosalia Kripke.
p. cm.
Includes bibliographical references and index.
ISBN 978-1-63927-708-7
1. Iron--Physiological effect. 2. Iron--Pathophysiology. 3. Iron in the body. 4. Iron--Metabolism.
5. Iron--Metabolism--Disorders. 6. Iron--Therapeutic use. 7. Iron--Health aspects. I. Kripke, Rosalia.
QP535.F4 P49 2023
612.392 4--dc23

American Medical Publishers,
41 Flatbush Avenue,
1st Floor, New York,
NY 11217, USA

ISBN 978-1-63927-708-7 (Hardback)

Contents

Preface VII

Chapter 1 **Iron and Chelation in Biochemistry and Medicine: New Approaches to Controlling Iron Metabolism and Treating Related Diseases** 1
George J. Kontoghiorghes and Christina N. Kontoghiorghe

Chapter 2 **Emerging and Dynamic Biomedical Uses of Ferritin** 44
Brian Chiou and James R. Connor

Chapter 3 **Reductive Mobilization of Iron from Intact Ferritin: Mechanisms and Physiological Implication** 62
Fadi Bou-Abdallah, John J. Paliakkara, Galina Melman and Artem Melman

Chapter 4 **Ferritin in Kidney and Vascular Related Diseases: Novel Roles for an Old Player** 76
József Balla, György Balla and Abolfazl Zarjou

Chapter 5 **Unraveling Hepcidin Plasma Protein Binding: Evidence from Peritoneal Equilibration Testing** 90
Laura E. Diepeveen, Coby M. Laarakkers, Hilde P.E. Peters, Antonius E. van Herwaarden, Hans Groenewoud, Joanna IntHout, Jack F. Wetzels, Rachel P.L. van Swelm and Dorine W. Swinkels

Chapter 6 **The Efficacy of Iron Chelators for Removing Iron from Specific Brain Regions and the Pituitary—Ironing out the Brain** 103
Robert R. Crichton, Roberta J. Ward and Robert C. Hider

Chapter 7 **Iron Release from Soybean Seed Ferritin Induced by Cinnamic Acid Derivatives** 116
Xuejiao Sha, Hai Chen, Jingsheng Zhang and Guanghua Zhao

Chapter 8 **Iron as a Therapeutic Target in *HFE*-Related Hemochromatosis: Usual and Novel Aspects** 126
Olivier Loréal, Thibault Cavey, François Robin, Moussa Kenawi, Pascal Guggenbuhl and Pierre Brissot

Chapter 9 **Iron in Friedreich Ataxia: A Central Role in the Pathophysiology or an Epiphenomenon?** 140
David Alsina, Rosa Purroy, Joaquim Ros and Jordi Tamarit

Chapter 10 **Twenty Years of Ferroportin Disease: A Review or An Update of Published Clinical, Biochemical, Molecular and Functional Features** 155
L. Tom Vlasveld, Roel Janssen, Edouard Bardou-Jacquet, Hanka Venselaar, Houda Hamdi-Roze, Hal Drakesmith and Dorine W. Swinkels

Chapter 11 **Mitochondrial Targeting in Neurodegeneration: A Heme Perspective** 184
Veronica Fiorito, Deborah Chiabrando and Emanuela Tolosano

Chapter 12 **Protective Role of Histidine Supplementation Against Oxidative Stress Damage in the Management of Anemia of Chronic Kidney Disease** 205
Mayra Vera-Aviles, Eleni Vantana, Emmy Kardinasari, Ngat L. Koh and Gladys O. Latunde-Dada

Chapter 13 **Deregulation of Hepatic Mek1/2–Erk1/2 Signaling Module in Iron Overload Conditions** 220
Naveen Kumar Tangudu, Nils Buth, Pavel Strnad, Ion C. Cirstea and Maja Vujić Spasić

Permissions

List of Contributors

Index

Preface

For human beings, iron is an important trace element. It is required for various bodily processes such as cell growth and division, oxygen transport, various catalytic reactions, and oxidative metabolism. Human body requires only a small amount of iron on a daily basis. It must be consumed in a strictly monitored manner because there is no mechanism for excreting excess iron out of the body. Erythropoiesis, i.e., the production of new blood cells, takes place in the bone marrow, which is the major consumer of iron. The reticuloendothelial system helps in recycling iron by erythrocyte phagocytosis. Various proteins are involved in iron metabolism. For instance, hepcidin is a liver-derived peptide hormone that works as a major regulator of iron metabolism. This book explores all the important aspects of the physiology and pathophysiology of iron in the present day scenario. It is a valuable compilation of topics, ranging from the basic to the most complex advancements. Those in search of information to further their knowledge will be greatly assisted by this book.

The researches compiled throughout the book are authentic and of high quality, combining several disciplines and from very diverse regions from around the world. Drawing on the contributions of many researchers from diverse countries, the book's objective is to provide the readers with the latest achievements in the area of research. This book will surely be a source of knowledge to all interested and researching the field.

In the end, I would like to express my deep sense of gratitude to all the authors for meeting the set deadlines in completing and submitting their research chapters. I would also like to thank the publisher for the support offered to us throughout the course of the book. Finally, I extend my sincere thanks to my family for being a constant source of inspiration and encouragement.

Editor

1

Iron and Chelation in Biochemistry and Medicine: New Approaches to Controlling Iron Metabolism and Treating Related Diseases

George J. Kontoghiorghes * and **Christina N. Kontoghiorghe**

Postgraduate Research Institute of Science, Technology, Environment and Medicine, CY-3021 Limassol, Cyprus
* Correspondence: kontoghiorghes.g.j@pri.ac.cy

Abstract: Iron is essential for all living organisms. Many iron-containing proteins and metabolic pathways play a key role in almost all cellular and physiological functions. The diversity of the activity and function of iron and its associated pathologies is based on bond formation with adjacent ligands and the overall structure of the iron complex in proteins or with other biomolecules. The control of the metabolic pathways of iron absorption, utilization, recycling and excretion by iron-containing proteins ensures normal biologic and physiological activity. Abnormalities in iron-containing proteins, iron metabolic pathways and also other associated processes can lead to an array of diseases. These include iron deficiency, which affects more than a quarter of the world's population; hemoglobinopathies, which are the most common of the genetic disorders and idiopathic hemochromatosis. Iron is the most common catalyst of free radical production and oxidative stress which are implicated in tissue damage in most pathologic conditions, cancer initiation and progression, neurodegeneration and many other diseases. The interaction of iron and iron-containing proteins with dietary and xenobiotic molecules, including drugs, may affect iron metabolic and disease processes. Deferiprone, deferoxamine, deferasirox and other chelating drugs can offer therapeutic solutions for most diseases associated with iron metabolism including iron overload and deficiency, neurodegeneration and cancer, the detoxification of xenobiotic metals and most diseases associated with free radical pathology.

Keywords: iron metabolism; iron proteins; iron diseases; metals; antioxidants; chelators; therapeutics; deferiprone; deferoxamine

---

1. Introduction

Iron, copper, zinc, cobalt, chromium, manganese, molybdenum and selenium are essential metal ions and nutrients, which play an important role in maintaining normal healthy living in humans. Deficiencies or excesses of these metal ions, as well as abnormalities in their metabolism may cause serious diseases and mortality.

The important role of these essential metal ions is an integral part of enzymes and proteins, as well as that of transcription factors and other co-factors which secure the normal growth and development of the body. These metal ions and especially iron play a central role in important physiological processes such as oxygen transport and utilization, respiration and also other processes involving the metabolism of proteins, lipids, carbohydrates and nucleic acids [1–6].

There are many diverse functions of the essential metal ions. For example, it is estimated that there are more than 300 catalytically active zinc metalloproteins, as well as more than 2000 zinc dependent transcription factors [1,2]. It can be envisaged that any changes in essential metal homeostasis as a result of dietary, metallomic, genomic, proteomic, metabolomic and other factors can cause metabolic changes which may lead to physiological and clinical abnormalities. For example, low levels of dietary zinc can cause zinc deficiency and can lead to abnormalities such as growth retardation, hair loss, delayed sexual maturation, impotence, skin lesions, weight loss, delayed healing of wounds and taste abnormalities [3]. In contrast, zinc overload can reduce immune function, alter iron metabolic function and cause anemia, neuronal injury, kidney disease, acute pancreatitis and in some cases multi-system organ failure [1–3]. Similarly, deficiency of copper or its abnormal distribution, e.g., in Menkes disease, can lead to side effects such as growth failure, nervous system deterioration and kinky hair. Copper overload, e.g., in Wilson's disease can lead to hepatitis, kidney diseases and neurological disorders [4].

Iron-containing proteins are at the crossroads of almost all physiological and metabolic pathways, including oxygen and electron transport. The health implications of the activity of iron-containing proteins are enormous, considering that these are also involved in the metabolic pathways of most natural and xenobiotic molecules, which include dietary molecules and drugs.

Abnormalities in iron homeostasis, iron-containing proteins and iron metabolic pathways can lead to diseases such as iron deficiency, which affects more than a quarter of the world's population and idiopathic hemochromatosis, which is a genetic disease affecting one in ten people of the Caucasian population [5–7]. Another major category of related diseases are the hemoglobinopathies, which are the most common group of genetic disorders in humans [8]. In particular, one of these disorders thalassemia has the highest morbidity and mortality rate in relation to iron or metal toxicity worldwide [8,9]. A rapidly expanding category of iron loaded patients currently estimated to about 0.5 million are those undergoing hematopoietic stem cell transplantation, which is a widely used form of treatment for many hematological malignancies and genetic disorders [10–14].

Iron and copper are the major catalysts of free radical (FR) and reactive oxygen species (ROS) production and chain reaction cascades in biologic systems [15–18]. If these processes are not controlled, they can cause biomolecular damage and lead to oxidative stress toxicity (OST) in cells [15]. Oxidative biomolecular damage due to oxidative stress has been implicated in tissue damage in most pathologic conditions, in cancer initiation/progression and in other disease processes [15,19–21].

Metal ions in biologic systems are always found bound to ligands with electron donating atoms such as oxygen, nitrogen and sulfur. Almost all biologic activities, as well as the biochemical, metabolic, toxicological and other processes involving metal ions, are mostly based and expressed through ligand and chelator complex formation. The diversity of activities, processes and functions of metal ions is generally based on bond formation with electron donor molecules of adjacent ligands and the overall properties of the metal complex including the primary, secondary, tertiary and quaternary structure protein formation [22–25].

Many factors can influence the structure and biochemical functions of protein or non-protein iron complexes in vivo, leading to changes in biologic activity. Some of these interactions may include other ligands, metal ions, anions, free radicals and other reactive oxygen or nitrogen species, chelators, etc. Similarly, some changes in the structure of the metal complex can affect the function and metabolic pathways of the metal ions and associated processes [22]. Within this context many molecules with chelating or metal binding properties can affect all processes involving metal ions. Most importantly, specific chelating drugs could be designed to offer therapeutic solutions to many diseases associated with metal metabolic imbalance and toxicity [22–26].

The diversity of the interactions of ligands and chelators with essential metal ions on the molecular level can be highlighted by the use and effects of chelating drugs and other chelators in vitro, in vivo and clinical studies. It should be emphasized that each such interaction has unique properties, characteristics and varies under different conditions [22].

The implications of the use and interactions of chelating drugs and other chelators on metal ions covers many other areas in metal biochemistry and medicine considering that microbes and cancer cells require iron and other essential metals for survival and proliferation. The biochemistry of essential metal ions is also affected by interactions with xenobiotic metal complexes which are used in medical diagnosis and in the treatment of cancer [22,26].

Chelating drugs can be used as the main, alternative or adjuvant therapy for the treatment of a large number of human diseases, including those associated with essential or xenobiotic metal detoxification, antioxidant, anticancer and anti-infective therapies and in the modulation of protein function or pathways associated with many diseases [22,26].

In this review, the molecular characteristics and properties of iron, chelators, chelating drugs, chelator metal complexes, as well as factors involved in modifying their activity, is discussed in the biochemical and clinical context with major emphasis on the prospects of understanding and treating relevant clinical conditions.

2. The Properties and Role of Iron and Iron Proteins in Human Health

The chemistry, biochemistry, physiology and medical fields in relation to iron are rapidly expanding and advancing, and include new discoveries such as new mutations of hemoglobin and other iron proteins. Similar advances are also reported on the pathologic implications of such mutations and also on other iron related diseases. Some of the molecular aspects of iron and iron-containing proteins will be discussed focusing on factors influencing different aspects related to health [22,27–29].

2.1. Basic Properties and Distribution of Iron in the Body

Each metal ion has its unique characteristics, chemical, biochemical, pharmacological and toxicological properties. The sources of essential metals for living organisms come from the soil, stones and their ores, usually composed of salts containing oxygen and sulfur. Very small quantities of metals are soluble and available for aquatic life. All metals are sparingly soluble in water at physiological pH and are more soluble at acidic pH. Metal ions are positively charged in aqueous solution and form ionic bonds with anions or molecules with electron donor atoms such as oxygen from water molecules [23–25].

Iron is one of the essential transition metal ions found in all organisms. It is the most important metal ion in aerobic organisms because it is required mainly for oxygen transport and utilization and energy transduction, as well as many other physiological processes. It is mainly found in the ferrous (Fe^{2+}) or ferric (Fe^{3+}) states under physiological conditions. In aqueous solutions, at physiological pH ferrous iron is oxidized to ferric iron. Under the same conditions soluble aqueous ferric iron is found in trace detectable levels (10^{-18} mol/L) since it mostly precipitates by forming insoluble polymeric ferric oxyhydroxide complexes with a high stability constant (log K = 38) [23–25].

Different mechanisms, pathways and proteins are involved in the uptake, distribution, utilization, recycling and excretion of iron in living organisms, including humans where each cell requires and utilizes different amounts of iron [5,6,29].

It is estimated that about 4.5–5.0 g iron is present and distributed in the human body of a 70–75-kg normal adult. Most of the iron is in the ferrous state in a complex form with a protoporphyrin ring (heme), which is mainly found in the proteins hemoglobin and myoglobin. In addition to heme iron in the form of hemoglobin (2.3–2.6 g) in red blood cells (RBC) and of myoglobin (0.32–0.40 g) in muscle, the remaining distribution of iron in the body is mainly in the form of polynuclear ferric oxyhydroxide phosphate complexes such as ferritin (0.7 g), hemosiderin (0.3 g) and non-heme enzymes (0.1 g). This totals to 1.1–1.5 g of iron in liver, spleen, muscle and bone marrow. Iron is also found in mitochondrial cytochromes (17 mg), catalase (5 mg) and transferrin (4 mg) [23–25].

2.2. Iron in Heme, Hemoglobin and Red Blood Cells

Most of the iron in the body is found in the form of heme in hemoglobin (58%) which is the major constituent of RBC and the component that carries oxygen and gives the red color to blood (Figure 1). The RBC is the vehicle that provides the continuous supply of oxygen to all cells and tissues of the body through blood circulation and ensures normal bodily function. It is estimated that hemoglobin occupies 95% of the RBC volume and amounts to about 670 g of the 25 kg dry body weight of an average adult human individual overall [30].

The quantitative molecular aspects in relation to oxygen transport by hemoglobin and the role of iron in heme to which oxygen is bound, is of primary importance for normal bodily function and survival. In this context, it is estimated that approximately 25 trillion RBC circulate in the bloodstream, each one packed with about 260 million hemoglobin molecules. Considering that one adult hemoglobin molecule is composed of two alpha and two beta globin protein subunits, to each of which one molecule of heme is embedded, the total amount of iron in the ferrous state as heme in one RBC is estimated to be 1.04 billion molecules. When the RBC are fully oxygenated the concentration of both iron and oxygen is estimated to reach 16 mM. No other cell in the body contains such a high concentration of iron in the ferrous state in heme and also so much oxygen. This high concentration of ferrous iron and oxygen can be a highly reactive mixture and can lead to FR/ROS and OST, especially in hemolytic and other conditions of RBC damage [5,20,30].

The production of RBC takes place in the bone marrow. Erythroblasts are the early stage RBC progenitors produced in the bone marrow which contain a nucleus. Erythroblasts progressively lose their nucleus and organelles before their release in the blood stream initially as reticulocytes without a nucleus and later as matured RBC with an average life span of 120 days. Heme production takes place in mitochondria and hemoglobin in the cytoplasm of erythroblasts and reticulocytes. Mature RBC cannot synthesize new proteins during their 120 day lifespan in the human bloodstream [30,31].

Aging RBC undergo progressive denaturing changes such as vesiculation, a process leading to the formation of vesicles [31,32]. Senescent RBC are more rigid and fragile than young RBC and are readily removed from the bloodstream via phagocytosis by macrophages of the reticuloendothelial system primarily in the spleen and also in the liver. The degradation process begins inside the macrophages and usually involves old and damaged RBC [30,31].

Owing to the high concentration and reactive nature of ferrous iron and oxygen, protective antioxidant mechanisms have been evolved to eliminate or reduce the associated oxidative damage inside and outside of the RBC. The presence of antioxidant molecules and enzymes such as reduced glutathione, glutathione peroxidase, glutathione S-transferase, glutathione reductase and superoxide dismutase, ensure the antioxidant protection inside the RBC [33]. Additional protection against oxidant damage is offered by other enzymes such as methemoglobin reductase. The removal of denatured hemoglobin or other aggregated species containing iron is accomplished by a vesiculation process [31–33].

Protection against oxidative and other damage caused by the release of heme and hemoglobin into the blood stream is provided by hemopexin and haptoglobin, respectively [34,35]. Hemopexin is a plasma protein expressed mainly in the liver and has a high affinity to heme binding. Similarly, haptoglobin in plasma binds free hemoglobin released from RBC forming a haptoglobin-hemoglobin complex, which is removed by the reticuloendothelial system in the spleen [34,35].

Hundreds of hemoglobin mutations are reported in humans [8,27,28]. Changes in the production and structure of hemoglobin can lead to abnormal function, toxic side effects and associated diseases. The hemoglobinopathies are the most common group of genetic disorders affecting millions of people [8,27,28]. There are many abnormalities in the function of hemoglobin, and these are related to changes in the globin structure and heme function. For example, patients with thalassemia have a low or absent production of the alpha globin (alpha-thalassemia) or beta globin (beta-thalassemia) or both globin chains of hemoglobin. Most beta-thalassemia patients are severely anemic and require RBC transfusions every 1–4 weeks from normal blood donors in order to survive [8,9]. The rate of body iron load in beta-thalassemia patients as a result of repeated RBC transfusions and consequently the overall rate of iron toxicity in organs is much faster than idiopathic hemochromatosis patients [6,8,9]. Another inherited hemoglobinopathy affecting millions of people worldwide is sickle cell disease. In this abnormal hemoglobin condition there is a single amino acid change from glutamic acid to valine in the beta globin chain resulting in hemoglobin polymerization, sickling of the RBC, anemia and other sickling crisis painful side effects [8,27].

Many non-genetic changes also occur in hemoglobin such as increased production of glycosylated hemoglobin in diabetes, carboxyhemoglobin formation due to carbon monoxide poisoning, S-nitrosohemoglobin formation from the reaction of hemoglobin cysteine with nitric oxide, etc. These and many other changes can affect normal hemoglobin function [36].

Similarly, changes in the concentration levels of iron, hemoglobin and RBC can cause many abnormalities and side effects. Most importantly in many such cases, associated diseases can be developed where there is insufficient transport of oxygen. Such changes have implications on the normal functioning of all cells, tissues and organs of the body in general, leading to physiological complications and requiring medical treatment.

2.3. *The Role and Function of Iron-Containing Proteins*

There are many iron-containing proteins in addition to hemoglobin which play a very important role in many biochemical pathways including the tricarboxylic acid cycle, DNA synthesis and the metabolism of proteins, lipids, carbohydrates and nucleic acids (Table 1). As is the case with hemoglobin, iron is in the active site of the protein and none of the iron-containing proteins are expected to function without the presence of iron.

Table 1. Examples of iron-containing proteins with the type of the iron complex prosthetic group and protein function.

Protein	Iron Complex Prosthetic Group	Function
Hemoglobin	Heme	Oxygen transport
Myoglobin	Heme	Oxygen transport
Cytochromes	Heme	Electron transport. Respiration
Cytochrome P450	Heme	Drug detoxification
Ribonucleotide reductase	Amino acids	DNA synthesis
Proline hydroxylase	Amino acids	Collagen synthesis
Phenylalanine hydroxylase	Amino acids	Degradation of phenylalanine
Tryptophan 2,3-dioxygenage	Heme	Degradation of tryptophan
Homogentisic acid 2,3-dioxygenase	Amino acids	Detection of alkaptonuria
Peroxidases	Heme	Decomposition of hydroperoxides
Catalase	Heme	Decomposition of hydrogen peroxide
Lipoxygenase	Amino acids	HPETE and leukotriene synthesis
Cyclooxygenase	Heme and Amino acids	Prostaglandin and thromboxane synthesis
Adrenodoxin	2Fe-2S	Electron transport. Oxidation/reduction
Aconitase	4Fe–4S	Tricarboxylic acid cycle
Succinate dehydrogenase	2Fe-2S, 4Fe–4S, 3Fe-4S	Tricarboxylic acid cycle
NADH dehydrogenase	Fe–S Clusters	Electron transport. Respiration
Xanthine oxidase	4x (2Fe-2S)	Conversion of xanthine to uric acid
Aldehyde oxidase	2x (2Fe-2S)	Metabolism of aldehydes
Transferrin	Amino Acids	Iron transport in plasma
Lactoferrin	Amino Acids	Iron binding in milk and secretions
Ferritin	Oxyhydroxide, phosphate Fe	Iron storage
Hemosiderin	Oxyhydroxide, phosphate Fe	Iron storage
Hephaestin	Not carrying or containing Fe	Ferroxidase and influx transmembrane iron transport
Ferroportin	Not carrying or containing Fe	Efflux transmembrane iron transporter in cells
Hepcidin	Not carrying or containing Fe	Regulatory protein affecting iron uptake and release

Myoglobin is another important hemoprotein that stores oxygen in muscle tissue. Oxygen is transported and utilized primarily by the mitochondria of muscle cells, where it can be used in cellular respiration to produce energy for body movement [37]. Abnormalities in the structure and function of myoglobin affect associated processes. For example, the release of myoglobin due to muscle damage can cause rhabdomyolysis, where redox activity by Fe^{4+} in heme is implicated [38]. Modulation of the redox activity of globin hemoproteins may have a major impact on the therapeutic targeting of diseases such as cancer and neurodegeneration [39].

Iron in the form of heme is also widely found in another big group of hemoproteins, namely the cytochromes, e.g., cytochrome c and cytochrome oxidase in mitochondria, which are involved in the respiratory electron transport chain for the production of energy in the form of ATP [40–46]. Many other metabolic functions are performed by other cytochromes, e.g., cytochrome P450 which has thousands of variants and is involved in oxidative, peroxidative and reductive metabolism of endogenous and xenobiotic substrates such as drugs, environmental pollutants, agrochemicals, steroids and fatty acids [47–50].

Another major group of iron-containing proteins involved in electron transfer and redox metabolic processes are those possessing iron–sulfur (Fe –S) clusters, which may vary in number in each protein and in composition (Table 1, Figure 1). Some of the Fe –S cluster proteins are involved in the tricarboxylic acid cycle, e.g., aconitase, in the respiratory chain, e.g., NADH dehydrogenase and in the metabolism of biochemical compounds, e.g., xanthine oxidase [5,6,51–53].

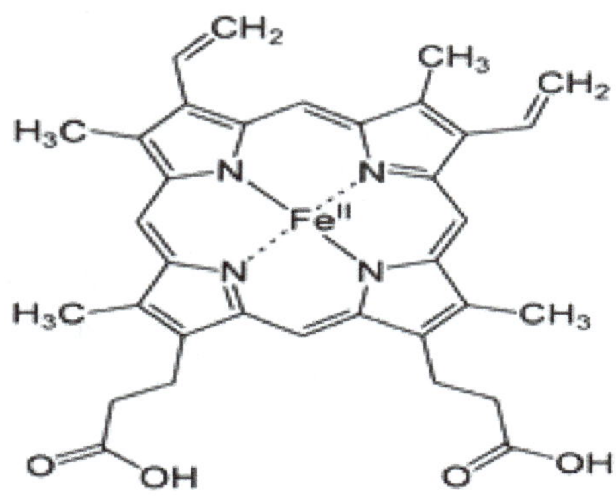

(a)

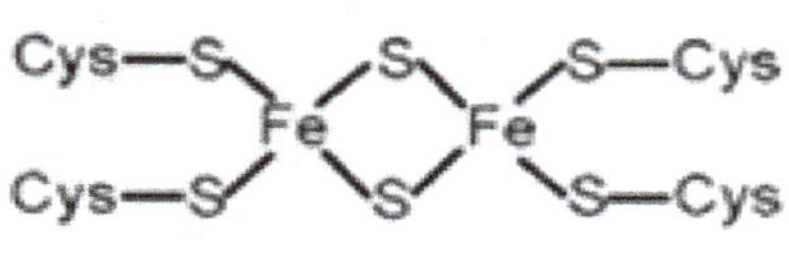

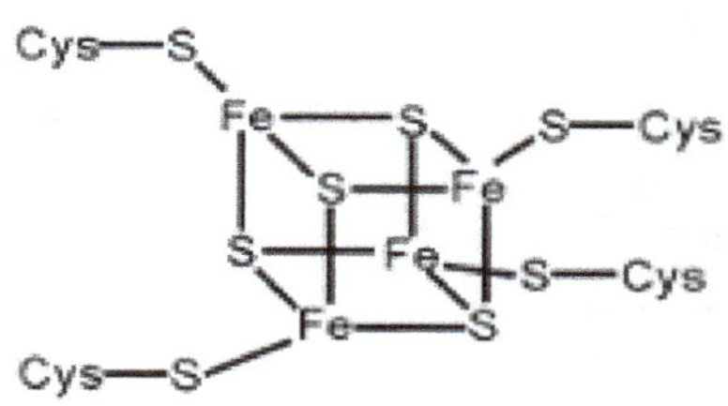

(b) (c)

Figure 1. Chemical structure of heme (**a**) shows the prosthetic groups in heme-containing proteins, involved mainly in oxygen and electron transport. The chemical structure of the (**b**) iron sulfur (2Fe-2S) and (**c**) cuboidal iron sulfur (4Fe-4S) prosthetic groups found in iron sulfur proteins are involved mainly in electron transport.

Many other iron-containing proteins may use iron in the active site, which is composed of amino acids and not heme or Fe–S clusters. Among these proteins is ribonucleotide reductase involved in DNA synthesis, proline hydroxylase involved in collagen synthesis and phenylalanine hydroxylase involved in the degradation of phenylalanine (Table 1) [54,55].

In general, most of the iron-containing proteins are participating in biochemical reactions involved in electron transfer and oxygen utilization. Some examples of such proteins include the respiratory electron transport chain cytochromes, the oxygenases, which are involved in the incorporation of oxygen in organic substrate, the hydroxylases (monooxygenases), which catalyze the incorporation of one atom of elemental oxygen in organic substrate and the oxidases, which are involved in the oxidation of organic substrate by the reduction of oxygen to peroxides. Decomposition of hydrogen peroxide to water and oxygen is accomplished by the heme protein catalase and decomposition of other peroxides by heme containing peroxidases [20,21].

Overall, the iron-containing proteins are involved in a variety of biochemical pathways, which are essential for the normal function and development of the organism. Within this context, there are many metabolic controls associated with the absorption, distribution and excretion of iron. Iron transport is mainly accomplished by the iron transport plasma protein transferrin. Iron storage in cells is accomplished by the ferritin and hemosiderin proteins. Several other proteins like ferroportin and hepcidin do not bind or carry iron but are key regulators in the movement of iron in and out of cells (Table 1) [5,6,29,51]. In particular hepcidin, a peptide hormone produced in the liver plays a central role in mammalian iron homeostasis by mediating the effects of erythropoiesis, hypoxia, inflammation and iron load on the levels of circulating iron. In this context, new emerging therapies and strategies for iron metabolic disorders have been proposed based on hepcidin agonists and antagonists [5,6,29,51,52].

Changes in the concentration, structure and function of iron-containing proteins and also of non-iron-containing regulatory proteins of iron metabolism can lead to many abnormalities in biologic functions and physiological complications and may require medical intervention.

2.4. *Factors Affecting Iron-Containing Proteins and Implications on Health*

The essentiality of iron-containing proteins and associated metabolic pathways highlights the importance of iron for the normal growth and development in humans and all other organisms. However, a variety of dietary, genetic, environmental, iatrogenic and other factors can lead to abnormal metabolic effects and a variety of diseases in relation to iron. Some of these abnormalities and associated diseases have been introduced in previous sections, e.g., iron deficiency anemia, hereditary hemochromatosis, hemoglobinopathies, etc. [7,8,27].

It is envisaged that any similar changes and factors involving different natural or synthetic molecules with iron binding ligands, may lead to abnormal biologic function, physiological changes, toxicity and disease. Similar effects can be observed in relation to structural and functional changes in iron proteins and also in the case of other factors affecting the rate of production of proteins, as well as metabolic changes in pathways associated to iron. There is a wide spectrum of diseases associated with iron metabolism especially when considering the large number of proteins and factors involved [5,6,29,51]. Some of these are associated with abnormal levels or distribution of iron. Similarly, almost all forms of tissue damage which are related to FR pathology are due to OST, which involves mainly the catalytic activity of iron in the formation of FR and other ROS, causing a vicious circle of biomolecular and cellular damage [20–22].

Most importantly, iron appears to play a key role as a target for new therapeutics in many diseases with a high morbidity and mortality rate, which have no effective treatments at present such as cancer, neurodegenerative and infectious diseases [56].

Appropriate therapeutic interventions could decrease the extent of unwanted negative health implications and may also treat diseases associated with abnormalities related to iron, iron-containing proteins and associated metabolic pathways. Such approaches require the characterizing the targets and determining the molecular interactions involving iron with the anticipated therapeutics [22,24,56]. The use of iron chelating drugs for controlling iron metabolic pathways in relation to associated abnormalities, toxicities and diseases can in many cases, offer therapeutic solutions. The therapeutic process however is more complex since metallomic, genomic, proteomic, metabolomic, pharmacogenomic and other factors can also influence the therapeutic outcome [57].

In general, it appears that the diversity of activities and functions of iron and any associated pathology is broadly based and related to its binding with different ligands. Similarly, the overall structure of the iron complex and its properties, including stability and redox activity at physiological conditions are important parameters in determining the mode of action and toxicity of iron related processes [22–24].

3. Ligands and Chelators Binding with Iron

Iron and all other essential metal ions are positively charged and found bound to ligands such as =O, -OH, -N and –SH, which usually contain the electron donor atoms O, N and S capable of donating a pair of electrons for the formation of a coordinated bond with the metal ion. These electron donor atoms can be found in ligands in almost all classes of biomolecules, e.g., amino acids, nucleic acids, carbohydrates, phosphates, etc. [22–25].

A molecule containing two of the ligands described above, which are adjacent to each other and can bind to a metal ion forming a ring structure with the metal ion as the closing member, is called a bidentate chelator, for a molecule with three such ligands a tridentate chelator, and with six such ligands a hexadentate chelator, etc. [22–25]. Ligands with electron donor atoms are found in the iron binding site of all the iron-containing proteins, including heme in hemoglobin and in the iron-sulfur cluster proteins. Similar ligands are also found in the transport and deposition or storage sites of iron in transferrin and ferritin, respectively and also many other proteins with domains containing iron, which are necessary for enzymatic activity (Table 1).

In hemoglobin iron (Fe^{2+}) in heme is bound by six ligands in an octahedral arrangement, four nitrogen atoms of a protoporphyrin planar ring and an imidazole nitrogen of a distant histidine amino acid (Figure 1). The sixth binding site of the octahedral structure arrangement is formed with one of the two oxygen atoms of the dioxygen molecule. In methemoglobin, ferric iron (Fe^{3+}) cannot bind oxygen, but instead an oxygen atom from a water molecule is bound in the sixth coordinating position. Carbon monoxide is poisonous because it can replace oxygen in the sixth coordinating site of heme in hemoglobin. Carbon dioxide is also partly carried by hemoglobin by binding to the globin protein structure, but not the heme part of the protein.

There is a variety of iron-sulfur cluster proteins, where the composition of the iron-sulfur clusters and the oxidation state of iron may vary. In most cases of the iron-sulfur cluster proteins, the iron centers are tetrahedral and four- coordinated, whereas the sulfide groups are either two- or three-coordinated. Similarly, in most cases, the terminal ligands attached to iron are from thiol groups from cysteinyl residues (Figure 1) [58–60].

There are two major iron chelating proteins in humans, namely transferrin found in blood plasma and responsible for the transport of iron in all cells of the body and its sister protein lactoferrin which is found in neutrophils and secretions including saliva, tears, milk, nasal and vaginal fluids. Both transferrin and lactoferrin have similar iron binding affinity, lower affinity for other metal ions and also ferroxidase activity [61–66]. Ferritin and hemosiderin are iron storage proteins, with the former found in all cells of the body and also in serum [67–70].

In the case of the iron chelator protein transferrin the two iron binding sites are almost identical and consist of four to five amino acids, two to three tyrosines, one histidine and one aspartic acid, as well as a bicarbonate synergistic anion in an octahedral hexacoordinated arrangement. The hydrogen of the phenolic –OH of tyrosines is displaced for binding iron (Fe^{3+}), releasing a proton (H^+) and the lone pair of electrons of oxygen are utilized for bond formation with iron (tyrosine-O- Fe^{3+}). The other bonds with iron are formed with an imidazole nitrogen of histidine, the oxygen anion of aspartic acid and bicarbonate. Furthermore, transferrin binds many other metal ions, but with lower affinity in comparison to iron [61–63,71,72].

At any time in the human body iron storage is available within ferritin and hemosiderin which accounts for 20–25% of the total body iron in physiological conditions. In contrast to other proteins of iron metabolism iron is not bound to amino acids or other organic groups but stored as polynuclear ferric oxyhydroxide phosphate complexes within the hollow spherical protein structure of ferritin, which is composed of 24 subunits [67–70,73–75]. Hemosiderin is considered a broken protein shell of ferritin structures stacked together with the iron cores exposed [68,73–75]. Iron in both ferritin and hemosiderin is bound to oxo ligands in an octahedral hexacoordinated arrangement.

Iron that is not incorporated into proteins and is instead in "transit" between different cellular compartments and organelles and also between the different proteins of iron transport, storage and utilization, is considered to be mostly bound to low molecular weight (LMWt) biomolecules with chelating sites, such as amino acids, nucleic acids, fatty acids, sugars, citrate, ascorbic acid, glutathione, ATP, FADH, NADH, etc., forming LMWt iron complexes, which constitute the low LMWt iron pool (Table 2). Proteins containing side chains with metal binding ligands such as –OH, -SH and -COOH can also form complexes with iron. The LMWt iron pool in "transit", composed of these LMWt iron complexes and is present intracellularly is considered to exchange iron with storage iron in ferritin and is utilized for incorporation into apoproteins with the final product being the iron-containing proteins [62,64,76].

Table 2. Examples of naturally occurring low molecular weight chelators affecting iron metabolism.

Phosphates	Pyridoxal phosphate, thiamine pyrophosphate, ribonucleoside and deoxyribonucleoside phosphates, phytic acid (IP6), Pyrophosphate, ATP, ADP, AMP, etc.
Amino acids	Aspartic acid, glutamic acid, histidine, cysteine, tyrosine, etc.
Carboxylic acids	Citric acid, aconitic acid, oxaloacetic acid, etc.
Mono- and di- saccharides	Fructose, glucose, lactose, etc.
Vitamins	Ascorbic acid, lipoic acid, riboflavin.
Fatty acids and phosphoglycerides	Oleic acid, linoleic acid, phosphatidic acid.
Other naturally occurring chelators	Catecholamines, pteridines, purines, spermine, spermidine. Glutathione. Folic acid.
Dietary molecules	In addition to food components containing the above molecules, there are also many plant products including most polyphenols and other phytochelators with iron chelating properties such as: gallic acid, caffeic acid, quercetin, ellagic acid, curcumin, catechin, maltol, etc.

There is variation in the affinity of iron-containing proteins, ligands and chelators for iron and other metal ions. The metal complexes formed are of variable stability depending on their concentration, pH, as well as a number of molecular, steric and electronic features. In this context, all interactions including competition of natural chelators or proteins with iron or other metal ions are governed by a number of physicochemical, thermodynamic and kinetic parameters, which have previously been reviewed [23–26]. Similarly, the competitive interactions with microbial and plant chelators for iron is of physiological, nutritional, pharmacological, toxicological and clinical importance [77,78].

3.1. Naturally Occurring Microbial Chelators (Siderophores)

There are many synthetic and naturally occurring chelators, which have high specificity and affinity for iron. Iron is required for the growth of microbes and other organisms invading the human body. The presence of transferrin in plasma deprives iron required for the growth and proliferation of microbes in blood.

The uptake of iron by microbes is controlled and accomplished by a variety of specifically produced chelators called siderophores (Figure 2). Major groups of siderophores which have high affinity for binding iron in bacteria mainly contain the catechol (Figure 2a) chelating site, whereas in fungi mainly contain the hydroxamate (Figure 2d) chelating site [23,24,77].

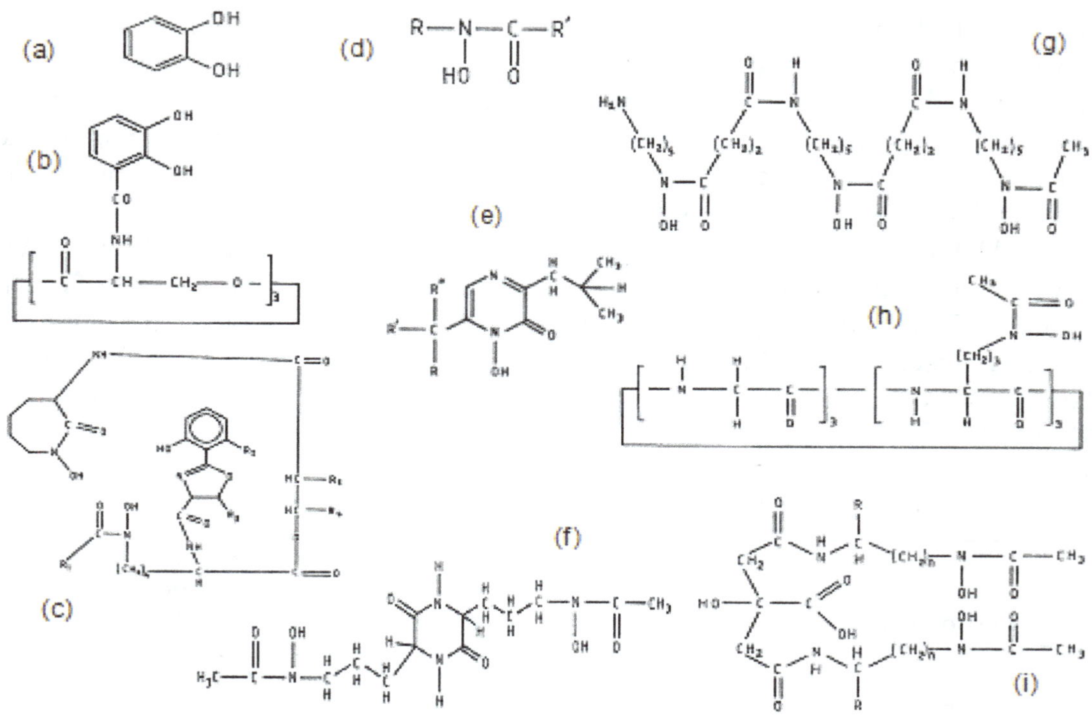

Figure 2. The chemical structure of different microbial siderophores. Many bacteria species produce (**a**) catechol structure-based siderophores such as (**b**) enterobactin. Many fungal species produce (**d**) hydroxamate-based structures such as (**g**) deferoxamine, (**h**) ferrichrome, (**i**) citrate hydroxamate and (**f**) rhodotorulic acid. Siderophores with different chelating structures include (**c**) mycobactin and (**e**) aspergillic acid. For more siderophore structures see references 13 and 14.

Bacterial siderophores are primarily produced by bacteria when the surrounding media is low in iron concentration. One of the most important siderophores with a high affinity for iron binding is enterobactin, a hexadentate chelator, which is produced by enteric bacteria and contains three 2,3-dihydroxy-N-benzoyl-serine units, forming a hexacoordinating octahedral complex with Fe^{3+} (Figure 2b) [23,24,77].

There are several hydroxamate-based siderophores found in fungi such as those of the ferrioxamine, ferrichrome, rhodotorulic acid and citrate hydroxamate families. Of particular importance is the iron chelating drug deferoxamine (DFO or DF) (Figure 2g), which is a hexadentate tris hydroxamate-based siderophore synthesized by *Streptomyces pylosus* that forms a hexacoordinating octahedral complex with Fe^{3+} (Figure 2) [23,24].

Many other siderophores have been identified in microorganisms in addition to catechol and hydroxamate-based chelating structures. For example, a cyclic heteroaromatic hydroxamate is the major chelating feature of the bidentate chelator aspergillic acid (Figure 2e) and also one of the chelating sites of mycobactin (Figure 2c) [23,24].

The competition among microbes and between microbes and other microorganisms for iron is not only an essential parameter for the growth and proliferation of pathogenic versus non-pathogenic species, but is also important for the control of infections and the design of antibacterial and antifungal agents for targeted therapeutic strategies [79,80].

3.2. Naturally Occurring Plant Chelators (Phytochelators)

The chemical structural characteristics and some of the iron binding properties of naturally occurring chelators found in plants (phytochelators) have been recently reviewed [78].

Although hundreds of phytochelators of different chemical structures have been described, no systematic investigations have yet been carried out to identify their role in iron and other metal metabolic pathways in plants and animals [78]. Similarly, many of these phytochelators such as ascorbic acid, quercetin, ellagic acid, gallic acid, silibinin, curcumin, etc. are used daily as nutraceuticals by millions of people and also in clinical trials [81–90]. Furthermore, many of the phytochelators are dietary components of vegetables and fruits which can play a significant role in iron and other metal metabolism related to human health (Table 2) [91–93]. Most of the phytochelators are included in the popular classification of 'polyphenols', which are widely reported in the mass media and scientific literature for their powerful antioxidant properties [94,95]. Most of these polyphenols have iron and other metal chelating properties [78].

One of the major classes of phytochelators are the polyphenols containing a catechol moiety metal chelating site which has a high affinity for iron, e.g., caffeic acid, gallic acid, protocatechuic acid and catechin. Other polyphenol groups not possessing adjacent hydroxyl groups like catechols have much weaker metal chelation properties. Among some of the catechol phytochelator characteristics is antioxidant activity via the inhibition of iron catalyzed FR reactions, which was identified in an in vitro FR model system more than 30 years ago [96].

Many other groups of polyphenols such as the flavonoids quercetin, kaempferol and fisetin contain catechol and other iron binding sites including alpha-ketohydroxy and beta-ketohydroxy iron chelating sites in multiple ring structures. Similarly, many other flavonoid, isoflavonoid and xanthonoid polyphenols contain chelating sites such as ellagic acid and mangiferin [78,97,98].

In addition to polyphenols, there are other groups of phytochelators containing different hydroxyl and phosphate chelating sites such as inositol and phytic acid. Phytochelators with thiol-containing chelating sites include glutathione, dihydrolipoic acid and phytochelatin [78].

The phytochelators with the highest affinity for iron are the alpha-ketohydroxy heteroaromatic chelators mimosine, maltol, kojic acid and the tropolones [78,99]. These alpha-ketohydroxy chelators and 8-hydroxyquinoline appear to be important phytochelators, affecting metabolic pathways including iron absorption, iron excretion and iron catalyzed FR reactions [78,96,100].

Many of the other properties of phytochelators such as antimicrobial and anticancer activity may also be related to iron chelation and also the biologic activities of their iron complexes. For example, the antibacterial and anticancer effects of the phytochelator mimosine and the antifungal and anticancer effects of pyridinethione (or omadine) appear to be related to their iron and other metal binding properties. Interestingly the iron complex of pyridinethione was identified to be a more potent anticancer molecule than pyridinethione itself [101,102].

3.3. Iron Chelating Drugs in Clinical Use

There are three iron chelating drugs in current clinical use, mostly for the treatment of thalassemia and other transfusional iron overloading conditions, namely DFO (Figure 3a), deferiprone (L1) (Figure 3b) and deferasirox (DFRA) (Figure 3c). Deferiprone is the smallest, a bidentate chelator forming a 3 L1:1 Fe^{3+} complex, DFRA is a tridentate chelator forming a 2 DFRA:1 Fe^{3+} complex and DFO is a hexadentate chelator forming a 1 DFO:1 Fe^{3+} complex at physiological pH (Table 3) [26]. Deferiprone and DFRA are orally active whereas DFO is not orally active and mostly administered subcutaneously or sometimes intravenously. Some of the structural, physicochemical, pharmacological, toxicological, metal binding and other properties of the three iron chelating drugs have been previously reviewed [26].

All three drugs have a different mode of chelation activity, efficacy, toxicity and interaction with the iron pools and iron-containing proteins, as well as differences in the process of excess iron removal from different organs (Tables 4–6) [103].

Table 3. The stability constants (log K) of essential metal ion complexes with the chelating drugs EDTA, DTPA, deferoxamine, deferiprone and deferasirox.

Ion	EDTA	DTPA	Deferoxamine	Deferiprone	Deferasirox
Fe^{3+}	25.1	28.6	30.6	35.0	27.0
Cu^{2+}	18.8	21.0	14.0	19.6	–
Zn^{2+}	16.5	18.4	11.1	13.5	–
Charge					
(pH 7)	−ve	−ve	+ve	neutral	−ve
MWt	292	393	561	139	373

Table 4. Molecular interactions and general effects of iron chelators in vitro.

Iron oxidation	Oxidation of Fe (II) to Fe (III) by L1, DFO or transferrin at pH 7.4 Oxidation of hemoglobin to methemoglobin by DFO Oxidation of cytochrome c by 2,3-dihydroxybenzoic acid
Iron reduction	Heme Fe (IV) to Fe (III) in myoglobin and hemoglobin by DFO and L1
Allosteric interactions	L1 and hemoglobin. Hydroxyurea and ribonucleotide reductase.
Competition with other metals	Order of stability constants of L1, DFO with metals: Fe>Al> Zn>Mg
Lipid / water partition coefficients (Kpar: n-octanol/water)	Order of hydrophilicity: DTPA and EDTA >DFO>L1>DFRA Order of lipophilicity: 8-hydroxyquinoline >tropolone>maltol
Inhibition or increase of iron induced free radical damage	L1 and DFO inhibit iron induced free radical damage to the DNA sugar deoxyribose. EDTA causes an increase in the iron induced free radical damage to deoxyribose.
Inhibition of iron-containing enzymes by iron chelating drugs	Lipoxygenase and cyclooxygenase inhibition by L1 and DFO. Catechol-O-methyltransferase, tyrosine and tryptophan hydroxylase inhibition by L1.
Promotion and inhibition of cell growth by iron binding and transport to cells	Maltol promotes cell growth. L1 and DFO inhibit cell growth.
Iron donors to transferrin	Ascorbate, citrate and L1 bound iron. DFO bound iron is not available to transferrin.
Iron mobilization from diferric transferrin and lactoferrin	L1 mobilizes iron preferentially from the C-terminal site and mimosine preferentially from the N-terminal site of transferrin. DFO and DFRA are not effective in transferrin or lactoferrin iron mobilization.
Differential rate of mobilization of iron species and forms by L1	Mononuclear> oligonuclear> polynuclear. Transferrin, lactoferrin > ferritin, hemosiderin.

Table 5. Metabolic and other effects of iron chelating drugs in patients.

Increase in iron excretion and route of elimination in iron loaded patients	L1: Urinary iron. DFRA: Fecal iron. DFO: Urinary and fecal iron.
Differential iron removal from various organs. Efficacy is dose related.	L1 preferential iron removal from the heart and DFRA from the liver. DFO from the liver and to lesser extent from the heart. L1 iron removal from focal iron deposits in the brain of patients with neurodegenerative diseases.
Iron removal from diferric transferrin in iron loaded patients	About 40% at L1 concentrations > 0.1 mM, but not by DFO or DFRA.
Iron redistribution	DFO and especially L1 redistribute iron from the reticuloendothelial system to the erythron in anemic rheumatoid arthritis patients. DFO in cell studies. DFRA may cause redistribution of iron from the liver to other organs in thalassemia and other iron loaded patients.
Increase excretion of metals other than iron, e.g., zinc (Zn) and aluminum (Al).	DTPA > L1 > DFO. (Order of increased Zn excretion in iron loaded patients). DFO and L1 cause increase Al excretion in renal dialysis patients. DFRA causes Al and other xenobiotic metal absorption.
Iron mobilization and excretion of chelator metabolite iron complexes	Several DFO metabolites have iron chelation potential and cause increase in iron excretion. No increase in iron excretion by the L1 glucuronide and DFRA glucuronide metabolites.
Combination chelation therapy	L1 and DFO or L1 and DFRA or other chelator combinations are likely to be more effective than monotherapy.
Chelating drug synergism with reducing agents	Ascorbic acid acts synergistically with DFO, but not with L1 or DFRA for increasing iron excretion.

Table 5. *Cont.*

Effects on iron absorption by lipophilic and hydrophilic chelators	Increase of iron absorption by maltol, 8-hydroxyquinoline and DFRA. Decrease of iron absorption by DFO, DTPA, EDTA and L1.
Chelating drugs minimizing toxicity of other drugs	L1 and ICRF187 (Dexrazoxane), but not DFRA, inhibit doxorubicin induced cardiotoxicity.
Chelator prodrugs	ICRF 187 (Dexrazoxane) is converted in vivo to an EDTA like chelator.
Chelators with enterohepatic circulation	DFRA and cholyl hydroxamic acid.

Table 6. Molecular and pharmacological differences between deferiprone and deferasirox.

	Deferiprone (L1)	Deferasirox (DFRA)
Molecular Differences		
Molecular weight of chelators	139	373
Molecular weight of iron complexes	470	798
Charge of chelators at pH 7.4	Neutral	Negative
Charge of iron complexes at pH 7.4	Neutral	Negative
Partition coefficient of chelators (Kpar: n-octanol/water)	0.19	6.3
Partition coefficient of iron complexes (Kpar: n-octanol/water)	0.05	Not reported
Stability constant (Log K) of chelator iron complexes– (Transferrin: 36)	35	27
Metabolic and Pharmacokinetic Differences		
Metabolite(s)	Glucuronide conjugate, which is cleared through the urine and have no iron chelation properties	Glucuronide conjugate cleared through the fecal route
T1/2 absorption	0.7–32 min	estimated within 1 h
T max of the chelator	Mostly within 1 h	1–3 h
T1/2 elimination of chelator	47–134 min at 35–71 mg/kg	19 +/− 6.5 h at 20 and 40 mg/kg
T1/2 elimination of the iron complex	Estimated within 47–134 min	17.2 +/− 7.8 h at 20 mg/kg and 17.7 +/− 5.1 h at 40 mg/kg
T max of the iron complex	Estimated within 1 h	at 20 mg/kg 1–6 h and at 40 mg/kg 4–8 h
T max of the metabolite	glucuronide: 1–3 h	glucuronide: Not known
Route of elimination of chelator and its iron complex	urine	Almost exclusively in feces and less than 0.1% of the administered dose in urine
Enterohepatic re-circulation	L1 and iron complex not shown or suspected	DFRA and iron complex suspected from pharmacokinetic data
Clinical Use and Dose Ranges		
Longest period of treatment	33 years	11 years
Time of experience of clinical use	33 years	16 years
Maximum dose in humans in 24 h	250 mg/kg	80 mg/kg
Maximum iron excretion in 24 h	325 mg	55 mg (estimated from the reported iron balance studies using 40 mg/kg)
Dose in current use in 24 h	75–110 mg/kg in divided doses	20–40 mg/kg single dose
Effective dose for iron balance in most thalassemia patients	>80 mg/kg/day	>40 mg/kg

The iron chelating drugs intended for the treatment of iron overload in thalassemia or other similar conditions are administered daily in order to remove the excess body iron intake from repeated RBC transfusions. The buildup of excess storage iron in the various body organs in the form of ferritin and hemosiderin, originates from the catabolism of hemoglobin from senescent RBC. It is estimated that an additional 100–125 g of iron, which is equivalent to about 500 transfused units of RBC can be stored in the body of regularly transfused thalassemia patients by the time they reach adulthood.

The role of the chelating drugs is to seek and bind the excess iron from various compartments causing its excretion. These compartments include mainly the iron storage proteins ferritin and hemosiderin, and to a lesser extent the intracellular transit iron pools and also extracellular iron such as transferrin and non–transferrin bound iron (NTBI) found in plasma [104]. A chelating drug used for iron removal in iron overload is only considered effective if it increases iron excretion in the urine, feces or through both of these routes at a rate higher than the rate of iron intake from RBC transfusions and gastrointestinal iron absorption [105].

All three iron chelating drugs can remove excess iron at different rates from different compartments and organs in iron loaded patients. The most effective chelating drug for the removal of excess iron from the heart is L1 (Table 5) [103,106]. The complete removal of excess iron from transfused iron loaded thalassemia patients can be achieved using selective combinations of L1 and DFO [107–111]. This combination also appears to be effective in the removal of excess iron in other categories of iron loaded patients and is also recommended as the safest and most effective combination protocol of intensive chelation for iron removal in heavily iron loaded patients [110,111]. Similar combinations of DFO and DFRA or L1 and DFRA, as well as other intensive chelation protocols have been tested. Unfortunately, as of now, neither improvements in safe iron removal, nor maintenance of iron at physiological levels have been reported yet, possibly due to iron-toxicity implications [112–119]. Overall, it appears that L1 is necessary for the achievement of the ultimate aim of iron chelation therapy, i.e., the achievement and maintenance of normal iron stores in regularly transfused and other categories of iron loaded patients [110,111,120].

Recently, therapeutic achievements in non-iron-loaded conditions with focal iron deposits, such as patients with neurodegenerative and renal diseases have been accomplished using L1, because of better BBB and other organ penetration, as well as lower toxicity than DFO and DFRA [121].

Chelating drugs such as L1 can also be used in other abnormalities of iron metabolism such as in the treatment of the anemia of chronic disease, where L1 appears to redistribute iron from the reticuloendothelial system directly or via transferrin to the erythropoietic tissues for increasing hemoglobin production [122,123]. Similar mechanisms are used in the redistribution of focal iron deposits from other tissues, such as the brain in pantothenate kinase-associated neurodegeneration (PKAN) and other cases of neurodegeneration with brain iron accumulation [124–127]. Overall, it appears that L1 has the ability to redistribute iron and act as a buffering agent for the achievement of balance and normal iron body levels in abnormal conditions related to gross body or focal iron deposits.

In contrast to the chelating drugs intended for the treatment of iron overload, the iron chelating drugs intended for the treatment of iron deficiency anemia should be able to increase iron absorption and increase hemoglobin production to normal physiological levels. The maltol iron complex, with international non-proprietary name (INN) feraccru is currently used for the treatment of iron deficiency anemia (Figure 3) [128–130]. Several lipophilic chelator iron complexes in addition to iron maltol have previously been shown to increase iron absorption in animals [131]. It also appears that lipophilic chelators such as 8-hydroxyquinoline can increase dietary iron absorption and cause iron overload in tissues following long term administration [132].

Two other chelating drugs, namely ethylenediaminetetraacetic acid (EDTA) (Figure 3f) and diethylenetriaminepentaacetic acid (DTPA) (Figure 3e) are used worldwide for general metal detoxification, but can also influence body iron balance, iron metabolic pathways and iron related redox changes (Table 3, Figure 3). In particular, intravenous EDTA is routinely used for xenobiotic metal detoxification in alternative medicine clinics by millions of patients worldwide and DTPA for the detoxification of radioactive metals such as plutonium (Pu) [133,134].

In addition to chelating drugs there are many other drugs with chelating metal binding sites and potential for metal complex formation such as hydroxyurea, tetracycline, bleomycin, ciclopirox and doxorubicin [135,136]. Treatment with these drugs may influence body iron balance levels, iron-containing proteins and metabolic pathways and also iron related redox changes. Similarly, the pharmacological activities of these drugs could also be influenced in the presence of excess iron, since their iron complexes have a different mode of action to their non-iron-bound drug forms. A similar influence on pharmacological activities could also be exerted by other metal ions such as copper, zinc and aluminum, which are competing with iron (Table 5) [137].

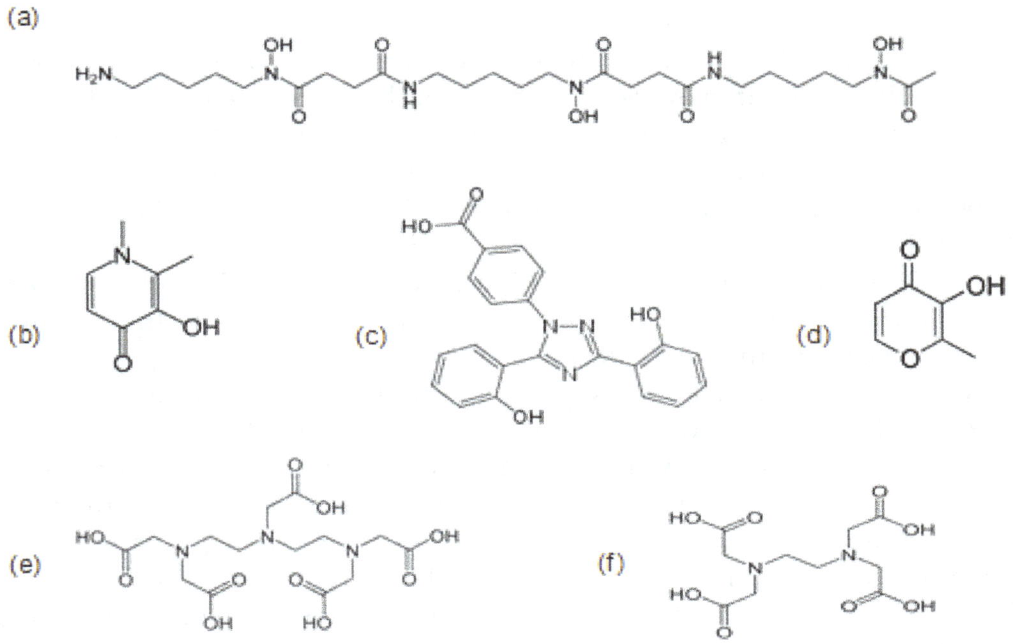

Figure 3. The chemical structure of the main chelating drugs in clinical use. The main iron chelating drugs which are commercially available for the treatment of transfusional iron overload are (**a**) deferoxamine, (**b**) deferiprone and (**c**) deferasirox. The (**d**) iron complex of maltol is used for iron deficiency. The other two chelating drugs (**e**) DTPA and (**f**) EDTA are mainly used for the detoxification of xenobiotic metals.

4. Biologic and Physiological Implications of Interactions with Iron Chelators

Iron binding by chelators in biologic systems is a complex process influenced by many factors and with specific, but variable characteristics. Metal complexation reactions in vitro can provide important basic information on the affinity of chelators for iron, other metals and the stability of the metal complexes (Table 3) [22–26]. Additional information on the interactions of chelators with iron-containing proteins and the iron metabolic pathways both in different cell types and in vivo could not only provide a better understanding of the physiological processes involved, but also better prospects for designing improved therapeutic approaches for different conditions.

There are generally many types of interactions and also many factors influencing the properties and roles of chelators in vivo. Some of these interactions are focused on in vitro and in vivo studies which are helpful in determining the mechanism of action of iron chelating drugs, naturally occurring chelators and also other drugs with chelation potential, all of which can have implications on health [22–26,78].

Characterization of the molecular mechanisms on iron chelation, as well as in vitro and in vivo studies and also following clinical findings could have an impact on determining the pathologic effects in serious diseases and could also possibly improve therapeutic approaches to their treatment.

4.1. *Effects of Chelator and Chelator Iron Complexes on Iron Absorption*

The interactions of natural or synthetic chelators with iron, appear to affect many normal physiological processes and have wide implications on human health. Some of these interactions may lead to metabolic abnormalities and diseases such as iron deficiency anemia and iron overload.

It is estimated that in normal individuals, about 1–1.4 mg of iron from a total of about 6–10 mg present in a typical western diet, is absorbed daily and the same amount is lost from the body, resulting in the maintenance of iron balance. This balance is reflected by normal range hemoglobin levels, as well as liver and other organ iron concentration levels following routine diagnostic tests. There are many abnormalities in relation to iron absorption such as iron deficiency anemia [7]. The prevalent groups affected by iron deficiency are vegetarians, due to insufficient quantities of iron in vegetarian meals, as well as menstruating females due to blood loss and children, due to increased iron requirements for rapid growth [138].

In contrast to iron deficiency anemia, there is an increase in dietary iron absorption, gradual increase in body iron levels and iron overload in idiopathic hemochromatosis [139]. Increase in dietary iron absorption and body iron levels have also been observed in Bantu siderosis as a result of the use of iron cooking utensils [140]. Rapid absorption of excess iron can be observed in iron poisoning cases. This is usually observed in children, due to the accidental ingestion of iron tablets and sometimes may lead to fatalities [141–143].

Overall, it appears that under normal conditions, the rate of iron absorption depends on several iron parameters and other factors in the gastrointestinal tract, such as the amount of iron, the nature of the iron complex form and the ferric or ferrous state of iron [138]. Heme, feraccru, other lipophilic iron complexes, e.g., with 8-hydoxyquinoline or DFRA, as well as ferrous iron formulations are readily absorbed in the gastrointestinal tract [138–142]. In contrast, hydrophilic and charged iron complexes formed for example with DFO, EDTA, L1, tannins and phosphates decrease iron absorption [131,144–148]. It is envisaged that chelators mobilizing iron in the gastrointestinal tract and forming non absorbable iron complexes can be used in the treatment of idiopathic hemochromatosis, in addition to the current treatment using venesection [131].

Interaction with iron and interference with iron absorption in the gastrointestinal tract is also expected with naturally occurring chelators such as phytochelators and drugs with chelating sites. Similarly, the absorption of natural and synthetic chelators including drugs with chelating sites from the gastrointestinal tract can be expected to be affected and be dependent on the quantity of iron and also the properties of the iron complex being formed [135,136,149].

Interference with iron absorption is also expected in the presence of other metal ions competing with iron for chelator metal complex formation and vice versa, i.e., lipophilic chelators such as DFRA are expected to increase other metal absorption such as aluminum [149,150].

Several therapeutic approaches could be designed to decrease the absorption of excessive and toxic iron formulations. In this context, the design of chelating drugs for preventing iron absorption in accidental iron poisoning could prevent or reduce the associated high mortality rate. Similarly, prevention or elimination of the oxidative and other toxic effects of iron complexes such as that of heme in meat and also nitroso heme derivatives found mostly in processed meat, could decrease the morbidity and mortality associated with these conditions. Both heme and nitroso heme derivatives are suspected to be major carcinogens in colorectal and other cancers [151].

4.2. Iron Removal by Chelators from Ferritin and Hemosiderin and Other Proteins

The interactions of the chelating drugs and also other chelators with proteins of iron metabolism, are directly related to the therapeutic mode of action of each chelator and the relevant outcome in each of the iron metabolic diseases (Table 1). In particular, the interactions of chelators with the iron transport and storage proteins, are of major importance since these are considered as major targets in relation to the chelation treatment of transfusional iron overloading diseases such as thalassemia [23–28,56].

The major chelator interactions with proteins of iron metabolism, may include protein iron removal, iron donation, allosteric effects, redox changes with iron centers, and the formation of mixed iron complexes. The extent of such interactions in vivo, will depend on the intracellular and extracellular compartmentalization of the chelators and their iron complexes, as well as their metabolic and other parameters (Tables 3 and 4) [25,26]. Indirect effects of chelators may also be observed through their interactions with iron in the intracellular LMWt iron pool, which is the linking pathway associated with iron delivery and turnover of the iron-containing proteins (Table 2) [55,56].

In relation to iron removal from proteins of iron storage, many chelators including L1 and DFO, have been shown to mobilize iron from hemosiderin and ferritin in vitro [24]. However, only L1 and some other similar alpha-ketohydroxy heteroaromatic chelators, but not DFO and DFRA appear to remove iron from transferrin and lactoferrin [24,72]. In contrast to iron removal from transferrin, lactoferrin, ferritin and hemosiderin, no iron removal has been shown by chelators or chelating drugs from other proteins of iron metabolism, which include hemoglobin, myoglobin, cyclooxygenase, lipoxygenase and ribonucleotide reductase [152].

Ferritin and hemosiderin iron removal is a primary target of chelation therapy in iron loaded diseases, where excess iron in the form of these proteins and especially hemosiderin is present at much higher concentrations and is stored in major organs such as the liver, heart, spleen and pancreas. Individuals with excess stored iron are usually diagnosed by high serum ferritin levels, magnetic resonance imaging (MRI) T2 or T2* measurements of signal intensity decreases due to polynuclear iron concentration increases, and also estimations of the iron concentration increases in liver biopsies [153–156]. MRI T2 and T2* are recently developed non-invasive diagnostic techniques, which are used for measuring excess iron deposition in the various organs of iron loaded patients [153–155]. It appears that in general there is a correlation between serum ferritin and liver iron concentration, but not between serum ferritin and cardiac iron concentration, where it could be misrepresentative in the diagnosis of cardiac iron load [157]. In other diseases of focal iron deposition, e.g., Friedreich's ataxia and PKAN, serum ferritin levels are within the normal range, but iron deposits can be detected in focal points in the brain using MRI T2 or T2* measurements [158].

Many factors influence the mobilization of iron from ferritin and hemosiderin by chelators [28,159]. The structure composition of the polynuclear iron core is also important in the mobilization process. In this context, it appears that the iron cores of ferritin and hemosiderin are not uniform and the outer oxohydroxy complexed iron is easier to mobilize by chelators than the oxo bridge complexed iron in the inner iron core (Figure 4). In this context, the "last in-first out" principle applies for iron release from ferritin and hemosiderin. Furthermore, in vitro studies have shown that iron mobilization by chelators is faster from freshly formed polynuclear iron precipitates than hemosiderin and even slower from ferritin [160].

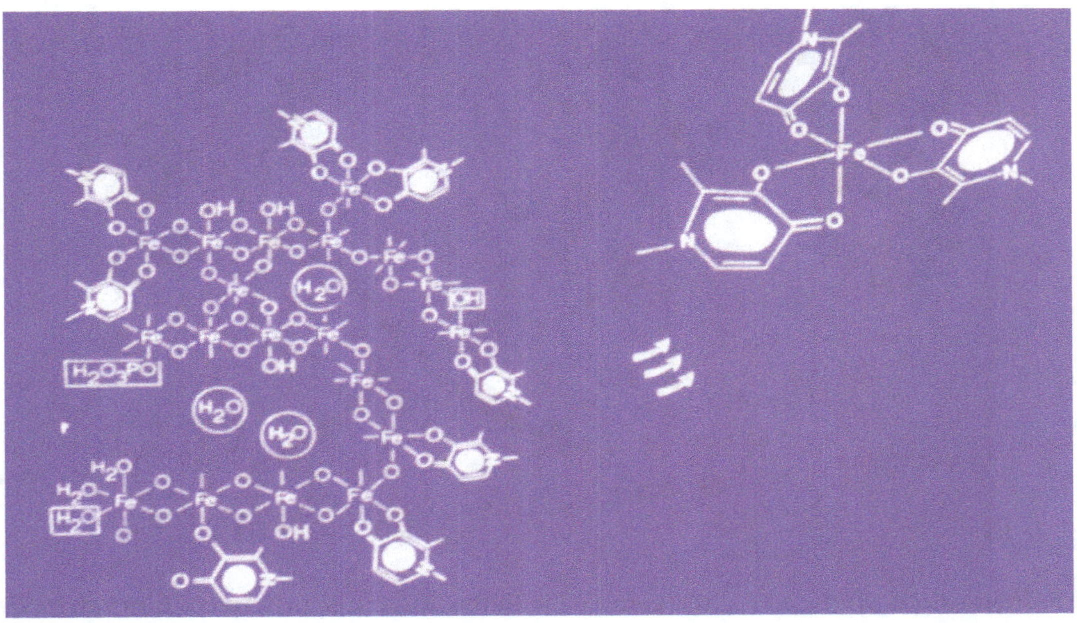

Figure 4. Iron mobilization from ferritin and hemosiderin by deferiprone (L1). Cartoon image of iron mobilization by L1, from the oxohydroxy polynuclear iron complex found in ferritin and hemosiderin. Iron binding by L1 begins from the outer surface of the iron core. Iron binding from the inner iron core is much more difficult to achieve due to lower accessibility by L1 and also because the polynuclear iron complex formation is much denser than the outer surface of the iron core.

The rate of iron mobilization from ferritin and hemosiderin by chelators is slow and may take several days to reach completion. In both cases, only a portion of the iron stored in the proteins is removed [159,160]. Similarly, only a portion of the chelator molecules are saturated with iron at the end of the reaction with both proteins, suggesting that there is a high affinity for iron in the oxohydroxide polynuclear complex, which competes with the chelator for iron [159–161]. This is also confirmed by further studies involving repeated chelator incubations of the same previously treated samples of ferritin or hemosiderin, where it has been shown that the lower the concentration of iron stored in these proteins, the smaller the amount of iron that can be mobilized by chelators [161].

It appears in general, that the amount of iron removed by chelators in vitro depends on the concentration of the chelators and the quantity of iron stored in the proteins (Figure 4) [159–161]. Similar findings are also observed during the chelation treatment of iron loaded patients, where the higher the chelating drug dose and iron load of the patient, the more iron is mobilized and excreted. Much less iron is excreted in normal individuals than iron loaded patients receiving the same chelating drug dose [162]. The slow iron mobilization process from ferritin and hemosiderin by chelators, is also in agreement with what is observed in the treatment of iron overloaded patients, where repeated daily doses are used for months in order for excess iron to be cleared out of the iron loaded organs [107,163].

4.3. Transferrin Iron Removal and Other Interactions by Chelators

Transferrin is the protein responsible for the transport of iron in plasma and its delivery to all cells of the body. It has two metal binding sites and can carry up to two molecules of iron (Figure 5). It can also carry many other essential and xenobiotic metals in addition to iron. Under normal conditions it is found in plasma in four forms, i.e., as apotransferrin, two monotransferrins and diferric transferrin, with about 25–35% saturation with iron overall [164]. Transferrin is recharged 6–10 times per day with iron and redistributes about 25 mg of iron in total among all cells of the body via transferrin receptors [5,28,165].

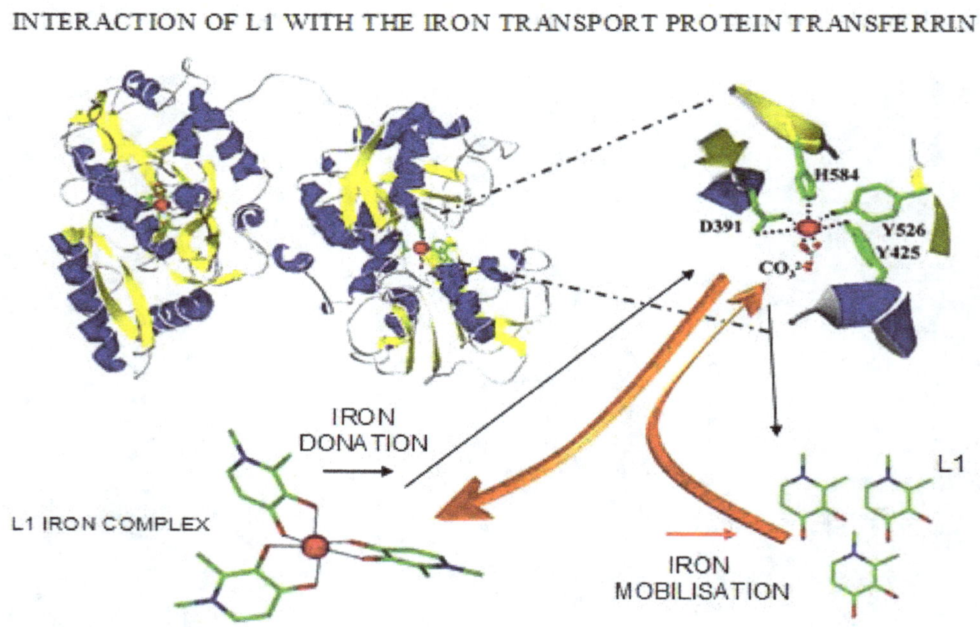

Figure 5. Interactions of L1 and L1 iron complex with the iron transport protein transferrin. Cartoon image of iron mobilization by L1 from diferric transferrin, which usually occurs in iron loaded patients and when high L1 concentration is present in plasma. In a reverse reaction, iron from the L1 iron complex can be donated to apo-transferrin increasing transferrin iron saturation. The latter reaction occurs in non-iron loaded patients with normal transferrin saturation treated with L1.

Transferrin plays an essential role in the transfer of iron between the sites of absorption, utilization, storage and redistribution. It is also regarded as a potent antioxidant and antimicrobial protein because of its ability to sequester iron (Fe^{2+} and Fe^{3+}) in plasma [72,166,167]. It has ferroxidase and iron scavenging activity, rapidly converting Fe^{2+} to Fe^{3+} and binding Fe^{3+}. Similar roles are attributed to transferrin's sister protein lactoferrin, found mainly in bodily secretions and macrophages [65,66,168,169].

In most iron overloaded patients with serum ferritin greater than about 1 mg/L the amount of excess iron causes the saturation of transferrin in plasma and the formation of diferric transferrin. Under these conditions, transferrin is estimated to carry 75 mg of iron per day, which makes it a major target for iron removal in chelation therapy. Iron overload and transferrin iron saturation favors the proliferation of infections and cancer cells [72].

In vitro studies of iron mobilization from diferric transferrin have shown that only L1 out of the three iron chelating drugs can remove iron efficiently. Similar results have been observed in studies with diferric lactoferrin [170,171]. The rate of iron removal from the two proteins was similar and took up to 2–3 h to reach completion [170,171]. Iron mobilization from diferric transferrin has also been shown in vitro using several L1-analogs and other alpha-ketohydroxypyridine chelators [172,173].

In contrast, it has been shown in similar studies that both DFO and DFRA are ineffective in the mobilization of iron from diferric transferrin and lactoferrin [170,171]. The lower efficiency observed by DFO and DFRA in comparison to L1 appears to be related to the lower efficacy and kinetic restrictions imposed by the structural features of DFO and DFRA and the two aforementioned proteins.

In further in vitro and in vivo studies of iron mobilization by L1 from transferrin it was found that the process is chelator concentration dependent and biphasic with iron being released preferentially from the C-terminal site of transferrin [174]. In contrast, under similar in vitro conditions iron was preferentially mobilized from the N-terminal site of the protein in studies using the alpha-ketohydroxypyridine plant amino acid chelator mimosine [174].

Similar iron removal effects from diferric transferrin have been observed in iron-loaded patients treated with L1 (Figure 5) [72,162]. Maximum levels of iron mobilization were observed when the concentration of L1 in the plasma of patients was also at its maximum, which was about 0.5–1.0 h following L1 administration (Table 6) [72,162].

It has also been observed that in the elimination phase of L1 from plasma, when the concentration of L1 is transiently decreasing, transferrin iron saturation progressively increases and transferrin becomes fully saturated with iron in about 2.5 hours, the period when L1 is almost cleared from plasma. The rapid turnover of transferrin iron suggests that iron can be continuously mobilized from transferrin by repeated administration of L1 at effective doses [72,162].

Non transferrin-bound iron (NTBI) is a more labile form of iron in comparison to diferric transferrin in iron loaded patients (Figure 6). In some patients, iron removal from transferrin may not be achieved if high quantities of NTBI are present in plasma. In these cases, L1 can rapidly bind NTBI forming L1 iron complex, thus reducing the non-iron bound L1 concentration to compete efficiently with transferrin for iron (Figures 5 and 6) [72,162,175].

The mobilization by L1 of both NTBI and transferrin-bound iron present in the plasma of iron loaded patients, is a further advantage of chelation therapy using L1, because it reduces the prospects of excess iron deposition and toxicity in the heart and other organs (Figure 6) [72,162,175]. The ability of L1 to remove other toxic metals such as Al and Pu from transferrin is a further advantage in its use for metal intoxication [176]. In these cases, L1 can reduce the prospect of toxic metal accumulation in the tissues, from where it is much more difficult to remove at a later stage. It is estimated that about forty metal ions have been shown to interact with transferrin and their metabolism may be influenced by L1 chelation therapy [72].

In contrast to the targeting of transferrin iron removal by chelators in iron overload, the uptake of iron by transferrin from chelator iron complexes and other iron complex forms is of metabolic and clinical significance (Figure 5). The uptake of iron by apo-transferrin and monoferric transferrin species is of physiological importance for the hemopoietic tissues and also of pharmacological importance for the treatment of iron deficiency anemia. It is also important for preventing microbial and cancer growth, for metal detoxification and some other clinical conditions [175].

In most cases the uptake of iron by transferrin in vitro requires that iron be presented in a mononuclear ferrous or ferric form. Oligonuclear and polynuclear forms of iron such as NTBI are not readily available for apo-transferrin binding. Iron donation to apo-transferrin can be achieved by many bidentate iron chelator complexes, e.g., of L1, maltol and nitrilotriacetic acid, but this is not readily achieved by EDTA nor DFO iron complexes (Figure 5).

Clinical investigations have shown that the administration of L1 to normal individuals causes a transient increase in transferrin iron saturation from about 20% to 80% within 6 hours, suggesting that L1 can mobilize iron from intracellular sites and donate it to apo-transferrin or mono-ferric transferrins (Figure 5) [177]. Iron redistribution by chelators is significant in the treatment of the anemia of chronic disease, e.g., in rheumatoid arthritis patients, where substantial amounts of iron are usually diverted to the reticuloendothelial system and are not supplied to hemopoietic tissues for erythropoiesis [122,123,177]. Iron redistribution is also significant in neurodegenerative and other diseases of focal iron toxicity, where L1 can progressively divert the excess focal iron deposits to apo-transferrin and/or cause its excretion [124,177].

It appears, that transferrin iron removal or donation by L1 and similar chelators in general, are chelator concentration dependent processes. In this context, many of the conflicting in vitro and clinical results are related to the use of inappropriate L1 or other similar chelator dose protocols (Figures 5 and 6) [178,179].

Overall, transferrin plays a central role in iron metabolism and pharmacology and also in treatments involving chelators and chelator metal complexes.

4.4. The Intracellular Low Molecular Weight Iron Pool Changes during Chelation

Under normal conditions, the classical pathway of cellular iron uptake involves binding of diferric transferrin or monoferric transferrin molecules onto the transferrin receptors at the cell membrane and their incorporation in an endosome intracellularly. Iron release from transferrin in the endosome is accomplished by a decrease in the pH to 5. Iron is then distributed intracellularly and detected in different intracellular compartments, including ferritin, heme and other iron-containing proteins (Figure 6) [72,76,180].

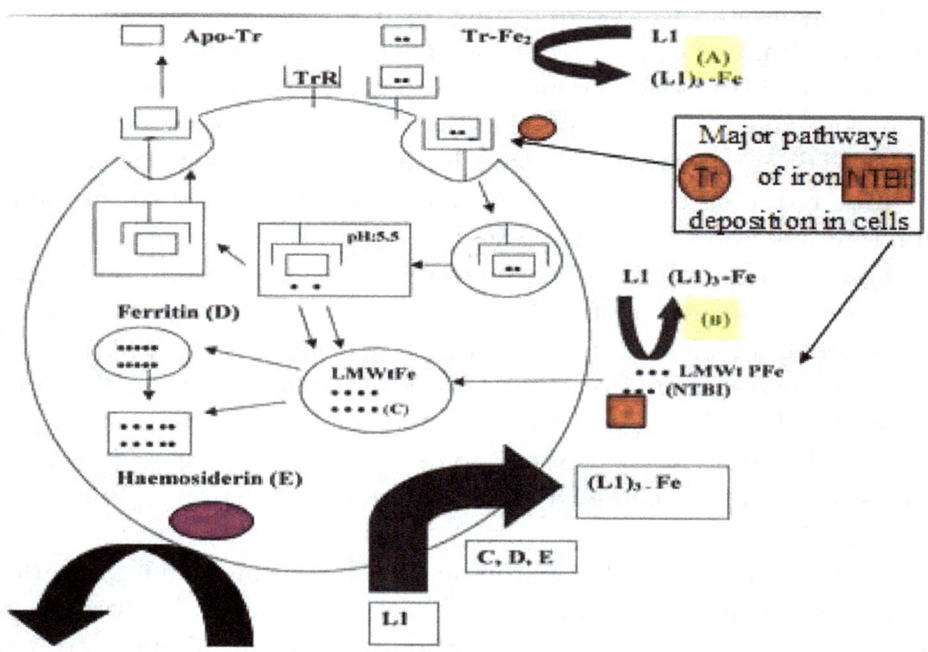

Figure 6. Iron mobilization by deferiprone (L1) from plasma and from cells in iron overloading conditions. Deferiprone can prevent iron accumulation in cells by mobilizing (**A**) transferrin bound iron (Tr-Fe2) and (**B**) non-transferrin bound iron (NTBI) found in plasma. Deferiprone can also mobilize intracellular iron from the (**C**) low molecular weight iron pool (LMWtFe), (**D**) ferritin and (**E**) hemosiderin. (Tr R: transferrin receptor; Apo-Tr: apotransferrin).

Transferrin returns to plasma following the intracellular iron release. During the period of cellular entry transferrin is not involved directly in the iron delivery to iron-containing proteins.

The mechanism of transport of iron intracellularly and subsequently its donation to iron storage proteins and apo-proteins can only be envisaged through the context of a labile, "transit" LMWt chelator iron complex pool (Table 2) [76]. The natural chelating molecules from the LMWt involved specifically in the transfer of iron and the formation of ternary iron complexes with apo-proteins or the incorporation of iron into the iron domains of proteins have not yet been specifically studied or identified. However, the iron uptake and release processes that are involved intracellularly to and from the naturally occurring chelators and their complexes, are expected to be governed by the same thermodynamic and kinetic parameters as for other chelators and their complexes [23–25]. The distribution of the natural chelator and chelator iron complexes into lipophilic and hydrophilic intracellular compartments, is expected to depend on their lipid/water partition coefficient and other physicochemical properties, similar to that of other chelators (Table 6) [180–183].

Similarly, it is envisaged that additional LMWt iron pools with different characteristics are expected to be present in different organelles. In particular, the mitochondrial LMWt iron pool appears to be of physiological and pathologic importance, especially in relation to iron transfer and deposition in mitochondrial ferritin and also the presence of hemosiderin-like deposits in the mitochondria of Friedreich's ataxia patients [184,185].

The importance of the LMWt iron pool is also relevant to the iron chelation therapy pathways. In particular, in vitro studies have shown that the mechanism of iron removal from cells, e.g., hepatocytes by L1 and DFO is thought to involve the stepwise mobilization of mostly ferritin and hemosiderin iron, resulting in the gradual formation of a large intracellular LMWt chelating drug iron complex pool, which is then diffused out of the cells [186].

In transfusional iron overload, each cell type and organ is affected variably by the three chelating drugs, due to differences in their physicochemical and other properties, including cell permeability and affinity for iron (Tables 4–6) [25,26]. Iron removal from the intracellular LMWt iron pool can be accomplished within minutes, provided the chelating drugs can cross the cell membrane and compete effectively with endogenous chelators. Such differences are relevant to the ability of the chelating drugs to remove iron from different organs and iron pools at variable rates [25,187].

Iron removal from the intracellular LMWt iron pool by chelating drugs and other chelators is an important targeting method for the inhibition of the turnover of iron-containing proteins (C in Figure 6). This inhibitory effect could be used as a therapeutic tool for pathways involving iron-containing proteins and metabolites associated with cancer, inflammation and other diseases [72,175].

In contrast to iron removal, iron donation to cells by lipophilic chelators could increase the size of the intracellular LMWt iron pool, ferritin iron levels and the production of heme in hemopoietic cells [180–182]. These non-transferrin iron delivery effects to cells could be used as therapeutic tools for pathways involving the low turnover of iron-containing proteins and especially in abnormal conditions related to low heme production and insufficient transferrin iron delivery, e.g., in the anemia of chronic disease [122,123].

In vitro findings suggest that there are no major differences in the distribution of iron delivery to cells by lipophilic chelators such as 8-hydroxyquinoline, tropolone and maltol [180]. Within this context none of the chelators showed exclusive delivery to or rejection of a particular cellular iron compartment such as ferritin or heme [180]. However, some lipophilic chelators appear to inhibit iron incorporation into heme originating from transferrin and similar interactions are anticipated with iron delivery for other iron-containing proteins [182]. Furthermore, such lipophilic chelators could probably be substituted for transferrin and be used to probe metabolic events. However, diverting iron by chelators under normal conditions may also have toxicity implications.

The interactions of chelators and chelator iron complexes with the intracellular LMWt iron pool is of physiological, pharmacological and toxicological significance. The targeting of the intracellular LMWt iron pool could also have important therapeutic implications.

4.5. Allosteric and Other Interactions of Chelating Drugs with Proteins

There are a number of interactions, including allosteric effects by both the chelating drugs and also other drugs involving proteins of iron metabolism, most of which may not involve the domain coordinating iron (Table 4). These effects have not yet been fully studied, but they may have implications on the therapeutic mode of action or the toxicity of drugs with chelating properties.

Examples include hemoglobin structural changes which have been observed in the presence of L1 and DFO. In particular, fluorescence and circular dichroism studies have shown that L1 can induce conformation changes in hemoglobin (Table 4) [188]. Similarly, L1 was found to prevent carbonyl formation and advanced glycation end products by the inhibition of structural changes in hemoglobin during the fructation process [189]. In other in vitro studies using RBC hemolysate incubation with chelators, DFO, but not L1 appeared to cause methemoglobin formation in a time dependent process [152]. Further studies are required to evaluate the biologic and clinical consequences of these protein allosteric interactions with L1 and DFO.

The interaction of DFRA and its iron complex, as well as other lipophilic drugs and complexes with plasma proteins, is important in the efficacy, pharmacokinetics and clearance of drugs. It appears that both DFRA and its iron complex are bound to albumin and have long plasma half-life in comparison to L1 and DFO, which are hydrophilic and form hydrophilic iron complexes (Table 6).

Allosteric interactions are also envisaged with other iron-containing proteins. For example, the mechanism of action of the anticancer drug hydroxyurea is thought to involve the inhibition of ribonucleotide reductase, a key iron-containing enzyme for DNA synthesis. The inhibition appears to proceed through the free radical nitroxide metabolite of hydroxyurea, which quenches the tyrosyl free radical at the active site of the M2 protein subunit of the enzyme [190,191]. Hydroxyurea is also used in the treatment of sickle cell anemia and thalassemia intermedia, by increasing fetal hemoglobin synthesis which reduces the polymerization of sickle cell hemoglobin and the level of RBC transfusions, respectively [192–200]. Hydroxyurea has been recently identified as a natural product with possible antiviral and other applications [201–203].

There are many other examples of allosteric changes due to substrate competition by different drugs, which may lead to inhibition of proteins of iron metabolism without involving the iron center of the protein. Such examples include the nonsteroidal anti-inflammatory drugs aspirin and ibuprofen which inhibit cyclooxygenase and are used in treating pain, fever and inflammation [204–207]. The inhibition of prostacyclin production and toxic FR generation by cyclooxygenase has also been shown in rat aorta using DFO, L1 and 1-ethyl-2-methyl (L1NEt)- and 1-propyl-2-methyl (L1NPr)-3-hydroxypyrid-4-ones in the same rank order of potency. The inhibition was thought to proceed through the removal or binding of iron in the LMWt pool linked to cyclooxygenase turnover activity and was associated with a hydrophilic cellular compartment [207].

The most complex interactions with iron-containing proteins are the drug metabolizing activities of the heme-containing cytochrome P450 group of enzymes. Drugs and other molecules of different sizes and physicochemical properties are used as substrates for cytochrome P450. In particular, the inhibition and activation of cytochrome P450 by different drugs is a major concern for safety since therapeutic protocols of drug co-administration may result in the accumulation of toxic metabolites and side effects [47–50,208]. Similar mechanisms of inhibition and activation apply for other iron-containing enzymes such as proline hydroxylase [209].

In general, the interactions of chelating and other drugs with iron-containing proteins can involve the iron centers or other parts of the proteins. These interactions are complex and diverse and may lead to therapeutic or toxicity effects. Further studies on such interactions may lead to a better understanding of the pharmacological, therapeutic and toxicity effects of chelating and other drugs in many diseases.

5. Interaction of Iron Proteins with Other Metal Ions and the Role of Chelators

Iron-containing proteins are on the crossroads of the metabolism and toxicity pathways of a large number of metabolites, endogenous and xenobiotic molecules including metals and metal complexes.

The utilization of these pathways has been exploited in medicine for the design of diagnostic and therapeutic products for many diseases including cancer.

There are many interactions of xenobiotic metals and their complexes with proteins of iron metabolism in relation to their use in medical diagnosis, therapeutic application and metal detoxification. Transferrin plays a major role in xenobiotic metal trafficking associated with these medical applications and their effects [72]. Specific chelator interventions and characteristics apply to each such interaction and could theoretically increase the prospects of improvements in therapies while minimizing toxicity in many clinical conditions.

The wide use of xenobiotic metals such as gadolinium (Gd), technetium (Tc), indium (In) and gallium (Ga) and their complexes in medical diagnosis is a rapidly evolving and growing area which is routinely used worldwide. Their application especially as contrast agents in MRI, but also in the labeling of cells and for detecting tumors, inflammatory sites, infections, etc., increases the prospect of medical diagnosis and the treatment of many diseases [22,210–214]. The diagnostic use, metabolism and toxicity of these xenobiotic metals are affected by proteins of iron metabolism and also chelating drugs or other chelators. In particular, the metabolism and transport of these metals is associated with transferrin [72].

Similarly, xenobiotic metals such as platinum (Pt), ruthenium (Ru) and Ga and their complexes which are used in therapeutic strategies primarily against cancer, interact with transferrin and other proteins of iron metabolism and also with chelating drugs. In particular, the antiproliferative effect of Ga in many types of cancer is due primarily to its ability to mimic ferric iron, which is required by ribonucleotide reductase for DNA synthesis [22]. Within this context, Ga transported by transferrin in plasma and competing with iron for ribonucleotide reductase could inhibit DNA production and cell division and be used in different types of cancer with a high number of transferrin receptors including hepatocellular carcinoma, breast and prostate cancers [215]. Different anticancer mechanisms apply in the case of Pt and Ru, although both of these metals also interact with transferrin and their efficacy, metabolism and toxicity depend on this interaction [22,216,217].

Many other interactions of proteins of iron metabolism with xenobiotic metals arising from environmental pollution, food and drug contamination, iatrogenic reasons, etc., may result in hematological and other metabolic changes and also toxic side effects. In these cases, the therapeutic strategies that have been used are similar to those used for the treatment of iron overload. For example, DFO and L1 are used in the detoxification of Al accumulation in aluminum-loaded renal dialysis patients [218,219]. Aluminum shares some of the properties and metabolic pathways of iron and is transported by transferrin. Similarly, L1 has been shown to be effective in the mobilization of Pu from transferrin and ferritin and also of other actinides used in the nuclear industry both in vitro and in vivo models [176,220,221].

Xenobiotic metal toxicity is also associated with FR and other ROS damage, which also involves metabolic pathways and proteins of iron metabolism including transport by transferrin. Specific chelator intervention can ameliorate their toxic side effects including oxidative damage.

6. Chelator Protein Interactions and Free Radical Pathology

The molecular interactions of chelators and proteins of iron metabolism in relation to FR toxicity and oxidative tissue damage in pathologic conditions has been previously reviewed [222,223].

In normal physiological conditions, FR such as superoxide, nitric oxide and hydroxyl radicals and other ROS such as hydrogen peroxide and other peroxides are naturally formed and participate in different physiological processes. These processes include the metabolism by cytochrome P450 of natural and xenobiotic compounds including drugs, food products, also cell signaling, circadian clock regulation, etc. [224–226].

Redox homeostasis is maintained by an innate antioxidant system involving many metabolic pathways, proteins and antioxidant molecules. Iron is the main catalyst of FR production in biologic systems and many iron-containing proteins play a key role in redox homeostasis [227].

Despite that the oxidative processes are strictly controlled by the antioxidant system under normal conditions, excess and uncontrollable FR and ROS production is observed in many pathologic conditions causing biomolecular, subcellular, cellular, tissue and organ damage [222,223].

There are many changes during FR/ROS toxicity including biochemical structural modification or breakdown of organic biomolecules. Such changes include the inactivation of enzymes, crosslinking of proteins, formation of toxic protein carbonyls, crosslinking of proteins and DNA, oxidation of glutathione to a glutathione dimer, lipid peroxidation, damage to sugars such as the breakdown of deoxyribose to malondialdehyde, nucleobase modifications in DNA such as the formation of 8-oxo-7,8-dihydro-2′-deoxyguanosine, etc. [222,223,228,229]. The molecular modifications due to oxidative toxicity can trigger the increased production of antioxidant enzymes and also the production of specific chemokines and other biomolecules involved in signaling processes and regulation of transcription factors for many other biochemical pathways [222,223].

The level of oxidative toxicity and damage can also be affected by dietary, genetic, metabolic and other factors or abnormalities, which can modify the regulation and activity of iron-containing and other enzymes associated with FR/ROS production. Included in this category of enzymes are superoxide dismutase, catalase, glutathione peroxidases, thioredoxin, NADPH oxidase, cyclooxygenase, lipoxygenase, cytochrome P450 enzymes, etc. [15,16,19,20,223].

Iron plays a catalytic and pivotal role in FR/ROS toxicity. In particular, cell death due to iron toxicity known as "ferroptosis", has specific characteristics and is different from apoptosis or other cell death pathways [230–233]. Ferroptosis has been identified in many conditions including cancer, acute kidney disease, stroke, etc. [230–233].

Under physiological conditions, oxidative FR/ROS toxicity can be confronted successfully by the antioxidant system, which is composed of antioxidant enzymes, endogenous antioxidants such as glutathione and also dietary antioxidants such as polyphenols, vitamins A, C and E. In addition, damaged cells due to oxidative stress can also be removed by repair systems involving macrophages [222,223].

In FR pathologic conditions, a vicious circle of FR/ROS toxicity is formed which cannot be confronted successfully by the antioxidant system leading to cellular and tissue damage. In each pathologic condition the oxidative FR/ROS toxicity is inflicted on different cellular and organ targets. Similarly, the toxicity in each case may have variations with respect to different causes, intensity and duration [222,223].

The design of optimal antioxidant therapeutic strategies is based on the identification of the target molecules and organs of oxidative toxicity and the application of efficacious antioxidant protocols, which include iron chelation [178].

It has been shown in in vivo and in vitro studies that there is a direct link between iron toxicity and decrease in glutathione levels. In contrast, iron chelation treatment causes replenishment in the levels of glutathione and other endogenous antioxidants [234,235].

The antioxidant effects of many dietary chelating polyphenols are via a mechanism of inhibition of oxidative damage involving both iron chelation and also scavenging of FR [98].

Deferiprone has been shown to be an effective antioxidant in in vitro, in vivo and clinical conditions [222,223]. The antioxidant effects of L1 in thalassemia patients includes the reversal and/or improvement of tissue damage of the heart, liver, kidney, pancreas and endocrine organs, as well as an improvement in the endothelial function, left ventricular ejection function, glucose metabolic disturbances and diabetes [222,223].

Similar antioxidant effects and therapeutic improvements have been recorded in patients treated with L1 in primary glomerulonephritis, diabetic nephropathy and healthy volunteers who received radiocontrast agents [236].

Many clinical trials using L1 have also been carried out in different categories of patients with neurodegeneration and brain damage [237–239]. These categories include patients with Alzheimer's and Parkinson's diseases, Friedreich's ataxia, PKAN and also other cases of neurodegeneration with brain iron accumulation [124–127].

In relation to the clinical effects in Friedreich's ataxia patients, treatment using L1 was accompanied by a reduction in the excess toxic iron in the brain, ataxic gait and neuropathy in general [124]. Similar effects of regression of symptoms were also observed in cases of neurodegeneration with brain iron accumulation [125–127].

The improvement in mitochondrial structure and function observed both in vitro and in vivo, in thalassemia and Friedreich's ataxia patients, is further evidence of the antioxidant potential of L1 at the clinical level, especially since mitochondrial abnormalities are related to cancer and many other diseases [240].

7. Prospects for the Clinical Use of Chelators in Infections and Cancer

Iron is essential in the growth of almost all living cells, including microbes and cancer cells [241]. Microbial infections are one of the most common causes of mortality in iron loaded patients. Similarly, iron overload as a result of transfusions can decrease the survival of cancer patients. Deprivation of iron has been a major target for the development of antimicrobial and anticancer therapeutics. Several other forms of interactions between chelators and iron, as well as related metabolic pathways in relation to microbes and cancer cells, may result in improved therapeutic approaches for these diseases.

7.1. Iron, Chelation and Therapeutic Strategies in Infections

Iron is essential for all microbial organisms but is also a major target for therapeutics for inhibiting the growth and proliferation of pathologic microorganisms involved in infectious diseases [242–244].

The interaction of chelators and iron with pathologic microbes, is of major significance to the development and progress of infections in many categories of patients [242–245]. The production of siderophores by microbes for the acquisition of iron from the surrounding media, is an illustration of the importance of iron for microbial survival [77]. The major roles played by transferrin and lactoferrin as antimicrobial agents in plasma and bodily secretions, respectively, further illustrates this link. Their antimicrobial activity is secured by the presence of non-iron-saturated transferrin and lactoferrin iron binding sites which can rapidly mobilize iron from the vicinity of the microbes and deprive them of iron required for their growth [71,72].

The chelating drugs and other chelators have variable effects on the growth of microbes. Antimicrobial drugs have specific targets for each microbial species and a major impact on the treatment of many associated diseases with high morbidity and mortality rates worldwide. Infectious diseases affect millions of people and are the major cause of death in developing counties, especially young children [245]. For example, malaria remains a major health hazard in developing countries [246,247]. In this context, all three iron chelating drugs L1, DFO and DFRA have been shown in in vitro, in vivo and clinical studies to have antimalarial effects [248–252].

In contrast to antimicrobial effects, some chelating drugs can exacerbate infections mainly by acting as siderophores for specific microbes. Among the established serious toxic side effects of DFO are yersiniosis and mucormycosis, which occur in iron loaded and renal dialysis patients, respectively. It appears that in both cases DFO acts as a siderophore and donates iron for the growth of *Yersinia enterocolitica* and *Zygomyces,* respectively [253,254].

Unlike DFO, both L1 and DFRA do not appear to promote the growth of either *Yersinia enterocolitica* or *Zygomyces*. There are many obstacles in the treatment of mucormycosis, which affects mainly patients in developed countries and in many cases can be fatal [254]. In contrast to DFO related toxicity effects, both L1 and DFRA have been tested for the treatment of mucormycosis with encouraging results [255,256].

Different effects on the growth of microbes have also been shown by other natural and synthetic chelators. The antibacterial activity of DFO, L1, maltol, mimosine and other experimental alpha-ketohydroxy heteroaromatic chelators appear to be chelator concentration dependent [257]. The alpha-ketohydroxypyridine chelating drug ciclopirox, has been developed for the treatment of external infections of the skin and nails and has also been tested for other clinical applications [258].

The chelator pyridinethione (omadine) and its salts have been used for over 50 years as antifungal agents. Pyridinethione was recently identified as a natural plant product [259].

The interaction of chelating drugs and siderophores with transferrin and lactoferrin for the acquisition of iron is an important area for investigation regarding the growth and proliferation of microbes and also for the design of antimicrobial therapeutic strategies. Pharmacological, thermodynamic, kinetic and other parameters can influence such interactions. Similarly, many other factors and limitations may also have to be considered regarding the design of antimicrobial therapeutic strategies including combination with other antimicrobial drugs, accessibility of the chelating drug in the site of the infection at therapeutic doses, the use of effective dose protocols and toxic side effects to name a few.

Some of the considerations and limitations in the antimicrobial activity of chelating drugs are particularly important in the design of antimicrobial therapies for fatal infections, which are currently untreatable. For example, L1 can be targeted to treat infections of the brain, such as meningitis, since transferrin and lactoferrin have no access to it and L1 is the only one of the three chelating drugs that can cross the BBB and mobilize iron associated with the growth and proliferation of the microbe *Neisseria* [121]. Very promising results were also shown in malaria infected patients from the use of the combination of L1 with the classical antimalarial drug chloroquine [252].

Further studies are needed to establish the potential therapeutic effects of iron chelating drugs on infections and also the implications of iron on infections from the use of drugs with metal chelating properties such as tetracycline and doxorubicin.

7.2. Iron, Chelation and Cancer Therapeutic Strategies

Cancer is a disease associated with high mortality and morbidity rates worldwide, despite continuous efforts for early diagnosis, prevention and therapeutic advances [245]. There is a need for the development of new approaches and therapeutics for cancer including those associated with iron metabolism and metal chelation.

The anticancer properties of chelators have been previously reviewed and new developments will be discussed in relation to the design of cancer targeting strategies based on new experimental and clinical findings [260,261].

Iron is essential for the growth and proliferation of all cancer cells, but each cancer cell type has different iron requirements. Iron chelators can affect the initiation, growth, proliferation and metastasis of cancer cells by targeting different stages of the progression of the disease, including related iron metabolic pathways and iron-containing proteins [262,263].

In relation to cancer targeting strategies by chelating drugs, many variables have to be considered, including the location of cancer in the body, the surrounding conditions, the anticancer mechanisms involved, as well as pharmacological and other parameters applied in each cancer type case.

The antioxidant activity of the chelating drugs is one of several modes of action utilized for anticancer strategies. The anticancer strategy is based on the mobilization of labile iron and the inhibition of the catalytic activity of FR/ROS production and oxidative damage, which is implicated at all stages of cancer progression to metastasis [263,264]. This therapeutic approach is in agreement with the wide publicity surrounding the use of antioxidants as a method of cancer prevention, which has been promoted for many years in the mass media, resulting in a substantial increase in the sale of antioxidant nutraceutical formulations over the counter.

In contrast to antioxidant effects, lipophilic redox active chelator iron or copper complexes such as omadine iron and di-2-pyridylketone thiosemicarbazone copper complexes have been designed and developed for specific targeting, uptake and destruction of cancer cells [100,101,265]. Some of these chelators, e.g., triapine and chelator metal complexes have reached the stage of clinical trials [266]. It seems that cancer cell death achieved by FR/ROS, copper and iron toxicity, shares a common pathway, which has specific characteristics and is different from apoptosis or other cell death pathways [230,233].

Ferroptotic cell death has been associated with neuroblastoma and other cancer types, all of which are targeted by new investigational therapeutics [230,233].

Different therapeutic approaches are needed for variable forms of iron induced carcinogenicity, some of which may be related to dietary and other habits and can be prevented. For example, iron in heme and the nitroso heme complexes have been implicated in the rise of different cancers [151]. Similar carcinogenic toxicity is suspected from other iron complexes formed during cigarette-smoking and in barbecuing.

The need for iron by cancer cells is another important strategy for anticancer targeting by chelators. In particular, some cancer types such as breast, prostate, bladder cancer and leukemias appear to have an increased number of transferrin receptors and requirements for iron [267]. Iron mobilization by L1 and DFO has been shown in in vitro studies to decrease DNA synthesis in cancer cells, through the inhibition of ribonucleotide reductase [268]. However, the allosteric inhibition of ribonucleotide reductase by the anticancer chelating drug hydroxyurea, appears to be more effective at lower doses than by L1 and DFO in cancer patients [190,191].

The use of Ga chelator complexes to compete with iron uptake and utilization by cancer cells, which is required by iron metabolic pathways is another form of anticancer targeting in different cancers-primarily hepatocellular carcinoma [22,215,269,270]. Platinum chelator complexes targeting other than iron metabolic pathways are routinely used for cancer chemotherapy and involves the treatment of about 50% of patients with different cancer types [22,217]. The anticancer activity of both Ga and Pt is mediated through transferrin transport in plasma, similar to the case of iron transport [72,165].

Another form of anticancer targeting applicable in some cancer types is the inhibition of cyclooxygenase activity. This inhibition may not be directly related to iron binding effects [205,206]. However, combination strategies involving cyclooxygenase inhibitors and iron chelators targeting cyclooxygenase turnover indirectly through the depletion of the LMWt iron pool may enhance anticancer activity [205–207,271].

The ability of L1 to remove iron from transferrin may increase the anticancer activity by minimizing cancer cell iron uptake [72]. Similarly, L1's ability to cross the BBB may have additional advantages over other anticancer drugs in neuroblastoma and other brain cancers [121,272].

Cancer is a multifactorial and diverse disease, caused partly by different carcinogens which include iron and other metal complexes [22]. The development and progression of different cancer types proceed at different rates. In many cases, cancer can be prevented or delayed by adopting healthy dietary and other habits, including the consumption of foods with variable chelating antioxidants. Iron chelating drugs and other chelators, as well as chelator metal complexes can play a significant role in the treatment of cancer by targeting specific metabolic pathways and proteins in cancer initiation, proliferation and metastasis. Drug combinations, including specific chelating drugs or chelator metal complexes with other anticancer drugs, may offer better therapeutic solutions than cancer monotherapy strategies, which are widely used at present [22].

8. Future Prospects

Chelators and biomolecules with metal binding ligands are essential in determining the solubility, transport, biochemical mode of action and metabolism of iron and other metals in biology and medicine [22–25]. Similarly, chelators and their metal complexes offer daily therapeutic solutions to millions of patients worldwide. Furthermore, their targeted use as main, alternative or adjuvant therapies can increase the prospect of treatment for many untreatable diseases with high mortality and morbidity rates such as thalassemia, cancer, acute kidney disease and neurodegeneration [191,236,273].

The interactions of chelators and other biomolecules possessing metal binding ligands with proteins involved in iron and other metal metabolism are very important in the turnover and inhibition/activation of enzymes involved in metabolic pathways associated with normal bodily functions, growth, development and immuno-protection [69,274–277]. The need for iron by cancer cells and pathogenic microbes make chelation a suitable tool for the design of anticancer and antimicrobial therapeutics [241,278].

The daily clinical use and chronic administration of iron chelating drugs in the treatment of transfusional iron overload is an indication of relatively low toxicity in comparison to other pharmaceuticals. In particular, the achievement of the complete treatment of iron overload and long term survival of thalassemia patients in the last decade using effective L1 and L1/DFO combinations highlights the importance of iron chelation in medicine [107–110]. Furthermore, it provides evidence of the importance of the design of therapeutic protocols based on information derived from biochemical studies and from findings on the target characteristics, as well as chelator therapeutic and toxicity effects [110,279]. In this context, biochemical studies are necessary for determining and understanding the modes of action of chelating and other drugs, which are particularly useful in the era of personalized medicine.

The characterization of the mode of action and the safety of L1 in iron loaded patients encouraged its application in many non-iron loaded conditions, especially those with no effective therapies at present [56]. In this context, L1 is currently regarded as one of the leading therapeutics in PKAN and Friedreich's ataxia, where neurodegenerative damage due to focal iron deposits has been identified by MRI in the brain of patients of both diseases [124,126,273,280]. The targeting of iron in many neurodegenerative diseases is the subject of ongoing clinical trials and other investigations involving L1 and other chelators [280–284].

Further encouraging results obtained from studies of L1 in HIV patients, and also in different models of prostate and other cancers and of mitochondrial injury, suggest that there are encouraging prospects for the use of L1 in many other diseases linked to iron metabolic pathways and also FR pathology [155,240,285–288]. The targeting of iron and copper for anticancer activity by chelators including L1 is the subject of specific strategies for different types of cancer [289–296]. Similar targeting has also been considered for cardiovascular and other diseases, where iron is implicated [297–299].

The approval of the use of the maltol iron complex (feraccru) for the treatment of iron deficiency anemia is another major development in the area of chelation. It has taken almost forty years to reach the clinical stage from the original discovery and from initial biochemical and other preclinical studies, which proposed the mechanisms of efficient iron delivery from iron complexes to cells, animals and humans [128–131]. Improvements have also been reported in the treatment of iron deficiency anemia using many other ferric and ferrous iron formulations and also different administration protocols [300–303].

The development of therapeutics based on essential or xenobiotic metal complexes with maltol and other similar chelators is in progress for other essential metal deficiencies and also in cancer [22,215,270,304,305]. The establishment of the use of chelators with radiotracers and similar metal complexes in diagnostic medicine and as theragnostic agents is another important development and also a rapidly expanding medical field [22,305,306].

There are many new challenges in the application of chelators and chelator metal complexes for improving human health. Metal detoxification is currently a major topic in medicine, since many toxic metals in food and environmental pollution have been identified as major causes of many diseases including hypertension, cancer and neurodegeneration [22,306–309]. The development of specific chelating drugs targeting such toxic metals and metal complexes, is likely to increase in the future since environmental pollution is steadily increasing worldwide [22,309].

Further investigations on the effect of chelators and chelator metal complexes on different cell types and model organisms, e.g., yeast, plants, *Drosophila* and *Caenorhabditis elegans* is not only of great importance to experimental research, but fundamental in identifying and understanding differences between organisms. The specificity of different chelators towards iron and/or other metals and of their metal complexes should also be investigated for membrane and cell-wall permeability, metabolic pathways and biologic effects, similar to previous studies in mammalian cells and cell lines [101,131,152,180,182,238]. In particular, iron and other metal donation by lipophilic phytochelators such as 8-hydroxyquinoline, tropolone and maltol should be compared in different types of cells and organisms. Similarly, the uptake, distribution and storage of iron in unicellular eukaryotes, such as *Saccharomyces cerevisiae* that lack ferritin also need to be investigated.

9. Conclusions

Iron is essential for living organisms, microbes and cancer cells. The diversity in the activity and function of iron and associated pathologies is broadly based on bond formation with adjacent ligands, overall molecular structure and redox properties. Abnormalities in the iron-containing proteins, the iron metabolic pathways and associated processes can lead to very common genetic and other diseases, such as the hemoglobinopathies, idiopathic hemochromatosis and iron deficiency.

Specific chelating drug protocols can offer therapeutic solutions for most diseases associated with iron. It has been shown recently that, L1 and selected combinations with DFO can completely clear transfusional iron overload in thalassemia and has converted thalassemia from a fatal to a chronic disease. Similarly, L1 is considered as one of the leading therapeutics in PKAN and Friedreich's ataxia patients, as well as other groups of patients with neurodegenerative disorders. It also has prospects for clinical use in cancer and HIV-AIDS patients and also patients with aluminum intoxication. In another new development, the maltol iron complex feraccru has been recently approved in the treatment of iron deficiency anemia. Similarly, the 1-hydroxypyrid-2-one chelating drug ciclopirox, which is used for treating fungal infections, may also be used in other diseases.

As Hippocrates suggested more than 2000 years ago prevention is better than cure in all diseases. In this context improvement in healthy habits including dietary changes and exercise could prevent or minimize many disease incidences including cancer, neurodegeneration, kidney, liver and cardiac diseases and also infections. New challenges and approaches using chelation and other methods could help to reach this target. For example, reduction in the consumption of red and processed meat could reduce carcinogenesis. These types of cancers appear to be promoted following chronic exposure to iron-based and also other forms of carcinogens in conjunction with insufficient antioxidant dietary intake.

Free radical toxicity caused by iron catalysis is implicated in tissue damage in most pathologic conditions. In most cases, chelating drugs can mitigate this form of toxicity. Further investigations and therapeutic advances on the use of iron and other chelators, as well as their metal complexes are in progress at all levels, including chemical synthesis of new chelators, cell studies and new applications.

Author Contributions: C.N.K. contributed to the literature background and critically reviewed the manuscript. G.J.K. conceived, designed and wrote the manuscript. All authors have read and agreed to the published version of the manuscript.

Acknowledgments: The study is dedicated to the memory of the distinguished academic colleagues Professors Erica Baker (Australia), Evgeny T. Denisov (Russia), Vladislav Eybl (Czech Republic), Premysl Ponka (Canada), David Taylor (UK) and Eugene D. Weinberg (USA), who recently passed away.

Abbreviations

BBB—blood-brain barrier; DFRA—deferasirox; DFO—deferoxamine; L1—deferiprone; EDTA—ethylenediaminetetraacetic acid; DTPA—diethylenetriaminepentaacetic acid; FR—free radicals; Gd—gadolinium; Ga—gallium; In—indium; INN—International non-proprietary name; Fe-S—iron-sulfur; LMWt—low molecular weight; MRI—magnetic resonance imaging; NTBI—non-transferrin bound iron; PKAN—pantothenate kinase-associated neurodegeneration; Pt—platinum; Pu—plutonium; Ru—ruthenium; Tc—technetium; OST—oxidative stress toxicity; ROS—reactive oxygen species; RBC—red blood cells.

References

1. Prasad, A.S. Zinc: An overview. *Nutrition* **1995**, *11*, 93–99. [PubMed]
2. E Coleman, J. Zinc Proteins: Enzymes, Storage Proteins, Transcription Factors, and Replication Proteins. *Annu. Rev. Biochem.* **1992**, *61*, 897–946. [CrossRef] [PubMed]
3. Prasad, A.S. Zinc deficiency. *BMJ* **2003**, *326*, 409–410. [CrossRef] [PubMed]
4. Daniel, K.G.; Harbach, R.H.; Guida, W.C.; Dou, Q.P. Copper storage diseases: Menkes, Wilsons, and cancer. *Front. Biosci* **2004**, *9*, 2652–2662. [CrossRef]
5. Galaris, D.; Pantopoulos, K. Oxidative Stress and Iron Homeostasis: Mechanistic and Health Aspects. *Crit. Rev. Clin. Lab. Sci.* **2008**, *45*, 1–23. [CrossRef]
6. Gozzelino, R.; Arosio, P. Iron Homeostasis in Health and Disease. *Int. J. Mol. Sci.* **2016**, *17*, 130. [CrossRef] [PubMed]
7. McLean, E.; Cogswell, M.; Egli, I.; Wojdyla, D.; De Benoist, B. Worldwide prevalence of anaemia, WHO Vitamin and Mineral Nutrition Information System, 1993–2005. *Public Heal. Nutr.* **2008**, *12*, 444. [CrossRef] [PubMed]
8. Community control of hereditary anaemias: Memorandum from a WHO meeting*. *Bull. World Heal. Organ.* **1983**, *61*, 63–80.
9. Zurlo, M.; De Stefano, P.; Borgna-Pignatti, C.; Di Palma, A.; Melevendi, C.; Piga, A.; Di Gregorio, F.; Burattini, M.; Terzoli, S. Survival and causes of death in thalassaemia major. *Lancet* **1989**, *334*, 27–30. [CrossRef]
10. Inamoto, Y.; Lee, S.J. Late effects of blood and marrow transplantation. *Haematologica* **2017**, *102*, 614–625. [CrossRef]
11. Gratwohl, A.; Pasquini, M.C.; Aljurf, M.; Atsuta, Y.; Baldomero, H.; Foeken, L.; Gratwohl, M.; Bouzas, L.F.; Confer, D.; Frauendorfer, K.; et al. Worldwide Network for Blood and Marrow Transplantation. (WBMT). One million haemopoietic stem-cell transplants: A retrospective observational study. *Lancet Haematol.* **2015**, *2*, e91–e100.
12. Shenoy, S.; Angelucci, E.; Arnold, S.D.; Baker, K.S.; Bhatia, M.; Bresters, D.; Dietz, A.C.; De La Fuente, J.; Duncan, C.; Gaziev, J.; et al. Current Results and Future Research Priorities in Late Effects after Hematopoietic Stem Cell Transplantation for Children with Sickle Cell Disease and Thalassemia: A Consensus Statement from the Second Pediatric Blood and Marrow Transplant Consortium International Conference on Late Effects after Pediatric Hematopoietic Stem Cell Transplantation. *Boil. Blood Marrow Transplant.* **2017**, *23*, 552–561. [CrossRef]
13. Germing, U.; Schroeder, T.; Kaivers, J.; Kündgen, A.; Kobbe, G.; Gattermann, N. Novel therapies in low- and high-risk myelodysplastic syndrome. *Expert Rev. Hematol.* **2019**, *12*, 893–908. [CrossRef] [PubMed]
14. Kontoghiorghes, G.J. How to manage iron toxicity in post-allogeneic hematopoietic stem cell transplantation? *Expert Rev. Hematol.* **2020**, *13*, 299–302. [CrossRef] [PubMed]
15. Kontoghiorghes, G.J.; Kontoghiorghe, C.N. Prospects for the introduction of targeted antioxidant drugs for the prevention and treatment of diseases related to free radical pathology. *Expert Opin. Investig. Drugs* **2019**, *28*, 593–603. [CrossRef] [PubMed]
16. Galaris, D.; Barbouti, A.; Pantopoulos, K. Iron homeostasis and oxidative stress: An intimate relationship. *Biochim. Biophys. Acta (BBA)-Bioenerg* **2019**, *1866*, 118535. [CrossRef]
17. Nakamura, T.; Naguro, I.; Ichijo, H.; Nakmura, T. Iron homeostasis and iron-regulated ROS in cell death, senescence and human diseases. *Biochim. Biophys. Acta (BBA)-Gen. Subj.* **2019**, *1863*, 1398–1409. [CrossRef]
18. Balsano, C.; Porcu, C.; Sideri, S. Is copper a new target to counteract the progression of chronic diseases? *Metallomics.* **2018**, *10*, 1712–1722. [CrossRef]
19. Denisov, E.T.; Afanas'Ev, I.B. *Oxidation and Antioxidants in Organic Chemistry and Biology*; CRC Press: Boca Raton, FA, USA, 2005.
20. Halliwell, B.; Gutteridge, J.M.; E Cross, C. Free radicals, antioxidants, and human disease: Where are we now? *J. Lab. Clin. Med.* **1992**, *119*, 598–620.
21. Kontoghiorghes, G.J. Free radicals, oxidant stress and drug action. In *Iron Chelation in Biochemistry and Medicine*; Rice-Evans, C., Ed.; Rechelieu Press: London, UK, 1978; pp. 277–303.
22. Kontoghiorghes, G.J. Advances on Chelation and Chelator Metal Complexes in Medicine. *Int. J. Mol. Sci.* **2020**, *21*, 2499. [CrossRef]

23. *Development of Iron Chelators for Clinical Use*; Anderson, F.W., Hiller, M.C., Eds.; DHEW Publication: Bethesda, MD, USA, 1975; pp. 1–275.
24. Kontoghiorghes, G.J. The Design of Orally Active Iron Chelators for the Treatment of Thalassaemia. Ph.D. Thesis, University of Essex, Colchester, UK, 1982; pp. 1–243. Available online: https://www.pri.ac.cy/files/KGJ_thesis_1982.pdf (accessed on 7 May 2020).
25. Kontoghiorghes, G.J.; Pattichis, K.; Neocleous, K.; Kolnagou, A. The design and development of deferiprone (L1) and other iron chelators for clinical use: Targeting methods and application prospects. *Curr. Med. Chem.* **2004**, *11*, 2161–2183. [CrossRef] [PubMed]
26. Kontoghiorghes, G.; Eracleous, E.; Economides, C.; Kolnagou, A. Advances in iron overload therapies. Prospects for effective use of deferiprone (L1), deferoxamine, the new experimental chelators ICL670, GT56-252, L1NAll and their combinations. *Curr. Med. Chem.* **2005**, *12*, 2663–2681. [CrossRef] [PubMed]
27. Weatherall, D.; Clegg, J.B. Inherited haemoglobin disorders: An increasing global health problem. *Bull. World Heal. Organ.* **2001**, *79*, 704–712.
28. Teawtrakul, N.; Chansung, K.; Sirijerachai, C.; Wanitpongpun, C.; Thepsuthammarat, K. The impact and disease burden of thalassemia in Thailand: A population-based study in 2010. *J. Med. Assoc. Thail.* **2012**, *95*, 95.
29. Cairo, G.; Bernuzzi, F.; Recalcati, S. A precious metal: Iron, an essential nutrient for all cells. *Genes Nutr.* **2006**, *1*, 25–39. [CrossRef]
30. Yoshida, T.; Prudent, M.; D'Alessandro, A. Red blood cell storage lesion: Causes and potential clinical consequences. *Blood Transfus.* **2019**, *17*, 27–52.
31. Asaro, R.J.; Zhu, Q.; Cabrales, P. Erythrocyte Aging, Protection via Vesiculation: An Analysis Methodology via Oscillatory Flow. *Front. Physiol.* **2018**, *9*, 9. [CrossRef]
32. Alaarg, A.; Schiffelers, R.M.; Van Solinge, W.W.; Van Wijk, R. Red blood cell vesiculation in hereditary hemolytic anemia. *Front. Physiol.* **2013**, *4*, 4. [CrossRef]
33. Jóźwik, M.; Jóźwik, M.; Józwik, M.; Szczypka, M.; Gajewska, J.; Laskowska-Klita, T. Antioxidant defence of red blood cells and plasma in stored human blood. *Clin. Chim. Acta* **1997**, *267*, 129–142. [CrossRef]
34. Tolosano, E.; Altruda, F. Hemopexin: Structure, Function, and Regulation. *DNA Cell Boil.* **2002**, *21*, 297–306. [CrossRef]
35. Shih, A.W.; McFarlane, A.; Verhovsek, M. Haptoglobin testing in hemolysis: Measurement and interpretation. *Am. J. Hematol.* **2014**, *89*, 443–447. [CrossRef] [PubMed]
36. Stamler, J.S. Blood Flow Regulation by S-Nitrosohemoglobin in the Physiological Oxygen Gradient. *Science* **1997**, *276*, 2034–2037. [CrossRef]
37. Postnikova, G.B.; Shekhovtsova, E.A. Myoglobin: Oxygen Depot or Oxygen Transporter to Mitochondria? A Novel Mechanism of Myoglobin Deoxygenation in Cells (review). *Biochemistry (Moscow)* **2018**, *83*, 168–183. [CrossRef]
38. Reeder, B.; Wilson, M.T. Hemoglobin and myoglobin associated oxidative stress: From molecular mechanisms to disease States. *Curr. Med. Chem.* **2005**, *12*, 2741–2751. [CrossRef] [PubMed]
39. Reeder, B.J. Redox and Peroxidase Activities of the Hemoglobin Superfamily: Relevance to Health and Disease. *Antioxid. Redox Signal* **2017**, *26*, 763–776. [CrossRef] [PubMed]
40. González-Arzola, K.; Velázquez-Cruz, A.; Guerra-Castellano, A.; Casado-Combreras, M.A.; Pérez-Mejías, G.; Díaz-Quintana, A.J.; Díaz-Moreno, I.; De La Rosa, M.A. New moonlighting functions of mitochondrial cytochrome c in the cytoplasm and nucleus. *FEBS Lett.* **2019**, *593*, 3101–3119. [CrossRef]
41. Grevel, A.; Pfanner, N.; Becker, T. Coupling of import and assembly pathways in mitochondrial protein biogenesis. *Boil. Chem.* **2019**, *401*, 117–129. [CrossRef] [PubMed]
42. Vringer, E.; Tait, S.W. Mitochondria and Inflammation: Cell Death Heats Up. *Front. Cell Dev. Boil.* **2019**, *7*, 100. [CrossRef]
43. Santucci, R.; Sinibaldi, F.; Cozza, P.; Polticelli, F.; Fiorucci, L. Cytochrome c: An extreme multifunctional protein with a key role in cell fate. *Int. J. Boil. Macromol.* **2019**, *136*, 1237–1246. [CrossRef]
44. Ramzan, R.; Vogt, S.; Kadenbach, B. Stress-mediated generation of deleterious ROS in healthy individuals-role of cytochrome c oxidase. *J. Mol. Med.* **2020**, *98*, 651–657. [CrossRef]
45. Timon-Gomez, A.; Nývltová, E.; Abriata, L.A.; Vila, A.J.; Hosler, J.; Barrientos, A. Mitochondrial cytochrome c oxidase biogenesis: Recent developments. *Semin. Cell Dev. Boil.* **2018**, *76*, 163–178. [CrossRef] [PubMed]
46. Llases, M.; Morgada, M.N.; Vila, A.J. Biochemistry of Copper Site Assembly in Heme-Copper Oxidases: A Theme with Variations. *Int. J. Mol. Sci.* **2019**, *20*, 3830. [CrossRef] [PubMed]

47. Kwon, D.; Kim, S.-M.; Correia, M.A. Cytochrome P450 endoplasmic reticulum-associated degradation (ERAD): Therapeutic and pathophysiological implications. *Acta Pharm. Sin. B* **2019**, *10*, 42–60. [CrossRef] [PubMed]
48. Manikandan, P.; Nagini, S.; Palrasu, M. Cytochrome P450 Structure, Function and Clinical Significance: A Review. *Curr. Drug Targets* **2018**, *19*, 1. [CrossRef] [PubMed]
49. Tornio, A.; Backman, J.T. Cytochrome P450 in Pharmacogenetics: An Update. *Adv. Pharmacol.* **2018**, 3–32. [CrossRef]
50. Danielson, P.B. The Cytochrome P450 Superfamily: Biochemistry, Evolution and Drug Metabolism in Humans. *Curr. Drug Metab.* **2002**, *3*, 561–597. [CrossRef]
51. Anderson, G.J.; Frazer, D.M. Current understanding of iron homeostasis. *Am. J. Clin. Nutr.* **2017**, *106*, 1559S–1566S. [CrossRef]
52. Kim, A.; Nemeth, E. New insights into iron regulation and erythropoiesis. *Curr. Opin. Hematol.* **2015**, *22*, 199–205. [CrossRef]
53. Miller, C.G.; Holmgren, A.; Arnér, E.S.J.; Schmidt, E.E. NADPH-dependent and -independent disulfide reductase systems. *Free. Radic. Boil. Med.* **2018**, *127*, 248–261. [CrossRef]
54. Puig, S.; Ramos-Alonso, L.; Romero, A.M.; Pastor, M.T.M. The elemental role of iron in DNA synthesis and repair. *Metallomics* **2017**, *9*, 1483–1500. [CrossRef]
55. Aye, Y.; Li, M.; Long, M.J.C.; Weiss, R.S. Ribonucleotide reductase and cancer: Biological mechanisms and targeted therapies. *Oncogene* **2014**, *34*, 2011–2021. [CrossRef] [PubMed]
56. Kontoghiorghes, G.J.; Neocleous, K.; Kolnagou, A. Benefits and risks of deferiprone in iron overload in Thalassaemia and other conditions: Comparison of epidemiological and therapeutic aspects with deferoxamine. *Drug Saf.* **2003**, *26*, 553–584. [CrossRef] [PubMed]
57. Patrinos, G.P.; Grosveld, F. Pharmacogenomics and Therapeutics of Hemoglobinopathies. *Hemoglobin* **2008**, *32*, 229–236. [CrossRef]
58. Beinert, H.; Holm, R.H.; Münck, E. Iron-Sulfur Clusters: Nature's Modular, Multipurpose Structures. *Science* **1997**, *277*, 653–659. [CrossRef] [PubMed]
59. Ciofi-Baffoni, S.; Nasta, V.; Banci, L. Protein networks in the maturation of human iron–sulfur proteins. *Metallomics* **2018**, *10*, 49–72. [CrossRef] [PubMed]
60. Cardenas-Rodriguez, M.; Chatzi, A.; Tokatlidis, K. Iron–sulfur clusters: From metals through mitochondria biogenesis to disease. *J. Boil. Inorg. Chem.* **2018**, *23*, 509–520. [CrossRef] [PubMed]
61. Kawabata, H. Transferrin and transferrin receptors update. *Free. Radic. Boil. Med.* **2019**, *133*, 46–54. [CrossRef]
62. Levina, A.; Lay, P.A. Transferrin Cycle and Clinical Roles of Citrate and Ascorbate in Improved Iron Metabolism. *ACS Chem. Boil.* **2019**, *14*, 893–900. [CrossRef]
63. Ott, D.B.; Hartwig, A.; Stillman, M.J. Competition between Al3+ and Fe3+ binding to human transferrin and toxicological implications: Structural investigations using ultra-high resolution ESI MS and CD spectroscopy. *Metallomics* **2019**, *11*, 968–981. [CrossRef]
64. Pratt, R.; Handelman, G.J.; Edwards, T.E.; Gupta, A. Ferric pyrophosphate citrate: Interactions with transferrin. *BioMetals* **2018**, *31*, 1081–1089. [CrossRef]
65. Wang, B.; Timilsena, Y.; Blanch, E.; Adhikari, B. Lactoferrin: Structure, function, denaturation and digestion. *Crit. Rev. Food Sci. Nutr.* **2017**, *59*, 580–596. [CrossRef] [PubMed]
66. Rosa, L.; Cutone, A.; Lepanto, M.; Paesano, R.; Valenti, P. Lactoferrin: A Natural Glycoprotein Involved in Iron and Inflammatory Homeostasis. *Int. J. Mol. Sci.* **2017**, *18*, 1985. [CrossRef] [PubMed]
67. Arosio, P.; Elia, L.; Poli, M. Ferritin, cellular iron storage and regulation. *IUBMB Life* **2017**, *69*, 414–422. [CrossRef] [PubMed]
68. Saito, H. Storage Iron Turnover from a New Perspective. *Acta Haematol.* **2019**, *141*, 201–208. [CrossRef] [PubMed]
69. La, A.; Nguyen, T.; Sauble, E.; Tu, D.; Gonzalez, A.; Kidane, T.Z.; Soriano, C.; Morgan, J.; Doan, M.; Tran, K.; et al. Mobilization of iron from ferritin: New steps and details. *Metallomics* **2018**, *10*, 154–168. [CrossRef]
70. Wang, W.; Knovich, M.A.; Coffman, L.; Torti, F.M.; Torti, S.V. Serum ferritin: Past, present and future. *Biochim. Biophys. Acta (BBA)-Gen. Subj.* **2010**, *1800*, 760–769. [CrossRef]
71. Sargent, P.J.; Farnaud, S.; Evans, R.W. Structure/function overview of proteins involved in iron storage and transport. *Curr. Med. Chem.* **2005**, *12*, 2683–2693. [CrossRef]

72. Kontoghiorghe, C.N.; Kolnagou, A.; Kontoghiorghes, G.J. Potential clinical applications of chelating drugs in diseases targeting transferrin-bound iron and other metals. *Expert Opin. Investig. Drugs* **2013**, *22*, 591–618. [CrossRef]
73. Mehlenbacher, M.; Poli, M.; Arosio, P.; Santambrogio, P.; Levi, S.; Chasteen, N.D.; Bou-Abdallah, F. Iron Oxidation and Core Formation in Recombinant Heteropolymeric Human Ferritins. *Biochemistry* **2017**, *56*, 3900–3912. [CrossRef]
74. Theil, E.C. Ferritin: The Protein Nanocage and Iron Biomineral in Health and in Disease. *Inorg. Chem.* **2013**, *52*, 12223–12233. [CrossRef]
75. Iancu, T.C. Ferritin and hemosiderin in pathological tissues. *Electron Microsc. Rev.* **1992**, *5*, 209–229. [CrossRef]
76. Jacobs, A. An intracellular transit iron pool. *Ciba Found. Symp.* **1976**, *51*, 91–106.
77. Neilands, J.B. Siderophores: Structure and Function of Microbial Iron Transport Compounds. *J. Boil. Chem.* **1995**, *270*, 26723–26726. [CrossRef] [PubMed]
78. Kontoghiorghe, C.N.; Kolnagou, A.; Kontoghiorghes, G.J. Phytochelators Intended for Clinical Use in Iron Overload, Other Diseases of Iron Imbalance and Free Radical Pathology. *Molecules* **2015**, *20*, 20841–20872. [CrossRef] [PubMed]
79. Wilson, B.R.; Bogdan, A.R.; Miyazawa, M.; Hashimoto, K.; Tsuji, Y. Siderophores in Iron Metabolism: From Mechanism to Therapy Potential. *Trends Mol. Med.* **2016**, *22*, 1077–1090. [CrossRef] [PubMed]
80. Page, M.G.P. The Role of Iron and Siderophores in Infection, and the Development of Siderophore Antibiotics. *Clin. Infect. Dis.* **2019**, *69*, S529–S537. [CrossRef]
81. Huang, H.; Liao, D.; Dong, Y.; Pu, R. Effect of quercetin supplementation on plasma lipid profiles, blood pressure, and glucose levels: A systematic review and meta-analysis. *Nutr. Rev.* **2020**, pii: nuz071. [CrossRef]
82. Hezaveh, Z.S.; Azarkeivan, A.; Janani, L.; Hosseini, S.; Shidfar, F. The effect of quercetin on iron overload and inflammation in β-thalassemia major patients: A double-blind randomized clinical trial. *Complement. Ther. Med.* **2019**, *46*, 24–28. [CrossRef]
83. Salehi, B.; Stojanović-Radić, Z.; Matejić, J.; Sharifi-Rad, J.; Kumar, N.V.A.; Martins, N.; Sharifi-Rad, J. The therapeutic potential of curcumin: A review of clinical trials. *Eur. J. Med. Chem.* **2019**, *163*, 527–545. [CrossRef]
84. Gillessen, A.; Schmidt, H.H.-J. Silymarin as Supportive Treatment in Liver Diseases: A Narrative Review. *Adv. Ther.* **2020**, *37*, 1279–1301. [CrossRef]
85. Xie, Y.; Zhang, D.; Zhang, J.; Yuan, J. Metabolism, Transport and Drug-Drug Interactions of Silymarin. *Molecules* **2019**, *24*, E3693. [CrossRef] [PubMed]
86. Liu, Y.; Yu, S.; Wang, F.; Yu, H.; Li, X.; Dong, W.; Lin, R.; Liu, Q. Chronic administration of ellagic acid improved the cognition in middle-aged overweight men. *Appl. Physiol. Nutr. Metab.* **2018**, *43*, 266–273. [CrossRef] [PubMed]
87. Kosuru, R.Y.; Roy, A.; Das, S.K.; Bera, S. Gallic Acid and Gallates in Human Health and Disease: Do Mitochondria Hold the Key to Success? *Mol. Nutr. Food Res.* **2017**, *62*, 1700699. [CrossRef] [PubMed]
88. Van Gorkom, G.N.; Lookermans, E.L.; Van Elssen, C.H.; Bos, G.M. The Effect of Vitamin C (Ascorbic Acid) in the Treatment of Patients with Cancer: A Systematic Review. *Nutrition* **2019**, *11*, 977. [CrossRef]
89. Hager, D.N.; Hinson, J.S.; Rothman, R.E. Vitamin C for Sepsis and Acute Respiratory Failure. *JAMA* **2020**, *323*, 791–792. [CrossRef]
90. Nielsen, T.K.; Højgaard, M.; Andersen, J.T.; Poulsen, H.E.; Lykkesfeldt, J.; Mikines, K.J. Elimination of Ascorbic Acid After High-Dose Infusion in Prostate Cancer Patients: A Pharmacokinetic Evaluation. *Basic Clin. Pharmacol. Toxicol.* **2014**, *116*, 343–348. [CrossRef] [PubMed]
91. Martín-Peláez, S.; Covas, M.I.; Fitó, M.; Kušar, A.; Pravst, I. Health effects of olive oil polyphenols: Recent advances and possibilities for the use of health claims. *Mol. Nutr. Food Res.* **2013**, *57*, 760–771. [CrossRef]
92. Visioli, F.; De La Lastra, A.; Andres-Lacueva, C.; Aviram, M.; Calhau, C.; Cassano, A.; D'Archivio, M.; Faria, A.; Favé, G.; Fogliano, V.; et al. Polyphenols and Human Health: A Prospectus. *Crit. Rev. Food Sci. Nutr.* **2011**, *51*, 524–546. [CrossRef]
93. Iriti, M.; Varoni, E.M. Chemopreventive Potential of Flavonoids in Oral Squamous Cell Carcinoma in Human Studies. *Nutrients* **2013**, *5*, 2564–2576. [CrossRef]
94. Leopoldini, M.; Russo, N.; Toscano, M. The molecular basis of working mechanism of natural polyphenolic antioxidants. *Food Chem.* **2011**, *125*, 288–306. [CrossRef]

95. Perron, N.R.; Brumaghim, J.L. A Review of the Antioxidant Mechanisms of Polyphenol Compounds Related to Iron Binding. *Cell Biochem. Biophys.* **2009**, *53*, 75–100. [CrossRef] [PubMed]
96. Kontoghiorghes, G.J.; Jackson, M.J.; Lunec, J. In Vitro Screening of Iron Chelators Using Models of Free Radical Damage. *Free. Radic. Res. Commun.* **1986**, *2*, 115–124. [CrossRef] [PubMed]
97. Nkhili, E.; Loonis, M.; Mihai, S.; El Hajji, H.; Dangles, O. Reactivity of food phenols with iron and copper ions: Binding, dioxygen activation and oxidation mechanisms. *Food Funct.* **2014**, *5*, 1186–1202. [CrossRef]
98. Korkina, L.G.; Afanas'Ev, I.B. Antioxidant and chelating properties of flavonoids. *Adv. Pharmacol.* **1997**, *38*, 151–163. [PubMed]
99. Kontoghiorghes, G.J. Design, properties and effective use of the oral chelator L1 and other α-ketohydroxypyridines in the treatment of transfusional iron overload in thalassaemia. *Ann. N.Y. Acad. Sci.* **1990**, *612*, 339–350. [CrossRef] [PubMed]
100. Chobot, V.; Drage, S.; Hadacek, F. Redox properties of 8-quinolinol and implications for its mode of action. *Nat. Prod. Commun.* **2011**, *6*, 597–602. [CrossRef] [PubMed]
101. Kontoghiorghes, G.J.; Piga, A.; Hoffbrand, A. Cytotoxic effects of the lipophilic iron chelator omadine. *FEBS Lett.* **1986**, *204*, 208–212. [CrossRef]
102. Kontoghiorghes, G.J.; Piga, A.; Hoffbrand, A.V. Cytotoxic and DNA-inhibitory effects of iron chelators on human leukaemic cell lines. *Hematol. Oncol.* **1986**, *4*, 195–204. [CrossRef]
103. Kontoghiorghe, C.N.; Kontoghiorghes, G.J. Efficacy and safety of iron-chelation therapy with deferoxamine, deferiprone, and deferasirox for the treatment of iron-loaded patients with non-transfusion-dependent thalassemia syndromes. *Drug Des. Dev. Ther.* **2016**, *10*, 465–481. [CrossRef]
104. Hershko, C.; Graham, G.; Bates, G.W.; Rachmilewitz, E.A. Non-Specific Serum Iron in Thalassaemia: An Abnormal Serum Iron Fraction of Potential Toxicity. *Br. J. Haematol.* **1978**, *40*, 255–263. [CrossRef]
105. Kontoghiorghes, G.J.; A Aldouri, M.; Hoffbrand, A.V.; Barr, J.; Wonke, B.; Kourouclaris, T.; Sheppard, L. Effective chelation of iron in beta thalassaemia with the oral chelator 1,2-dimethyl-3-hydroxypyrid-4-one. *BMJ* **1987**, *295*, 1509–1512. [CrossRef] [PubMed]
106. Baksi, A.J.; Pennell, D. Randomized controlled trials of iron chelators for the treatment of cardiac siderosis in thalassaemia major. *Front. Pharmacol.* **2014**, *5*, 5. [CrossRef] [PubMed]
107. Kolnagou, A.; Kleanthous, M.; Kontoghiorghes, G.J. Reduction of body iron stores to normal range levels in thalassaemia by using a deferiprone/deferoxamine combination and their maintenance thereafter by deferiprone monotherapy. *Eur. J. Haematol.* **2010**, *85*, 430–438. [CrossRef] [PubMed]
108. Farmaki, K.; Tzoumari, I.; Pappa, C.; Chouliaras, G.; Berdoukas, V. Normalisation of total body iron load with very intensive combined chelation reverses cardiac and endocrine complications of thalassaemia major. *Br. J. Haematol.* **2010**, *148*, 466–475. [CrossRef] [PubMed]
109. Kolnagou, A.; Kontoghiorghe, C.N.; Kontoghiorghes, G.J. Prevention of Iron Overload and Long Term Maintenance of Normal Iron Stores in Thalassaemia Major Patients using Deferiprone or Deferiprone Deferoxamine Combination. *Drug Res.* **2017**, *67*, 404–411. [CrossRef]
110. Kolnagou, A.; Kontoghiorghes, G.J. Chelation protocols for the elimination and prevention of iron overload in thalassaemia. *Front. Biosci.* **2018**, *23*, 1082–1098. [CrossRef]
111. Kontoghiorghes, G.J.; Kleanthous, M.; Kontoghiorghe, C.N. The History of Deferiprone (L1) and the Paradigm of the Complete Treatment of Iron Overload in Thalassaemia. *Mediterr. J. Hematol. Infect. Dis.* **2020**, *12*, e2020011. [CrossRef] [PubMed]
112. Pepe, A.; Meloni, A.; Pistoia, L.; Cuccia, L.; Gamberini, M.R.; Lisi, R.; D'Ascola, D.G.; Rosso, R.; Allò, M.; Spasiano, A.; et al. MRI multicentre prospective survey in thalassaemia major patients treated with deferasirox versus deferiprone and desferrioxamine. *Br. J. Haematol.* **2018**, *183*, 783–795. [CrossRef]
113. Lin, C.-H.; Chen, X.; Wu, C.-C.; Wu, K.-H.; Song, T.-S.; Weng, T.-F.; Hsieh, Y.-W.; Peng, C.-T. Therapeutic mechanism of combined oral chelation therapy to maximize efficacy of iron removal in transfusion-dependent thalassemia major – a pilot study. *Expert Rev. Hematol.* **2019**, *12*, 265–272. [CrossRef]
114. Eghbali, A.; Shokri, P.; Afzal, R.R.; Bagheri, B. A 1-year randomized trial of deferasirox alone versus deferasirox and deferoxamine combination for the treatment of iron overload in thalassemia major. *Transfus. Apher. Sci.* **2019**, *58*, 429–433. [CrossRef]
115. Karimi, M.; Haghpanah, S.; Bahoush, G.; Ansari, S.; Azarkeivan, A.; Shahsavani, A.; Bazrafshan, A.; Jangjou, A. Evaluation of efficacy, safety, and satisfaction taking deferasirox twice daily versus once daily in patients with transfusion-dependent thalassemia. *J. Pediatrics Hematol.* **2020**, *42*, 23–26. [CrossRef] [PubMed]

116. Binding, A.; Ward, R.; Tomlinson, G.; Kuo, K.H.M. Deferiprone exerts a dose-dependent reduction of liver iron in adults with iron overload. *Eur. J. Haematol.* **2019**, *103*, 80–87. [CrossRef] [PubMed]
117. Khan, I.; Muhammad, M.; Patel, J. Deferasirox-a rarer cause of Fanconi syndrome. *J. Community Hosp. Intern. Med. Perspect.* **2019**, *9*, 358–359. [CrossRef]
118. Badeli, H.; Baghersalimi, A.; Eslami, S.; Saadat, F.; Rad, A.H.; Basavand, R.; Papkiadeh, S.R.; Darbandi, B.; Kooti, W.; Peluso, I. Early kidney damage markers after deferasirox treatment in patients with thalassemia major: A case-control study. *Oxidative Med. Cell. Longev.* **2019**, *2019*, 5461617-8. [CrossRef] [PubMed]
119. Parakh, N.; Chandra, J.; Sharma, S.; Dhingra, B.; Jain, R.; Mahto, D. Efficacy and safety of combined oral chelation with deferiprone and deferasirox in children with β-thalassemia major. *J. Pediatrics Hematol.* **2017**, *39*, 209–213. [CrossRef] [PubMed]
120. Kontoghiorghes, G.J. The aim of iron chelation therapy in thalassaemia. *Eur. J. Haematol.* **2017**, *99*, 465–466. [CrossRef]
121. Fredenburg, A.M.; Sethi, R.K.; Allen, D.D.; Yokel, R.A. The pharmacokinetics and blood-brain barrier permeation of the chelators 1,2 dimethly-, 1,2 diethyl-, and 1-[ethan-1'ol]-2-methyl-3-hydroxypyridin-4-one in the rat. *Toxicology* **1996**, *108*, 108–191. [CrossRef]
122. Vreugdenhil, G.; Kontoghiorghes, G.J.; Van Eijk, H.G.; Swaak, A.J. Impaired erythropoietin responsiveness to the anaemia in rheumatoid arthritis. A possible inverse relationship with iron stores and effects of the oral iron chelator 1,2-dimethyl-3-hydroxypyrid-4-one. *Clin. Exp. Rheumatol.* **1991**, *9*, 35–40.
123. Vreughtenhil, G.; Kontoghiorghes, G.J.; Van Eijk, H.G.; Swaak, A.J.G. Efficacy and safety of the oral chelator L1 in anaemic rheumadoit arthritis patients. *Lancet* **1989**, *II*, 1398–1399. [CrossRef]
124. Boddaert, N.; Sang, K.-H.L.Q.; Rötig, A.; Leroy-Willig, A.; Gallet, S.; Brunelle, F.; Sidi, D.; Thalabard, J.-C.; Munnich, A.; Cabantchik, Z.I. Selective iron chelation in Friedreich ataxia: Biologic and clinical implications. *Blood* **2007**, *110*, 401–408. [CrossRef]
125. Martin-Bastida, A.; Ward, R.J.; Newbould, R.; Piccini, P.; Sharp, D.; Kabba, C.; Patel, M.C.; Spino, M.; Connelly, J.; Tricta, F.; et al. Brain iron chelation by deferiprone in a phase 2 randomised double-blinded placebo controlled clinical trial in Parkinson's disease. *Sci. Rep.* **2017**, *7*, 1398. [CrossRef] [PubMed]
126. Zorzi, G.; Zibordi, F.; Chiapparini, L.; Bertini, E.; Russo, L.; Piga, A.; Longo, F.; Garavaglia, B.; Aquino, D.; Savoiardo, M.; et al. Iron-related MRI images in patients with pantothenate kinase-associated neurodegeneration (PKAN) treated with deferiprone: Results of a phase II pilot trial. *Mov. Disord.* **2011**, *26*, 1755–1759. [CrossRef] [PubMed]
127. Forni, G.; Balocco, M.; Cremonesi, L.; Abbruzzese, G.; Parodi, R.C.; Marchese, R. Regression of symptoms after selective iron chelation therapy in a case of neurodegeneration with brain iron accumulation. *Mov. Disord.* **2008**, *23*, 904–907. [CrossRef] [PubMed]
128. Harvey, R.S.J.; Reffitt, D.M.; Doig, L.A.; Meenan, J.; Ellis, R.D.; Thompson, R.P.H.; Powell, J.J. Ferric trimaltol corrects iron deficiency anaemia in patients intolerant of iron. *Aliment. Pharmacol. Ther.* **1998**, *12*, 845–848. [CrossRef] [PubMed]
129. Reffitt, D.M.; Burden, T.J.; Seed, P.T.; Wood, J.; Thompson, R.P.; Powell, J.J. Assessment of iron absorption from ferric trimaltol. *Ann. Clin. Biochem.* **2000**, *37*, 457–466. [CrossRef] [PubMed]
130. Gasche, C.; Ahmad, T.; Tulassay, Z.; Baumgart, D.C.; Bokemeyer, B.; Büning, C.; Howaldt, S.; Stallmach, A. Ferric maltol is effective in correcting iron deficiency anemia in patients with inflammatory bowel disease. *Inflamm. Bowel Dis.* **2015**, *21*, 579–588. [CrossRef]
131. Kontoghiorghes, G.J. Chelators affecting iron absorption in mice. *Arzneimittelforschung* **1990**, *40*, 1332–1335.
132. Yamamoto, R.S.; Williams, G.M.; Frankel, H.H.; Weisburger, J.H. 8-hydroxyquinoline: Chronic toxicity and inhibitory effect on the carcinogenicity of N-2- fluorenylacetamide. *Toxicol. Appl. Pharmacol.* **1971**, *19*, 687–698. [CrossRef]
133. Born, T.; Kontoghiorghe, C.N.; Spyrou, A.; Kolnagou, A.; Kontoghiorghes, G.J. EDTA chelation reappraisal following new clinical trials and regular use in millions of patients: Review of preliminary findings and risk/benefit assessment. *Toxicol. Mech. Methods* **2012**, *23*, 11–17. [CrossRef]
134. Taylor, D.M.; Hodgson, S.A.; Stradling, N. Treatment of human contamination with plutonium and americium: Would orally administered Ca- or Zn-DTPA be effective? *Radiat. Prot. Dosim.* **2007**, *127*, 469–471. [CrossRef]
135. Djaldetti, M.; Fishman, P.; Notti, I.; Bessler, H. The effect of tetracycline administration on iron absorption in mice. *Biomedicine* **1981**, *35*, 35–150.

136. Konstantinou, E.; Pashalidis, I.; Kolnagou, A.; Kontoghiorghes, G.J. Interactions of hydroxycarbamide (hydroxyurea) with iron and copper: Implications on toxicity and therapeutic strategies. *Hemoglobin* **2011**, *35*, 237–246. [CrossRef] [PubMed]
137. Sheppard, L.N.; Kontoghiorghes, G.J. Competition between deferiprone, desferrioxamine and other chelators for iron and the effect of other metals. *Arzneimittelforschung* **1993**, *43*, 659–663. [PubMed]
138. Kontoghiorghes, G.J.; Kolnagou, A. Molecular factors and mechanisms affecting iron and other metal excretion or absorption in health and disease: The role of natural and synthetic chelators. *Curr. Med. Chem.* **2005**, *12*, 2695–2709. [CrossRef]
139. Worwood, M. Inborn errors of metabolism: Iron. *Br. Med Bull.* **1999**, *55*, 556–567. [CrossRef]
140. Senba, M.; Nakamura, T.; Itakura, H. Relationships among iron accumulation, cirrhosis, and hepatitis B virus infection in Bantu siderosis. *Ann. Soc. Belg. Med. Trop.* **1989**, *69*, 77–78.
141. Robertson, A.; Tenenbein, M. Hepatotoxicity in acute iron poisoning. *Hum. Exp. Toxicol.* **2005**, *24*, 559–562. [CrossRef]
142. Baranwal, A.; Singhi, P. Acute iron poisoning: Management guidelines. *Indian Pediatrics* **2003**, *40*, 534–540.
143. Wu, M.-L.; Tsai, W.-J.; Ger, J.; Deng, J.-F. Clinical experience of acute ferric chloride poisoning. *Veter-Hum. Toxicol.* **2003**, *45*, 243–246.
144. Dresow, B.; Fischer, R.; Nielsen, P.; Gabbe, E.E.; Piga, A. Effect of oral iron chelator L1 on iron absorption in man. *Ann. N. Y. Acad. Sci.* **1998**, *850*, 466–468. [CrossRef]
145. Berkovitch, M.; Livne, A.; Lushkov, G.; Segal, M.; Talmor, C.; Bentur, Y.; Klein, J.; Koren, G. The efficacy of oral deferiprone in acute iron poisoning. *Am. J. Emerg. Med.* **2000**, *18*, 36–40. [CrossRef]
146. Iyengar, V.; Pullakhandam, R.; Nair, K.M. Dietary ligands as determinants of iron-zinc interactions at the absorptive enterocyte. *J. Food Sci.* **2010**, *75*. [CrossRef] [PubMed]
147. Petry, N.; Egli, I.; Zeder, C.; Walczyk, T.; Hurrell, R. Polyphenols and phytic acid contribute to the low iron bioavailability from common beans in young women. *J. Nutr.* **2010**, *140*, 1977–1982. [CrossRef] [PubMed]
148. Sotelo, A.; González-Osnaya, L.; Sánchez-Chinchillas, A.; Trejo, A. Role of oxate, phytate, tannins and cooking on iron bioavailability from foods commonly consumed in Mexico. *Int. J. Food Sci. Nutr.* **2009**, *61*, 29–39. [CrossRef]
149. Campbell, N.; Hasinoff, B. Iron supplements: A common cause of drug interactions. *Br. J. Clin. Pharmacol.* **1991**, *31*, 251–255. [CrossRef]
150. Jaramillo, A.; Briones, L.; Andrews, M.; Arredondo, M.; Olivares, M.; Brito, A.; Pizarro, F. Effect of phytic acid, tannic acid and pectin on fasting iron bioavailability both in the presence and absence of calcium. *J. Trace Elements Med. Boil.* **2015**, *30*, 112–117. [CrossRef]
151. Bouvard, V.; Loomis, D.; Guyton, K.Z.; Grosse, Y.; Ghissassi, F.E.; Benbrahim-Tallaa, L.; Guha, N.; Mattock, H.; Straif, K.; International Agency for Research on Cancer Monograph Working Group. Carcinogenicity of consumption of red and processed meat. *Lancet Oncol.* **2015**, *16*, 1599–1600. [CrossRef]
152. Kontoghiorghes, G.J. Orally active alpha-ketohydroxypyridine iron chelators: Effects on iron and other metal mobilisations. *Acta Haematol.* **1987**, *78*, 212–216. [CrossRef]
153. Mavrogeni, S.I.; Gotsis, E.D.; Markussis, V.; Tsekos, N.; Politis, C.; Vretou, E.; Kermastinos, D. T2 relaxation time study of iron overload in b-thalassemia. *MAGMA* **1998**, *6*, 7–12. [CrossRef]
154. Mavrogeni, S.I.; Markussis, V.; Kaklamanis, L.; Tsiapras, D.; Paraskevaidis, I.; Karavolias, G.; Karagiorga, M.; Douskou, M.; Cokkinos, D.V.; Kremastinos, D.T. A comparison of magnetic resonance imaging and cardiac biopsy in the evaluation of heart iron overload in patients with beta-thalassemia major. *Eur. J. Haematol.* **2005**, *75*, 241–247. [CrossRef]
155. Kolnagou, A.; Kontoghiorghe, C.N.; Kontoghiorghes, G.J. New targeted therapies and diagnostic methods for iron overload diseases. *Front. Biosci.* **2018**, *10*, 1–20. [CrossRef]
156. Villeneuve, J.-P.; Bilodeau, M.; Lepage, R.; Côté, J.; Lefebvre, M. Variability in hepatic iron concentration measurement from needle-biopsy specimens. *J. Hepatol.* **1996**, *25*, 172–177. [CrossRef]
157. Kolnagou, A.; Natsiopoulos, K.; Kleanthous, M.; Ioannou, A.; Kontoghiorghes, G.J. Liver iron and serum ferritin levels are misleading for estimating cardiac, pancreatic, splenic and total body iron load in thalassemia patients: Factors influencing the heterogenic distribution of excess storage iron in organs as identified by MRI T2*. *Toxicol. Mech. Methods* **2012**, *23*, 48–56. [CrossRef] [PubMed]
158. Wilson, R.B.; Lynch, D.R.; Fischbeck, K.H. Normal serum iron and ferritin concentrations in patients with Friedreich's ataxia. *Ann Neurol.* **1998**, *44*, 132–134. [CrossRef]

159. Kontoghiorghes, G.J. Iron mobilization from ferritin using α-oxohydroxy heteroaromatic chelators. *Biochem. J.* **1986**, *233*, 299–302. [CrossRef]
160. Kontoghiorghes, G.J.; Chambers, S.; Hoffbrand, A.V. Comparative study of iron mobilization from haemosiderin, ferritin and iron(III) precipitates by chelators. *Biochem. J.* **1987**, *241*, 87–92. [CrossRef]
161. Kontoghiorghes, G.J. Decrease solubilisation of ferritin iron and fresh iron(III) precipitate following repeated chelator treatments. *Inorg. Chim. Acta* **1987**, *138*, 35–39. [CrossRef]
162. Kontoghiorghes, G.J.; Goddard, J.G.; Bartlett, A.N.; Sheppard, L. Pharmacokinetic studies in humans with the oral iron chelator 1,2-dimethyl-3-hydroxypyrid-4-one. *Clin. Pharmacol. Ther.* **1990**, *48*, 255–261. [CrossRef]
163. Olivieri, N.F.; Koren, G.; Matsui, D.; Liu, P.P.; Blendis, L.; Cameron, R.; McClelland, R.A.; Templeton, D.M. Reduction of tissue iron stores and normalization of serum ferritin during treatment with the oral iron chelator L1 in thalassemia intermedia. *Blood* **1992**, *79*, 2741–2748. [CrossRef]
164. Makey, D.G.; Seal, U.S. The detection of four molecular forms of human transferrin during the iron binding process. *Biochim. Biophys. Acta (BBA)-Protein Struct.* **1976**, *453*, 250–256. [CrossRef]
165. Gomme, P.T.; McCann, K.B.; Bertolini, J. Transferrin: Structure, function and potential therapeutic actions. *Drug Discov. Today* **2005**, *10*, 267–273. [CrossRef]
166. Pantopoulos, K. TfR2 links iron metabolism and erythropoiesis. *Blood* **2015**, *125*, 1055–1056. [CrossRef] [PubMed]
167. Luna, B.M.; Ershova, K.; Yan, J.; Ulhaq, A.; Nielsen, T.B.; Hsieh, S.; Pantapalangkoor, P.; Vanscoy, B.; Ambrose, P.; Rudin, S.; et al. Adjunctive transferrin to reduce the emergence of antibiotic resistance in Gram-negative bacteria. *J. Antimicrob. Chemother.* **2019**, *74*, 2631–2639. [CrossRef] [PubMed]
168. Fernandes, K.E.; Weeks, K.; Carter, D.A. Lactoferrin Is Broadly Active against Yeasts and Highly Synergistic with Amphotericin B. *Antimicrob. Agents Chemother.* **2020**, *64*, pii: e02284. [CrossRef]
169. González-Chávez, S.A.; Arévalo-Gallegos, S.; Rascón-Cruz, Q. Lactoferrin: Structure, function and applications. *Int. J. Antimicrob. Agents* **2009**, *33*, 301.e1–301.e8. [CrossRef]
170. Kontoghiorghes, G.J. The study of iron mobilisation from transferrin using α-ketohydroxy heteroaromatic chelators. *Biochim. Biophys. Acta (BBA)-Protein Struct. Mol. Enzym.* **1986**, *869*, 141–146. [CrossRef]
171. Kontoghiorghes, G.J. Iron mobilisation from lactoferrin by chelators at physiological pH. *Biochim. Biophys. Acta (BBA)-Gen. Subj.* **1986**, *882*, 267–270. [CrossRef]
172. Kontoghiorghes, G.J.; Sheppard, L. Simple synthesis of the potent iron chelators 1-alkyl-3-hydroxy-2-methylpyrid-4-ones. *Inorg. Chim. Acta* **1987**, *136*, L11–L12. [CrossRef]
173. Kontoghiorghes, G.J.; Barr, J.; Nortey, P.; Sheppard, L. Selection of a new generation of orally active α-ketohydroxypyridine iron chelators intended for use in the treatment of iron overload. *Am. J. Hematol.* **1993**, *42*, 340–349. [CrossRef]
174. Kontoghiorghes, G.J.; Evans, R.W. Site specificity of iron removal from transferrin by α-ketohydroxypyridine chelators. *FEBS Lett.* **1985**, *189*, 141–144. [CrossRef]
175. Kontoghiorghes, G.J. Iron mobilization from transferrin and non-transferrin bound iron by deferiprone. Implications in the treatment of thalassaemia, anaemia of chronic disease, cancer and other conditions. *Hemoglobin* **2006**, *30*, 183–200. [CrossRef] [PubMed]
176. Taylor, D.M.; Kontoghiorghes, G.J. Mobilisation of plutonium and iron from transferrin and ferritin by α-oxohydroxypyridine chelators. *Inorg. Chim. Acta Bioinorg Chem.* **1986**, *125*, L35–L38. [CrossRef]
177. Evans, R.W.; Sharma, M.; Ogwang, W.; Patel, K.J.; Bartlett, A.N.; Kontoghiorghes, G.J. The effect of α-ketohydroxypyridine chelators on transferrin saturation in vitro and in vivo. *Drugs Today* **1992**, *28* (Suppl. A), 9–23.
178. Kontoghiorghes, G.J. A New Era in Iron Chelation Therapy: The Design of Optimal, Individually Adjusted Iron Chelation Therapies for the Complete Removal of Iron Overload in Thalassemia and other Chronically Transfused Patients. *Hemoglobin* **2009**, *33*, 332–338. [CrossRef] [PubMed]
179. Kontoghiorghe, C.N.; Kontoghiorghes, G.J. New developments and controversies in iron metabolism and iron chelation therapy. *World J. Methodol.* **2016**, *6*, 1–19. [CrossRef]
180. Kontoghiorghes, G.J.; May, A. Uptake and intracellular distribution of iron from transferrin and chelators in erythroid cells. *BioMetals* **1990**, *3*, 183–187. [CrossRef]
181. White, G.P.; Jacobs, A.; Grady, R.W.; Cerami, A. The effect of chelating agents on iron mobilization in Chang cell cultures. *Blood* **1976**, *48*, 923–929. [CrossRef]

182. Forsbeck, K.; Nilsson, K.; Kontoghiorghes, G.J. Variation in iron accumulation, transferrin membrane binding and DNA synthesis in the K-562 and U-937 cell lines induced by chelators and their iron complexes. *Eur. J. Haematol.* **1987**, *39*, 318–325. [CrossRef]
183. Kontoghiorghes, G.J. Structure/red blood cell permeability. Activity of iron(III) chelator complexes. *Inorg. Chim. Acta* **1988**, *151*, 101–106. [CrossRef]
184. Arosio, P.; Levi, S. Cytosolic and mitochondrial ferritins in the regulation of cellular iron homeostasis and oxidative damage. *Biochim. Biophys. Acta (BBA)-Gen. Subj.* **2010**, *1800*, 783–792. [CrossRef]
185. Yang, H.; Yang, M.; Guan, H.; Liu, Z.; Zhao, S.; Takeuchi, S.; Yanagisawa, D.; Tooyama, I. Mitochondrial ferritin in neurodegenerative diseases. *Neurosci. Res.* **2013**, *77*, 1–7. [CrossRef] [PubMed]
186. Mostert, L.J.; Van Dorst, J.; Koster, J.; Van Eijk, H.G.; Kontoghiorghes, G.J. Free radical and cytotoxic effects of chelators and their iron complexes in the hepatocyte. *Free. Radic. Res. Commun.* **1987**, *3*, 379–388. [CrossRef]
187. Kolnagou, A.; Kleanthous, M.; Kontoghiorghes, G.J. Efficacy, compliance and toxicity factors are affecting the rate of normalization of body iron stores in thalassemia patients using the deferiprone and deferoxamine combination therapy. *Hemoglobin* **2011**, *35*, 186–198. [CrossRef] [PubMed]
188. Chakraborty, D.; Bhattacharyya, M. Deferiprone (L1) induced conformation change of hemoglobin: A fluorescence and CD spectroscopic study. *Mol. Cell. Biochem.* **2000**, *204*, 17–20. [CrossRef] [PubMed]
189. Sattarahmady, N.; Heli, H.; Moosavi-Movahedi, A.A.; Karimian, K. Deferiprone: Structural and functional modulating agent of hemoglobin fructation. *Mol. Boil. Rep.* **2014**, *41*, 1723–1729. [CrossRef]
190. Offenbacher, A.R.; Minnihan, E.C.; Stubbe, J.; Barry, B.A. Redox-linked changes to the hydrogen-bonding network of ribonucleotide reductase β2. *J. Am. Chem. Soc.* **2013**, *135*, 6380–6383. [CrossRef]
191. Iman, M.; Khansefid, Z.; Davood, A. Modeling and proposed molecular mechanism of hydroxyurea through docking and molecular dynamic simulation to curtail the action of ribonucleotide reductase. *Recent Patents Anti-Cancer Drug Discov.* **2016**, *11*, 461–468. [CrossRef]
192. Lavelle, D.; Engel, J.D.; Saunthararajah, Y. Fetal hemoglobin induction by epigenetic drugs. *Semin. Hematol.* **2018**, *55*, 60–67. [CrossRef]
193. Ehsani, M.A.; Hedayati-Asl, A.A.; Bagheri, A.; Zeinali, S.; Rashidi, A. Hydroxyurea-induced hematological response in transfusion-independent beta-thalassemia intermedia: Case series and review of literature. *Pediatrics Hematol. Oncol.* **2009**, *26*, 560–565. [CrossRef]
194. Ballas, S.K.; Darbari, D.S. Review/overview of pain in sickle cell disease. *Complement. Ther. Med.* **2020**, *49*, 102327. [CrossRef]
195. Shah, F.; Dwivedi, M. Pathophysiology and recent therapeutic insights of sickle cell disease. *Ann. Hematol.* **2020**, *99*, 925–935. [CrossRef] [PubMed]
196. Nardo-Marino, A.; Brousse, V.; Rees, D.C. Emerging therapies in sickle cell disease. *Br. J. Haematol.* **2020**. [CrossRef] [PubMed]
197. Carden, M.A.; Little, J.A. Emerging disease-modifying therapies for sickle cell disease. *Haematologica* **2019**, *104*, 1710–1719. [CrossRef] [PubMed]
198. Lal, A.; Bansal, D. Thalassemia: Common clinical queries in management. *Indian J. Pediatrics* **2019**, *87*, 75–81. [CrossRef]
199. Shah, S.; Sheth, R.; Shah, K.; Patel, K. Safety and effectiveness of thalidomide and hydroxyurea combination in β-thalassaemia intermedia and major: A retrospective pilot study. *Br. J. Haematol.* **2019**, *188*, e18–e21. [CrossRef]
200. Fraser, D.I.; Liu, K.T.; Reid, B.J.; Hawkins, E.; Sevier, A.; Pyle, M.; Robinson, J.W.; Ouellette, P.H.R.; Ballantyne, J.S. Widespread natural occurrence of hydroxyurea in animals. *PLoS ONE* **2015**, *10*, e0142890. [CrossRef]
201. Manaresi, E.; Gallinella, G. Advances in the development of antiviral strategies against parvovirus B19. *Viruses* **2019**, *11*, 659. [CrossRef]
202. Tremblay, D.; Mascarenhas, J.O. Novel therapies in polycythemia vera. *Curr. Hematol. Malign-Rep.* **2020**, *15*, 133–140. [CrossRef]
203. Rainsford, K.D. Ibuprofen: Pharmacology, efficacy and safety. *Inflammopharmacology* **2009**, *17*, 275–342. [CrossRef]
204. Dos Santos, P.R.; Pich, C.T.; Back, D.; Smiderle, F.; Dumas, F.; Moura, S. Synthesis, chemical characterization and DNA interaction study of new diclofenac and ibuprofen zinc (II)-nicotinamide ternary complexes as cyclooxygenase inhibitor prototypes. *J. Inorg. Biochem.* **2020**, *206*, 111046. [CrossRef]

205. Vane, J.; Botting, R. The mechanism of action of aspirin. *Thromb. Res.* **2003**, *110*, 255–258. [CrossRef]
206. Dubois, R.N.; Abramson, S.B.; Crofford, L.; Gupta, R.A.; Simon, L.S.; Van De Putte, L.B.A.; Lipsky, P.E. Cyclooxygenase in biology and disease. *FASEB J.* **1998**, *12*, 1063–1073. [CrossRef] [PubMed]
207. Jeremy, J.Y.; Kontoghiorghes, G.J.; Hoffbrand, A.V.; Dandona, P. The iron chelators desferrioxamine and 1-alkyl-2-methyl-3-hydroxypyrid-4-ones inhibit vascular prostacyclin synthesis in vitro. *Biochem. J.* **1988**, *254*, 239–244. [CrossRef] [PubMed]
208. Villeneuve, J.-P.; Pichette, V. Cytochrome P450 and liver diseases. *Curr. Drug Metab.* **2004**, *5*, 273–282. [CrossRef] [PubMed]
209. Speer, R.E.; Karuppagounder, S.S.; Basso, M.; Sleiman, S.F.; Kumar, A.; Brand, D.; Smirnova, N.; Gazaryan, I.; Khim, S.J.; Ratan, R.R. Hypoxia-inducible factor prolyl hydroxylases as targets for neuroprotection by "antioxidant" metal chelators: From ferroptosis to stroke. *Free. Radic. Boil. Med.* **2013**, *62*, 26–36. [CrossRef] [PubMed]
210. Goldsmith, S.J.; Vallabhajosula, S. Clinically Proven Radiopharmaceuticals for Infection Imaging: Mechanisms and Applications. *Semin. Nucl. Med.* **2009**, *39*, 2–10. [CrossRef]
211. Zak, O.; Aisen, P. Spectroscopic and thermodynamic studies on the binding of gadolinium(III) to human serum transferrin. *Biochemistry* **1988**, *27*, 1075–1080. [CrossRef]
212. Smith, T.; Perkins, A.C.; Walton, P.H. 99mTc-labelled human serum transferrin for tumour imaging: An in vitro and in vivo study of the complex. *Nucl. Med. Commun.* **2004**, *25*, 387–391. [CrossRef]
213. Tsopelas, C. A study of radiogallium aqueous chemistry: In vitro and in vivo characterisation of 67 Ga-hydrolysed-stannous fluoride particles. *J. Label. Compd. Radiopharm.* **2016**, *59*, 197–204. [CrossRef]
214. E Dahlqvist, G.; Jamar, F.; Zech, F.; Geubel, A.P. In-111 transferrin scintigraphy in cirrhosis with hypoalbuminemia: Evidence for protein-losing enteropathy in a small group of selected cases. *Scand. J. Gastroenterol.* **2012**, *47*, 1247–1252. [CrossRef]
215. Collery, P.; Keppler, B.K.; Madoulet, C.; Desoize, B. Gallium in cancer treatment. *Crit. Rev. Oncol.* **2002**, *42*, 283–296. [CrossRef]
216. Sava, G.; Pacor, S.; Bregant, F.; Ceschia, V. Metal complexes of ruthenium: A potential class of selective anticancer drugs. *Anticancer. Res.* **1991**, *11*, 1103–1107. [PubMed]
217. Peng, H.; Jin, H.; Zhuo, H.; Huang, H. Enhanced antitumor efficacy of cisplatin for treating ovarian cancer in vitro and in vivo via transferrin binding. *Oncotarget* **2017**, *8*, 45597–45611. [CrossRef] [PubMed]
218. Brown, D.; Ham, K.; Dawborn, J.; Xipell, J. Treatment of dialysis osteomalacia with desferrioxamine. *Lancet* **1982**, *320*, 343–345. [CrossRef]
219. Kontoghiorghes, G.J.; Barr, J.; Baillod, R.A. Studies of aluminium mobilisation in renal dialysis patients using the oral chelator 1, 2-dimethyl-3-hydroxypyrid-4-one. *Arzn Forsch Drug Res* **1994**, *44*, 522–526.
220. Volf, V.; Kontoghiorghes, G.J. Retention of injected plutonium and americium in mice and rats after oral treatment with DTPA, desferrioxamine and alpha-ketohydroxypyridines. *Drugs Today* **1992**, *28* (Suppl. A), 169–172.
221. Pashalidis, I.; Kontoghiorghes, G.J. Effective complex formation in the interaction of I,2-dimethyl-3-hydroxypyrid-4-one (Deferiprone or L1) with Uranium (VI). *J. Radioanalyt. Nucl. Chem.* **1999**, *242*, 181–184. [CrossRef]
222. Kontoghiorghes, G.J. Prospects for introducing deferiprone as potent pharmaceutical antioxidant. *Front. Biosci. (Elite Ed)* **2009**, *1*, 161–178.
223. Kontoghiorghe, C.N.; Kolnagou, A.; Kontoghiorghes, G.J. Antioxidant targeting by deferiprone in diseases related to oxidative damage. *Front. Biosci. (Landmark Ed)* **2014**, *19*, 862–885. [CrossRef]
224. Forman, H.J. Redox signaling: An evolution from free radicals to aging. *Free Radic Biol Med.* **2016**, *97*, 398–407. [CrossRef]
225. Stangherlin, A.; Reddy, A.B. Regulation of circadian clocks by redox homeostasis. *J. Boil. Chem.* **2013**, *288*, 26505–26511. [CrossRef] [PubMed]
226. Arevalo, J.A.; Vazquez-Medina, J.P. The role of peroxiredoxin 6 in cell signaling. *Antioxidants.* **2018**, *7*, 172. [CrossRef] [PubMed]
227. Ďuračková, Z. Some current insights into oxidative stress. *Physiol. Res.* **2009**, *59*, 459–469. [PubMed]
228. Gutteridge, J.M. Lipid peroxidation and antioxidants as biomarkers of tissue damage. *Clin. Chem.* **1995**, *41*, 1819–1828. [CrossRef]

229. Stadtman, E.R.; Levine, R.L. Free radical-mediated oxidation of free amino acids and amino acid residues in proteins. *Amino Acids* **2003**, *25*, 207–218. [CrossRef]
230. Feng, H.; Stockwell, B.R. Unsolved mysteries: How does lipid peroxidation cause ferroptosis? *PLoS Boil.* **2018**, *16*, e2006203. [CrossRef]
231. Shah, R.; Shchepinov, M.S.; Pratt, D.A. Resolving the role of lipoxygenases in the initiation and execution of ferroptosis. *ACS Central Sci.* **2018**, *4*, 387–396. [CrossRef]
232. Lewerenz, J.; Ates, G.; Methner, A.; Conrad, M.; Maher, P. Oxytosis/ferroptosis—(re-) emerging roles for oxidative stress-dependent non-apoptotic cell death in diseases of the central nervous system. *Front. Mol. Neurosci.* **2018**, *12*, 214. [CrossRef]
233. Hao, S.; Liang, B.; Huang, Q.; Dong, S.; Wu, Z.; He, W.; Shi, M. Metabolic networks in ferroptosis. *Oncol. Lett.* **2018**, *15*, 5405–5411. [CrossRef]
234. Eybl, V.; Caisová, D.; Koutenský, J.; Kontoghiorghes, G.J. Influence of iron chelators, 1,2-dialkyl-3-hydroxypyridin-4-ones, on the lipid peroxidation and glutathione level in the liver of mice. *Arch. Toxicol. Suppl.* **1991**, *14*, 185–187. [CrossRef]
235. Maher, P.; Kontoghiorghes, G.J. Characterization of the neuroprotective potential of derivatives of the iron chelating drug deferiprone. *Neurochem. Res.* **2015**, *40*, 609–620. [CrossRef] [PubMed]
236. Rajapurkar, M.M.; Hegde, U.; Bhattacharya, A.; Alam, M.G.; Shah, S.V. Effect of deferiprone, an oral iron chelator, in diabetic and non-diabetic glomerular disease. *Toxicol. Mech. Methods* **2012**, *23*, 5–10. [CrossRef] [PubMed]
237. Wallis, L.I.; Paley, M.N.; Graham, J.M.; Grünewald, R.A.; Wignall, E.L.; Joy, H.M.; Griffiths, P.D. MRI assessment of basal ganglia iron deposition in Parkinson's disease. *J. Magn. Reson. Imaging* **2008**, *28*, 1061–1067. [CrossRef] [PubMed]
238. Brar, S.; Henderson, D.; Schenck, J.; Zimmerman, E.A. Iron accumulation in the substantia nigra of patients with Alzheimer disease and parkinsonism. *Arch. Neurol.* **2009**, *66*, 371–374. [CrossRef] [PubMed]
239. Waldvogel, D.; van Gelderen, P.; Hallett, M. Increased iron in the dentate nucleus of patients with Friedrich's ataxia. *Ann Neurol.* **1999**, *46*, 123–125. [CrossRef]
240. Chan, S.; Lian, Q.; Chen, M.-P.; Jiang, D.; Ho, J.T.; Cheung, Y.-F.; Chan, G.C.-F. Deferiprone inhibits iron overload-induced tissue factor bearing endothelial microparticle generation by inhibition oxidative stress induced mitochondrial injury, and apoptosis. *Toxicol. Appl. Pharmacol.* **2018**, *338*, 148–158. [CrossRef]
241. Weinberg, E.D. Iron depletion: A defense against intracellular infection and neoplasm. *Life Sci.* **1992**, *50*, 1289–1297. [CrossRef]
242. Andrews, S.C.; Robinson, A.K.; Rodríguez-Quiñones, F. Bacterial iron homeostasis. *FEMS Microbiol. Rev.* **2003**, *27*, 215–237. [CrossRef]
243. Kontoghiorghes, G.; Weinberg, E. Iron: Mammalian defense systems, mechanisms of disease, and chelation therapy approaches. *Blood Rev.* **1995**, *9*, 33–45. [CrossRef]
244. Kontoghiorghes, G.J.; Kolnagou, A.; Skiada, A.; Petrikkos, G. The role of iron and chelators on infections in iron overload and non iron loaded conditions: Prospects for the design of new antimicrobial therapies. *Hemoglobin* **2010**, *34*, 227–239. [CrossRef]
245. Kontoghiorghe, C.N.; Andreou, N.; Constantinou, K.; Kontoghiorghes, G.J. World health dilemmas: Orphan and rare diseases, orphan drugs and orphan patients. *World J. Methodol.* **2014**, *4*, 163–188. [CrossRef] [PubMed]
246. Lynch, M.; Korenromp, E.; Eisele, T.; Newby, H.; Steketee, R.; Kachur, S.P.; Nahlen, B.; Bhattarai, A.; Yoon, S.; MacArthur, J.; et al. New global estimates of malaria deaths. *Lancet* **2012**, *380*, 559. [CrossRef]
247. Uhlemann, A.-C.; Fidock, D.A. Loss of malarial susceptibility to artemisinin in Thailand. *Lancet* **2012**, *379*, 1928–1930. [CrossRef]
248. Gordeuk, V.R.; Thuma, P.E.; Brittenham, G.M.; Zulu, S.; Simwanza, G.; Mhangu, A.; Flesch, G.; Parry, D. Iron chelation with desferrioxamine B in adults with asymptomatic P. Falciparum parasitemia. *Blood* **1992**, *79*, 308–312. [CrossRef]
249. Heppner, D.G.; Hallaway, P.E.; Kontoghiorghes, G.J.; Eaton, J.W. Antimalarial properties of orally active iron chelators. *Blood* **1988**, *72*, 358–361. [CrossRef] [PubMed]
250. Mastrandrea, S.; Carvajal, J.L.; Kaeda, J.S.; Kontoghiorghes, G.J.; Luzzato, L. Growth inhibition of Plasmodium Falciparum by orally active iron chelators. *Drugs Today.* **1992**, *28* (Suppl. A), 25–27.

251. Goudeau, C.; Loyevsky, M.; Kassim, O.O.; Gordeuk, V.R.; Nick, H. Assessment of antimalarial effect of ICL670A on in vitro cultures of Plasmodium falciparum. *Br. J. Haematol.* **2001**, *115*, 918–923. [CrossRef]
252. Mohanty, D.; Ghosh, K.; Pathare, A.V.; Karnad, D. Deferiprone (L1) as an adjuvant therapy for Plasmodium falciparum malaria. *Indian J. Med Res.* **2002**, *115*, 17–21. [PubMed]
253. Robins-Browne, R.; Prpic, J. Desferrioxamine and systemic yersiniosis. *Lancet* **1983**, *322*, 1372. [CrossRef]
254. Boelaert, J.R.; Fenves, A.Z.; Coburn, J.W. Deferoxamine therapy and mucormycosis in dialysis patients: Report of an international registry. *Am. J. Kidney Dis.* **1991**, *18*, 660–667. [CrossRef]
255. Ibrahim, A.S.; Edwards, J.E.; Fu, Y.; Spellberg, B. Deferiprone iron chelation as a novel therapy for experimental mucormycosis. *J. Antimicrob. Chemother.* **2006**, *58*, 1070–1073. [CrossRef] [PubMed]
256. Ibrahim, A.S.; Gebermariam, T.; Fu, Y.; Lin, L.; Husseiny, M.I.; French, S.W.; Schwartz, J.; Skory, C.D.; Edwards, J.E.; Spellberg, B.J. The iron chelator deferasirox protects mice from mucormycosis through iron starvation. *J. Clin. Investig.* **2007**, *117*, 2649–2657. [CrossRef] [PubMed]
257. Brock, J.H.; Licéaga, J.; Kontoghiorghes, G.J. The effect of synthetic iron chelators on bacterial growth in human serum. *FEMS Microbiol. Immunol.* **1988**, *1*, 55–60. [CrossRef] [PubMed]
258. Jue, S.; Jue, S.G.; Dawson, G.W.; Brogden, R.N. Ciclopirox olamine 1% cream a preliminary review of its antimicrobial activity and therapeutic use. *Drugs* **1985**, *29*, 330–341. [CrossRef] [PubMed]
259. Schwartz, J.R. Zinc pyrithione: A topical antimicrobial with complex pharmaceutics. *J. Drugs Dermatol.* **2016**, *15*, 140–144. [PubMed]
260. Kontoghiorghes, G.J.; Efstathiou, A.; Ioannou-Loucaides, S.; Kolnagou, A. Chelators controlling metal metabolism and toxicity pathways: Applications in cancer prevention, diagnosis and treatment. *Hemoglobin* **2008**, *32*, 217–227. [CrossRef] [PubMed]
261. Voest, E.E.; Vreugdenhil, G.; Marx, J.J.M. Iron-chelating agents in non-iron overload conditions. *Ann. Intern. Med.* **1994**, *120*, 490–499. [CrossRef] [PubMed]
262. Manz, D.H.; Blanchette, N.L.; Paul, B.T.; Torti, F.M.; Torti, S.V. Iron and cancer: Recent insights. *Ann. N. Y. Acad. Sci.* **2016**, *1368*, 149–161. [CrossRef]
263. Lui, G.Y.L.; Kovacevic, Z.; Richardson, V.; Merlot, A.M.; Kalinowski, D.S.; Richardson, D.R. Targeting cancer by binding iron: Dissecting cellular signaling pathways. *Oncotarget* **2015**, *6*, 18748–18779. [CrossRef]
264. Valko, M.; Rhodes, C.; Moncol, J.; Izakovic, M.; Mazur, M. Free radicals, metals and antioxidants in oxidative stress-induced cancer. *Chem. Interact.* **2006**, *160*, 1–40. [CrossRef]
265. Park, K.C.; Fouani, L.; Jansson, P.; Wooi, D.; Sahni, S.; Lane, D.; Palanimuthu, D.; Lok, H.C.; Kovacevic, Z.; Huang, M.L.-H.; et al. Copper and conquer: Copper complexes of di-2-pyridylketone thiosemicarbazones as novel anti-cancer therapeutics. *Metallomics* **2016**, *8*, 874–886. [CrossRef] [PubMed]
266. Nutting, C.; Van Herpen, C.M.L.; Miah, A.B.; Bhide, S.A.; Machiels, J.-P.; Buter, J.; Kelly, C.; De Raucourt, D.; Harrington, K.J. Phase II study of 3-AP Triapine in patients with recurrent or metastatic head and neck squamous cell carcinoma. *Ann. Oncol.* **2009**, *20*, 1275–1279. [CrossRef] [PubMed]
267. Richardson, D.R. Molecular mechanisms of iron uptake by cells and the use of iron chelators for the treatment of cancer. *Curr. Med. Chem.* **2005**, *12*, 2711–2729. [CrossRef] [PubMed]
268. Ganeshaguru, K.; Lally, J.M.; Piga, A.; Hoffbrand, A.V.; Kontoghiorghes, G.J. Cytotoxic mechanisms of iron chelators. *Drugs Today* **1992**, *28* (Suppl. A), 29–34.
269. Eybl, V.; Svihovcova, P.; Koutensky., J.; Kontoghiorghes, G.J. Interaction of L1, L1NAll and desferoxamine with Gallium in vivo. *Drugs Today.* **1992**, *28* (Suppl. A), 173–175.
270. Chitambar, C.R. Gallium-containing anticancer compounds. *Futur. Med. Chem.* **2012**, *4*, 1257–1272. [CrossRef]
271. Jeremy, J.Y.; Gill, J.; Prior, T.; Sifaksi, G.; Barradas, M.A.; Kontoghiorghes, G.J. Inhibition of cycloxygenase and lipoxygenase activity by iron chelators:possible use in the treatment of eicosanoid-related disorders. *Drugs Today.* **1992**, *28* (Suppl. A), 35–43.
272. Donfrancesco, A.; De Bernardi, B.; Carli, M.; Mancini, A.; Nigro, M.; De Sio, L.; Casale, F.; Bagnulo, S.; Helson, L.; Deb, G. Deferoxamine followed by cyclophosphamide, etoposide, carboplatin, thiotepa, induction regimen in advanced neuroblastoma: Preliminary results. *Eur. J. Cancer* **1995**, *31*, 612–615. [CrossRef]
273. Kolnagou, A.; Kontoghiorghe, C.N.; Kontoghiorghes, G.J. Transition of Thalassaemia and Friedreich ataxia from fatal to chronic diseases. *World J. Methodol.* **2014**, *4*, 197–218. [CrossRef] [PubMed]
274. Timoshnikov, V.A.; Kobzeva, T.; Polyakov, N.E.; Kontoghiorghes, G.J. Redox interactions of vitamin C and iron: Inhibition of the pro-oxidant activity by deferiprone. *Int. J. Mol. Sci.* **2020**, *21*. [CrossRef]

275. Badu-Boateng, C.; Naftalin, R.J. Ascorbate and ferritin interactions: Consequences for iron release in vitro and in vivo and implications for inflammation. *Free. Radic. Boil. Med.* **2019**, *133*, 75–87. [CrossRef] [PubMed]
276. Dziuba, N.; Hardy, J.; Lindahl, P.A. Low-molecular-mass iron complexes in blood plasma of iron-deficient pigs do not originate directly from nutrient iron. *Metallomics* **2019**, *11*, 1900–1911. [CrossRef] [PubMed]
277. Dichtl, S.; Haschka, D.; Nairz, M.; Seifert, M.; Volani, C.; Lutz, O.; Weiss, G. Dopamine promotes cellular iron accumulation and oxidative stress responses in macrophages. *Biochem. Pharmacol.* **2018**, *148*, 193–201. [CrossRef]
278. Parquet, M.D.C.; Savage, K.A.; Allan, D.S.; Davidson, R.J.; Holbein, B. Novel iron-chelator DIBI inhibits Staphylococcus aureus growth, suppresses experimental MRSA infection in mice and enhances the activities of diverse antibiotics in vitro. *Front. Microbiol.* **2018**, *9*, 1–11. [CrossRef]
279. Kolnagou, A.; Economides, C.; Eracleous, E.; Kontoghiorghes, G.J. Long term comparative studies in thalassemia patients treated with deferoxamine or a deferoxamine/deferiprone combination. identification of effective chelation therapy protocols. *Hemoglobin* **2008**, *32*, 41–47. [CrossRef] [PubMed]
280. Klopstock, T.; Tricta, F.; Neumayr, L.; Karin, I.; Zorzi, G.; Fradette, C.; Kmieć, T.; Büchner, B.; E Steele, H.; Horvath, R.; et al. Safety and efficacy of deferiprone for pantothenate kinase-associated neurodegeneration: A randomised, double-blind, controlled trial and an open-label extension study. *Lancet Neurol.* **2019**, *18*, 631–642. [CrossRef]
281. Selim, M.H.; Foster, L.D.; Moy, C.S.; Xi, G.; Hill, M.D.; Morgenstern, L.B.; Greenberg, S.M.; James, M.L.; Singh, V.; Clark, W.M.; et al. Deferoxamine mesylate in patients with intracerebral haemorrhage (i-DEF): A multicentre, randomised, placebo-controlled, double-blind phase 2 trial. *Lancet Neurol.* **2019**, *18*, 428–438. [CrossRef]
282. Agrawal, S.; Fox, J.; Thyagarajan, B.; Fox, J.H. Brain mitochondrial iron accumulates in Huntington's disease, mediates mitochondrial dysfunction, and can be removed pharmacologically. *Free. Radic. Biol. Med.* **2018**, *120*, 317–329. [CrossRef] [PubMed]
283. Tosato, M.; Di Marco, V. Metal Chelation Therapy and Parkinson's Disease: A Critical Review on the Thermodynamics of Complex Formation between Relevant Metal Ions and Promising or Established Drugs. *Biomolecules* **2019**, *9*, 269. [CrossRef] [PubMed]
284. Ndayisaba, A.; Kaindlstorfer, C.; Wenning, G.K. Iron in neurodegeneration–cause or consequence? *Front. Neurosci.* **2019**, *13*, 180. [CrossRef] [PubMed]
285. Saxena, D.; Spino, M.; Tricta, F.; Connelly, J.; Cracchiolo, B.M.; Hanauske, A.-R.; Gandolfi, D.D.; Mathews, M.B.; Karn, J.; Holland, B.; et al. Drug-based lead discovery: The novel ablative antiretroviral profile of deferiprone in HIV-1-infected cells and in HIV-infected treatment-naive subjects of a double-blind, placebo-controlled, randomized exploratory trial. *PLoS ONE* **2016**, *11*, e0154842. [CrossRef] [PubMed]
286. Leftin, A.; Zhao, H.; Turkekul, M.; De Stanchina, E.; Manova, K.; Koutcher, J.A. Iron deposition is associated with differential macrophage infiltration and therapeutic response to iron chelation in prostate cancer. *Sci. Rep.* **2017**, *7*, 11632. [CrossRef] [PubMed]
287. Brock, J.H.; Licéaga, J.; Arthur, H.M.; Kontoghiorghes, G.J. Effect of novel 1-alkyl-3-hydroxy-2-methylpyrid-4-one chelators on uptake and release of iron from macrophages. *Am. J. Hematol.* **1990**, *34*, 21–25. [CrossRef] [PubMed]
288. Poprac, P.; Jomova, K.; Simunkova, M.; Kollar, V.; Rhodes, C.J.; Valko, M. Targeting free radicals in oxidative stress-related human diseases. *Trends Pharmacol. Sci.* **2017**, *38*, 592–607. [CrossRef] [PubMed]
289. Gaur, K.; Vázquez, A.M.; Duran-Camacho, G.; Dominguez-Martinez, I.; Benjamín-Rivera, J.A.; Fernández-Vega, L.; Sarabia, L.C.; García, A.C.; Pérez-Deliz, F.; Román, J.M.; et al. Iron and Copper Intracellular Chelation as an Anticancer Drug Strategy. *Inorganics* **2018**, *6*, 126. [CrossRef]
290. Kuang, Y.; Wang, Q. Iron and lung cancer. *Cancer Lett.* **2019**, *464*, 56–61. [CrossRef] [PubMed]
291. Wang, Y.; Yu, L.; Ding, J.; Chen, Y. Iron Metabolism in Cancer. *Int. J. Mol. Sci.* **2018**, *20*, 95. [CrossRef]
292. Heffeter, P.; Pape, V.F.; Enyedy, É.A.; Keppler, B.K.; Szakacs, G.; Kowol, C.R.; Szakas, G. Anticancer thiosemicarbazones: Chemical properties, interaction with iron metabolism, and resistance development. *Antioxid. Redox Signal.* **2019**, *30*, 1062–1082. [CrossRef]
293. Mody, K.; Mansfield, A.S.; Vemireddy, L.; Nygren, P.; Gulbo, J.; Borad, M. A phase I study of the safety and tolerability of VLX600, an iron chelator, in patients with refractory advanced solid tumors. *Investig. New Drugs* **2018**, *37*, 684–692. [CrossRef]

294. De Luca, A.; Barile, A.; Arciello, M.; Rossi, L. Copper homeostasis as target of both consolidated and innovative strategies of anti-tumor therapy. *J. Trace Elem. Med. Boil.* **2019**, *55*, 204–213. [CrossRef]
295. Huang, Y.-F.; Kuo, M.T.; Liu, Y.-S.; Cheng, Y.-M.; Wu, P.-Y.; Chou, C.-Y. A Dose escalation study of trientine plus carboplatin and pegylated liposomal doxorubicin in women with a first relapse of epithelial ovarian, tubal, and peritoneal cancer within 12 months after platinum-based chemotherapy. *Front. Oncol.* **2019**, *9*, 437. [CrossRef] [PubMed]
296. Timoshnikov, V.A.; Kobzeva, T.; Selyutina, O.Y.; Polyakov, N.E.; Kontoghiorghes, G.J. Effective inhibition of copper-catalyzed production of hydroxyl radicals by deferiprone. *J. Boil. Inorg. Chem.* **2019**, *24*, 331–341. [CrossRef] [PubMed]
297. Hagn, G.; Westhofen, R.; Burkovskiy, I.; Holbein, B.; Zhou, J.; Lehmann, C. Iron chelation as novel treatment for interstitial cystitis. *Pharmacology* **2019**, *103*, 159–162. [CrossRef]
298. Kobayashi, M.; Suhara, T.; Baba, Y.; Kawasaki, N.K.; Higa, J.K.; Matsui, T. Pathological roles of iron in cardiovascular disease. *Curr. Drug Targets* **2018**, *19*, 1068–1076. [CrossRef] [PubMed]
299. Zhang, C.; Rawal, S. Dietary iron intake, iron status, and gestational diabetes. *Am. J. Clin. Nutr.* **2017**, *106*, 1672S–1680S. [CrossRef] [PubMed]
300. Patil, P.; Geevarghese, P.; Khaire, P.; Joshi, T.; Suryawanshi, A.; Mundada, S.; Pawar, S.; Farookh, A. Comparison of therapeutic efficacy of ferrous ascorbate and iron polymaltose complex in iron deficiency anemia in children: A randomized controlled trial. *Indian J. Pediatrics* **2019**, *86*, 1112–1117. [CrossRef]
301. Chandra, J. Treating iron deficiency anemia. *Indian J. Pediatrics* **2019**, *86*, 1085–1086. [CrossRef]
302. Węgier, L.P.; Kubiak, M.; Liebert, A.; Clavel, T.; Montagne, A.; Stennevin, A.; Roye, S.; Boudribila, A. Ferrous sulfate oral solution in young children with iron deficiency anemia. *Pediatrics Int.* **2020**. [CrossRef]
303. Stoffel, N.U.; Zeder, C.; Brittenham, G.M.; Moretti, D.; Zimmermann, M.B. Iron absorption from supplements is greater with alternate day than with consecutive day dosing in iron-deficient anemic women. *Haematologica* **2019**, *105*, 1232–1239. [CrossRef]
304. Enyedy, É.A.; Dömötör, O.; Bali, K.; Hetényi, A.; Tuccinardi, T.; Keppler, B.K. Interaction of the anticancer gallium(III) complexes of 8-hydroxyquinoline and maltol with human serum proteins. *J. Boil. Inorg. Chem.* **2014**, *20*, 77–88. [CrossRef]
305. Tanzey, S.S.; Thompson, S.; Scott, P.J.; Brooks, A.F. Gallium-68: Methodology and novel radiotracers for positron emission tomography (2012–2017). *Pharm. Pat. Anal.* **2018**, *7*, 193–227. [CrossRef] [PubMed]
306. Yang, Z.; Lin, H.; Huang, J.; Li, A.; Sun, C.; Richmond, J.; Gao, J. A gadolinium-complex-based theranostic prodrug for in vivo tumour-targeted magnetic resonance imaging and therapy. *Chem. Commun.* **2019**, *55*, 4546–4549. [CrossRef] [PubMed]
307. Blanusa, M.; Varnai, V.M.; Piasek, M.; Kostial, K. Chelators as antidotes of metal toxicity: Therapeutic and experimental aspects. *Curr. Med. Chem.* **2005**, *12*, 2771–2794. [CrossRef] [PubMed]
308. Flora, S.J.S.; Mittal, M.; Mehta, A. Heavy metal induced oxidative stress & its possible reversal by chelation therapy. *Indian J. Med Res.* **2008**, *128*, 501–523. [PubMed]
309. Kontoghiorghes, G.J. Regulatory molecules and chelators used for the control of essential and toxic metals in health and disease: From molecular interactions to clinical effects and applications. *Curr. Med. Chem.* **2005**, *12*, 2661–2662. [CrossRef]

2

Emerging and Dynamic Biomedical Uses of Ferritin

Brian Chiou and James R. Connor *

Department of Neurosurgery, Penn State College of Medicine, Hershey, PA 17033, USA; bbc5138@psu.edu
* Correspondence: jconnor@pennstatehealth.psu.edu

Abstract: Ferritin, a ubiquitously expressed protein, has classically been considered the main iron cellular storage molecule in the body. Owing to the ferroxidase activity of the H-subunit and the nucleation ability of the L-subunit, ferritin can store a large amount of iron within its mineral core. However, recent evidence has demonstrated a range of abilities of ferritin that extends well beyond the scope of iron storage. This review aims to discuss novel functions and biomedical uses of ferritin in the processes of iron delivery, delivery of biologics such as chemotherapies and contrast agents, and the utility of ferritin as a biomarker in a number of neurological diseases.

Keywords: ferritin; iron; iron delivery; nanotechnology; nanocage; drug delivery; inflammation; serum biomarker

---

1. Ferritin Introduction

Ferritin, a protein originally identified in 1937 by Vilém Laufberger [1], is a ubiquitously expressed iron storage protein most commonly characterized by its ability to accumulate and store up to 4500 atoms of iron [2]. Ferritin consists of 24 subunits, typically comprised of different ratios of the H and L chain subunit. The ratios vary by organ and even by cell type. Importantly, the different subunits have divergent functions—H-ferritin utilizes ferroxidase activity that is necessary for the oxidation of ferrous (Fe^{2+}) to ferric (Fe^{3+}) iron while L-ferritin contains acidic residues on the surface cavity of the protein that facilitate ferroxidase turnover and are crucial for the nucleation of ferric iron within the core of the fully formed protein. Historically, the primary function of the 24-mer protein has been to sequester extracellular and cytosolic iron and store this iron within its core for future use by the cell. This functionally prevents the formation of harmful reactive oxygen species (ROS) created through Fenton chemistry. Many reviews in the past few decades have focused on various aspects of the normal biological function of ferritin and its regulation pertaining to iron homeostasis [3–6]. In this review, we will outline novel and dynamic functions of ferritin that have recently come to light, specifically focusing on the novel uses for ferritin as an iron delivery protein, a delivery agent for numerous other biologics, and as a biomarker for various diseases.

Although traditionally characterized as a cytosolic protein, ferritin has also been found in mitochondria [7], plant plastids [8], the nucleus [9–11], and extracellularly in serum [12] and cerebrospinal fluid [13]. The different subcellular localizations of ferritin suggest a unique function for it in a variety of cell types. For example, nuclear ferritin reportedly binds to and protects DNA from UV-induced damage [9] as well as iron-induced damage [11]. The presence of ferritin in nuclei led to a series of studies by our group on the role of ferritin in cancer cells that revealed knockdown of ferritin increases sensitivity to radiation and chemotherapy in cancer cells [14]. Mitochondrial ferritin, while coded by a different gene than either L- or H-ferritin, shares 79% homology to H-ferritin and forms the classic ferritin shell [15]. In the mitochondria, free iron can cause potentially devastating effects; mitochondrial ferritin serves to sequester potentially harmful iron using ferroxidase activity [4].

2. Ferritin as an Iron Delivery Protein

Iron delivery throughout the body is a vitally important process that is very tightly regulated. Iron deficiency may result in a number of longstanding and severe phenotypes such as anemia [16]. Similarly, iron overload, known as hemochromatosis, may result in organ failure [17] or significant inflammatory conditions [18]. Moreover, iron dyshomeostasis in the brain may result in significant neurodegeneration [19–21]. Excess organ and cellular accumulation in disease states occurs because the regulation of iron uptake is altered. The primary mechanism for iron uptake has historically been thought to be through the action of transferrin (Tf) delivering iron through transferrin receptor (TfR) (Figure 1). However, this paradigm may not address times of extreme iron need, such as during development and growth. While transferrin typically delivers two atoms of iron at a time, ferritin can potentially deliver a much more substantial amount of iron at a single time, allowing for rapid growth and iron utilization.

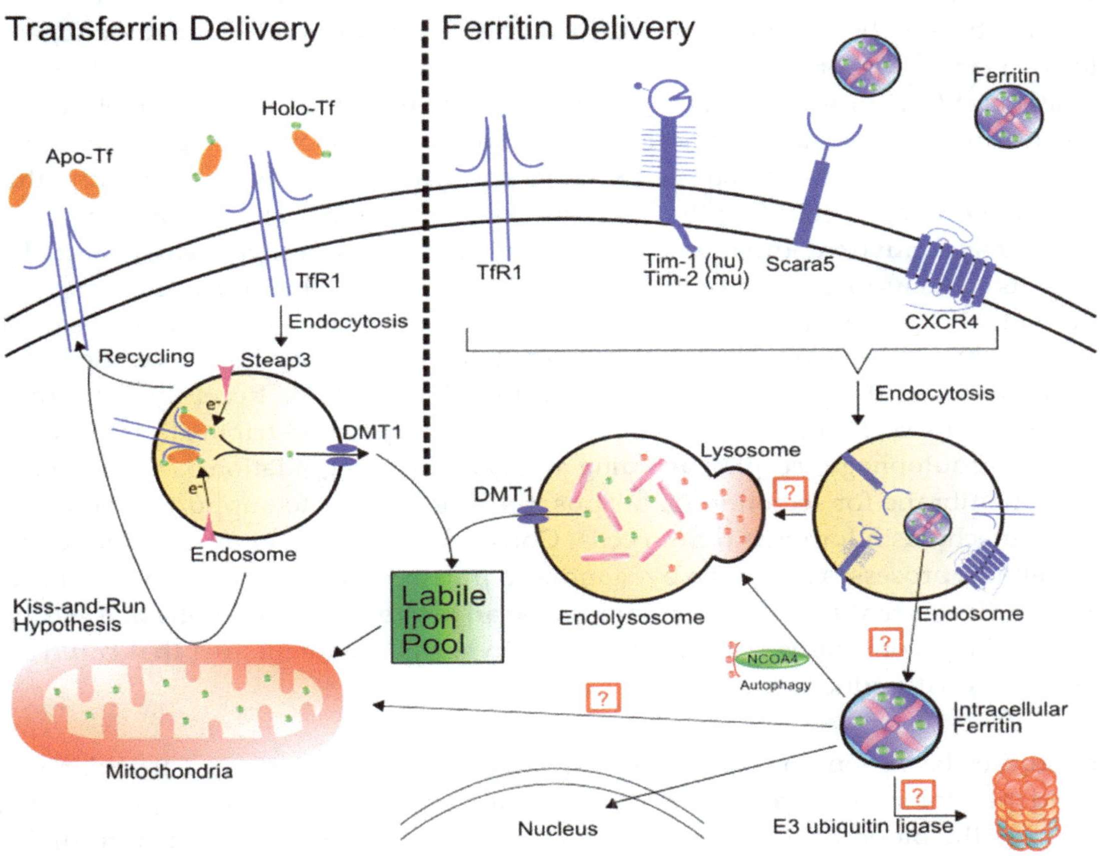

Figure 1. Schematic of transferrin and ferritin uptake and intracellular destiny. Left: Holo-Tf can bind to TfR1 and deliver iron into the labile iron pool through the endosome via DMT1. TfR1 can also be recycled to the cell surface, depositing apo-Tf into the extracellular matrix. An alternative hypothesis termed "kiss-and-run" results in endosomal delivery of iron to the mitochondria by brief interactions between the endosome and the mitochondria. Right: Ferritin binding has been shown for TfR1, Tim-1, Tim-2, Scara5, and CXCR4. After binding, ferritin is endocytosed. Note, while not all receptors are simultaneously required for endocytosis of ferritin, the schematic is demonstrating that all of the receptors in question have been found in the endosome. Ferritin trafficking after endocytosis has yet to be fully elucidated. Hypotheses include trafficking to the lysosome for protein degradation or for ferritin to leave the endosome through another means. Once ferritin is cytosolic, it can be shuttled to the lysosome via NCOA4 or it may be transported to the nucleus. There are a number of other potential hypotheses as well: (1) Ferritin may be poly-ubiquitinated and degraded by the proteasome or (2) ferritin may be shuttled to the mitochondria to deliver iron.

In particular, serum ferritin represents an important consideration in iron delivery; saturation of serum ferritin can range wildly depending on a number of factors, such as inflammation or development, with values ranging between 5% and 50% saturated [22]. It remains to be determined the extent to which serum ferritin functions to deliver iron; iron saturation of ferritin is largely ignored in the clinic. This is particularly important as around 90% of patients that present in the clinic with hyperferritinemia do not have iron overload [23]. While serum ferritin reportedly has a lower level of iron saturation than liver ferritin [24], the iron contained within serum ferritin was still a relatively higher amount than transferrin iron. Cohen et al. found that while liver ferritin contained 2074 atoms of iron per molecule of ferritin, serum ferritin contained 689 atoms of iron per molecule of ferritin [24]. Thus, despite the common tendency to refer to serum ferritin as "iron poor" that one consistently sees in the literature, it stands that if serum ferritin participates in iron delivery it is a significant source of iron.

In order for ferritin to serve as an iron delivery protein, it must be released from cells (Figure 2). Secretion of ferritin has been demonstrated in many cell types, such as macrophages [18,25,26], hepatocytes [27], and Kupffer cells of the liver [28], in both healthy and disease settings. While the exact mechanism of ferritin secretion is still very much open for debate, the lack of glycosylation of extracellular ferritin suggests a non-classical secretion route. Cohen et al. have demonstrated the secretion of ferritin through the lysosomal secretory pathway, a cell-specific directed pathway that is not the product of damaged cells [24]. In this pathway, specialized secretory lysosomal granules are created both as degradative/modulatory compartments as well as storage areas, eventually followed by secretion of its contents to the extracellular milieu [29]. Subsequently Truman-Rosentsvit et al. found that in addition to the lysosomal secretory pathway, ferritin can also be secreted via the multivesicular body-exosome pathway [30]. Consistent with the secretion in membrane bound vesicles, Mrowczynski et al. has demonstrated the presence of H-ferritin in exosomes [31]. Recently, Kimura et al. have further described this secretion mechanism as dependent upon the tripartite motif containing 16 (TRIM16) secretory autophagy receptor, avoiding autolysosomal degradation by pivoting ferritin cargo to the plasma membrane for secretion [32]. Thus, the data appear to support an active rather than passive release mechanism for ferritin from cells. Consequently, the amount of serum ferritin may be reflective of cellular processes and not a by-stander to inflammation and non-specific product of cell damage. This indicates that ferritin secretion may be an active response to physiological conditions and identifying those conditions that promote ferritin secretion are an area that could lead to new knowledge about ferritin function and iron requirements.

Recent studies have demonstrated ferritin ability for iron delivery. In particular, studies have provided evidence for H-ferritin uptake into the brain parenchyma [33], regulation of H-ferritin trafficking across the blood-brain barrier (BBB) [34–38], and H-ferritin uptake into the developing mouse brain (Unpublished Observations). In these experiments, radioactive ^{59}Fe loaded into H-ferritin was used to track the transport of iron directly across the BBB in vitro [34] or directly into the brain in vivo [33]. This was further corroborated by inductively coupled plasma mass spectrometry (ICP-MS) studies of iron delivery by H-ferritin [35]. Todorich et al. demonstrate the importance of H-ferritin-mediated iron delivery to the brain, demonstrating that H-ferritin can replace transferrin as an obligate iron source for oligodendrocytes in vitro [39]. Further evidence has demonstrated both H- and L-ferritin binding and endocytosis in a number of different cell types, including hepatocytes [40], reticulocytes [41], lymphoid cells [42], and erythroid precursors [26,43,44]. In all of these cell types, binding and endocytosis of ferritin results in increased intracellular iron levels. The ability of ferritin to deliver a significantly higher amount of iron relative to transferrin suggests the existence of a more efficient iron delivery system perhaps especially in times of high iron demand, such as neural development and rapid growth [45].

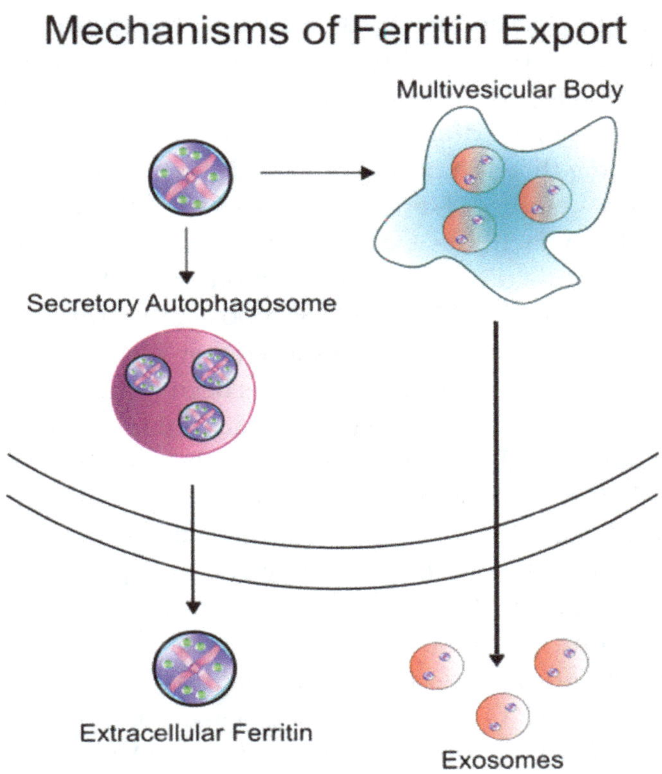

Figure 2. Schematic of iron export mechanisms. Ferritin has been hypothesized to be secreted in two different paradigms: (1) Ferritin is trafficked from the cell via secretory autophagy or (2) ferritin encapsulated in exosomes is released extracellularly from multivesicular bodies.

There is considerable debate regarding the mechanism for ferritin uptake. While previous studies have demonstrated clathrin-dependent endocytosis of ferritin [46], there is not yet a consensus on the specific receptor mediating the uptake. Further complicating matters is the report that both H-ferritin and L-ferritin utilize different receptors. As previously stated, ferritin typically exists in a ratio of H- and L-ferritin; the ratio of H- to L-subunits may dictate the specific receptor preferred. While L-ferritin has been shown to bind to Scara5 [47], H-ferritin has thus far been shown to bind to Tim-2 in rodents [48–50], Tim-1 in humans [34,51], as well as CXCR4 [52] and TfR1 [53] (Figure 1). There is discrepant literature describing the ability for ferritin binding to saturate to Tim-2; one study found ferritin binding to be saturable [49] while another found it is not [50]. Importantly, we are not aware of any literature testing for respective contributions of ferritin binding between the TfR1 and Tim receptors. To this point, most cells in the studies studying TfR1 binding to ferritin did not assay for Tim-1/2 as a second uptake receptor. It is likely that both systems exist side-by-side and display different expressions for TfR1 and Tim-1/2 depending on cell type. This suggests that in cells that do not have TfR1, such as mature oligodendrocytes [54], ferritin internalization is dependent on Tim-1/2. Furthermore, it is well known that Tf receptors are saturated to almost 100% capacity when Tf saturation is normal (30%)—further suggesting that ferritin binding to Tim-1/2 may represent the preferred method for uptake of ferritin into the cell.

While binding and endocytosis of ferritin have been previously demonstrated, the eventual downstream fate of endocytosed ferritin has yet to be studied. An important consideration for ferritin uptake is that ferritin can transport anywhere from 100 to 1000 times as much iron as transferrin and therefore improper delivery and regulation of this delivery may have devastating consequences for the cell. As such, it is clearly critical to cell viability to have a route for handling iron release after exogenous ferritin uptake. For example, does ferritin get moved to the endosome and/or lysosome after uptake? If so, what happens to the iron contained within ferritin after ferritin degradation? Li et al. have previously demonstrated H-ferritin delivery to a human T lymphoblast cell line (MOLT-4), showing H-ferritin trafficking to the endosome as well as to the lysosome [53]. It remains to be seen if this delivery route is the same for all cell types, especially in cells lacking TfR1 such as mature myelinating oligodendrocytes [54]. It may also possible for ferritin to leave the endosome without being transported to the lysosome; the diameter of ferritin is only 12 nm, leading to a hypothesis that ferritin may leave the endosome through pores created under cellular stress [55] (Figure 1).

Previous characterization of the Tf-TfR axis has shown the ability for endosomal divalent metal transporter 1 (DMT1) to facilitate exit of iron from the endosome to be utilized by the cell [36,38]. Furthermore, previous studies have also demonstrated that H-ferritin transport is affected by pharmacological inhibition of DMT1 [34]. A second possibility for the fate of ferritin after uptake can be seen again in the Tf-TfR axis. Das et al. have shown that Tf may deliver iron to the mitochondria after uptake while still in the endosome, a process that has been termed "endosomal kiss-and-run" [56]. It is likely that this process, namely the delivery of extracellular iron to the mitochondria, is highly upregulated especially in times of high iron demand. Thus, the possibility exists for ferritin to perform a similar function as Tf to deliver a substantially higher amount of iron directly to the mitochondria either through "kiss-and-run" activity or through a directed transport mechanism (Figure 1).

Once ferritin is within the cytosol either via exogenous (uptake) or endogenous (translation) means, the fate of the protein itself and the iron contained within has been the subject of many studies, but the literature is inconsistent. Some studies suggest that intracellular ferritin is transported to the lysosome to be degraded and the iron inside the ferritin core to be recycled [27]. In particular, nuclear receptor coactivator 4 (NCOA4) was found to be essential in the transport of cytosolic ferritin to the lysosome, a process termed "ferritinophagy" [57]; NCOA4 knockout cells had reductions in ferritin degradation as well as lower intracellular labile iron [57,58]. These studies demonstrated that NCOA4 binds specifically to H-ferritin, but not L-ferritin, at the Arg23 residue [58]. Furthermore, NCOA4 is importantly recognized by the HECT-type E3 ubiquitin ligase HERC2 which itself is iron-sensitive, suggesting NCOA4 is degraded under conditions of iron excess. However, since NCOA4 only recognizes H-ferritin, there is still the question of how L-ferritin is degraded. Other literature suggests that ferritin in general is largely degraded in the proteasome and this degradation can be regulated based on proteasomal activity [59]. Still, others suggest that both lysosomal-mediated and proteasome-mediated degradation of cytosolic ferritin are indeed important contributors to overall ferritin homeostasis [60]. In 2010, Zhang et al. examined the degradation pathway by inhibiting either the lysosome or the proteasome and found that lysosomal proteolysis is the major contributor to ferritin degradation, with proteasomal-mediated degradation conferring a smaller proportion of the degradation [61]. Whether this finding is relevant to all cell types or only the mouse B cell line used in the Zhang et al. study is unclear.

3. Ferritin as a Delivery Agent

In addition to iron, ferritin has the unique ability to encapsulate and deliver other molecules. Indeed, ferritin is a highly preferred molecule in the field of nanotechnology owing to its self-assembly properties, precise cage alignment, and the ability to modify the surface of the fully formed protein with various conjugates to increase specificity and functionality. Importantly, despite the rigid structure under normal physiological conditions, ferritin can be disassembled when the pH becomes very acidic (pH 2–3) or very basic (pH 11–12) [62]. This process can be reversed by changing the pH back to neutral conditions, spontaneously forming ferritin into the full 24-mer [62] (Figure 3). Many researchers have utilized these assembly properties to load various compounds and molecules within the ferritin core. This flexibility in loading and assembly allows for numerous non-classical uses of ferritin. Moreover, even though ferritin has a high molecular weight (~474 kDa), the total diameter of the assembled 24-mer is roughly 12 nm. This diameter is easily smaller than many nanoparticles that are currently in development as drug delivery vehicles; the small diameter of ferritin permits wide movement across membranes, including into the nucleus and potentially out of endosomes [10]. Furthermore, while typically containing a negative surface charge, the charge on ferritin can vary depending on subunit composition, which allows for further flexibility when targeting ferritin molecules across different membranes [63]. Taken together, the unique characteristics of ferritin allow for robust nanocage assembly and targeted delivery.

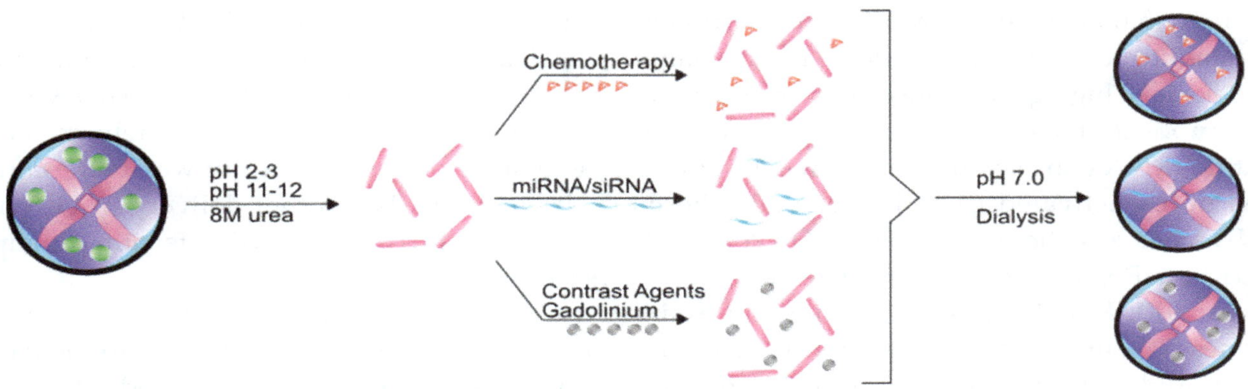

Figure 3. Schematic of encapsulation paradigms for ferritin. Fully formed 24-mer ferritin molecules can be disassembled using 8 M urea or acidic (pH 2–3) or basic (pH 11–12) conditions. A number of different molecules can be mixed with the disassembled ferritin, including chemotherapies, siRNAs/miRNAs, and contrast agents. Upon returning the ferritin mixture to neutral conditions (pH 7.0) coupled with dialysis, ferritin will spontaneously form the 24-mer around the molecule of interest. Free molecules can be dialyzed away from solution.

One prominent area of investigation in the application of ferritin nanocages is in the treatment of cancer. Taking advantage of the fact that cancer cells require a higher amount of iron, many researchers have begun to use ferritin nanocages with encapsulated chemotherapies as delivery agents both in vitro [64,65] and in vivo [65,66] to great effect. Typically, chemotherapeutics such as doxorubicin, are modified by either forming a complex of the drug with transition metals such as Cu(II) [67] or by adding a charged accessory molecule such as poly-L-aspartic acid [68]. Not only does this complex facilitate entry into the ferritin core, but it also allows the transition metal or accessory molecule to stay associated with the ferritin protein while the drug is gradually released from ferritin [68]. For several chemotherapies that target the nucleus or DNA, the ability of ferritin to translocate into the nucleus represents a potential added benefit therapeutically [9,10]. Though the mechanism for drug release from ferritin either in the cytosol or in the nucleus has not yet been elucidated, there is strong evidence that delivery of chemotherapies via ferritin is an effective method that results in reduced non-specific cytotoxicity [69,70]. These reduced off-target effects suggest that cancer cells preferentially take up the ferritin nanocages in an attempt to obtain more iron from circulating ferritin. To further promote the uptake of ferritin by cancer cells, Li et al. conjugated epidermal growth factor (EGF) to H-ferritin as a way to target epidermal growth factor receptor (EGFR)-overexpressing breast cancers in mice [71].

While many studies of ferritin delivery of chemotherapies reveal strong efficacy in non-central nervous system (CNS) cancers [72–74], the use of ferritin nanocages is even more promising for therapeutics targeting brain cancers. Owing to the BBB, effective chemotherapeutic treatment of brain cancers has been extremely difficult. However, as previously described, new evidence suggests ferritin can traffic across the human BBB through Tim-1 [34], potentially allowing for the delivery of directed therapeutics into the brain parenchyma. In diseases such as neuroblastoma or glioblastoma that are extremely aggressive and have a severe phenotype with limited treatment options, ferritin nanocages represent a highly exciting and novel delivery route (Figure 2). As an example, Chen et al. have recently demonstrated that apoferritin loaded with doxorubicin can reliably cross the BBB and deposit the chemotherapy specifically within the tumor in a mouse model resulting in increased survival [75]. This example again demonstrates the preferential uptake of ferritin by cancer cells, likely in an attempt to obtain more iron.

In addition to loading the ferritin molecule with chemotherapies such as doxorubicin, the ferritin molecule may allow for delivery of small interfering RNAs (siRNAs) in a number of different biological paradigms. For example, Li et al. have demonstrated a simple method for encapsulating siRNA and using this ferritin-siRNA combination to perform high efficiency transfections of human primary mesenchymal stem cells (hMSCs) and peripheral blood mononuclear cells (PBMCs) in vitro when compared to commercially available Lipofectamine [70]. This study demonstrated that ferritin-siRNA could achieve high gene expression silencing with a low siRNA concentration of 10 nM. This work has large implications in the treatment of various immune-related disorders, as in vivo delivery of this ferritin-siRNA complex did not show any immune activation of the PBMCs but was preferentially taken up by activated B- and T-cells. Furthermore, it has been shown that delivery of H-ferritin siRNA sensitizes glioma to radiation [14,76] which brings up the possibility of using ferritin containing H-ferritin siRNA in order to sensitize various cancers to radiation.

In 2013, Kanekiyo et al. detailed an exciting use for ferritin as a natural delivery agent for vaccines [77]. In this study, the authors fused the influenza virus haemagglutinin (HA) to the ferritin protein and immunized mice with this fusion protein. As a result, mice produced broad-scale neutralizing antibodies against common and vulnerable targets of universal influenza vaccines. Furthermore, the HA-ferritin fusion protein elicited ten times as high of a response as the naïve vaccine, demonstrating increased potency and breadth of influenza immunity. Kanekiyo and colleagues have also extended this approach to the creation of a potential vaccine for Epstein-Barr Virus [78]. This seminal study spawned other studies such as one by Han and colleagues—priming of dendritic cells using ferritin nanocages conjugated to ovalbumin antigenic peptides OT-1 and OT-2 [79]. In this study, the dendritic cell-based vaccine was developed by putting OT-1 and OT-2 on the exterior surface and interior cavity, respectively, resulting in effective priming of $CD4^+$ and $CD8^+$ T cells after antigen presentation by the dendritic cell. Immunization of mice with this vaccine resulted in differentiation and proliferation of $CD4^+$ and $CD8^+$ T cells specifically targeting OT-1 and OT-2.

4. Ferritin as a Mineralization Chamber

Magnetic resonance imaging (MRI) is a powerful diagnostic technique with extensive uses in the detection of tumor development [80], white matter development and injury [81,82], and aberrant vascularization [83,84]. To create a clinically useful image that is both highly sensitive and accurate, contrast agents are typically used to aid the visual interpretation of MRI scans. The most common contrast agents used are different formulations of gadolinium (Gd), owing to the strong paramagnetism of Gd from seven unpaired electrons. However, a significant problem with Gd is that it nonspecifically labels all highly vascularized tissues, resulting in false positives and a loss of spatial resolution.

Ferritin represents a viable alternative to Gd labeling for MRI. Both endogenous and exogenous ferritin have found great utility in improving MRI contrast capabilities and disease monitoring [85]. In particular, an increased amount of iron within the ferritin core directly correlates with T2* contrast power. It has been shown that Gd can also be loaded within the ferritin core and used as a more prominent imaging agent [72,86] (Figure 2). This function of improved contrast has many applications, especially in the diagnosis or monitoring of cancer progression. Other functionalities of ferritin use in MRI rely on preferential uptake of ferritin by resident macrophages within a cancer tumor [73] or by the tumor cells themselves either by native uptake or by enhancing uptake with further conjugations [87]

An interesting use of ferritin on an industrial process-scale level is the use of thermostable ferritin from *Pyrococcus furiosus* as a water treatment biologic [88]. In this example, ferritin is used to sequester excess phosphate and arsenate due to the high phosphate and arsenate content of seawater and industry waste. While current phosphate removal methods use a system that is heavily reliant on calcium and aluminum sulfates or bacteria that adsorb calcium, the removal of phosphates by ferritin represents a lower maintenance cost and a method that can be recycled [88].

5. Ferritin as a Marker for Inflammation

There are three main regulatory pathways for the expression of ferritin: The iron response proteins (IRPs)/iron responsive element (IRE) system [89], the regulation of transcription through NF-κB [90], and transcriptional regulation through the hypoxia inducible factor 1 alpha (HIF-1α) binding to a HIF responsive element (HRE) upstream of the IRE system [91]. The IRP/IRE system functions by the binding of IRPs to the IRE at the 5′ untranslated region (UTR) of ferritin mRNA under conditions of low iron, inhibiting its translation. However, in conditions of high iron, IRP binding to the IRE is decreased, leading to increased ferritin expression. Similarly, ferritin gene transcription is upregulated in conditions of inflammation where inflammatory cytokines such as tumor necrosis factor alpha (TNF-α) and interleukin-2 (IL-2) signal to increase binding of NF-κB to the transcription enhancer FER2 upstream of the IRE and coding region [90]. It has been shown that the NF-κB pathway is highly responsive to inflammation [92]. Evidence for this pathway stems from activation of toll-like receptor 2 (TLR2) in macrophages resulting in IRP-independent upregulation of H-ferritin, as well as direct pharmacological activation of the NF-κB pathway [93]. Similarly, it has been shown that H-ferritin expression is also responsive to tumor necrosis factor alpha (TNF-α) [94], interleukin-2 (IL-2) [95], and IL-10 [96]. Consequently, the elevated presence of ferritin in serum has long been considered in clinical settings to be an acute phase inflammatory marker, as elevated serum ferritin levels have been correlated with increased levels of pro-inflammatory cytokines [97,98]. Potential sources of serum ferritin during inflammation include secretion by macrophages [24,25] and/or release from cells due to tissue damage [99], both indicators of inflammation or infection. Importantly, there is disagreement in the literature about whether serum ferritin is a pro-inflammatory marker [100], an anti-inflammatory marker [101,102], or is simply a byproduct of release during the course of infection by damaged cells [99]. Understanding mechanisms of release of ferritin and how those mechanisms are influenced at the cellular level could provide insights into the biological and clinical meaning of ferritin in serum.

Serum ferritin has also been routinely interpreted in the clinic as a surrogate measure of iron storage in the body [103]. There are numerous studies that examine the correlation between serum ferritin and iron deficiency anemia or hemochromatosis in which serum ferritin levels are decreased or elevated, respectively [104]. However, inflammation or infection is known to drastically change the amount of serum ferritin present [105]. Accordingly, in an individual with acute or chronic inflammation, the extent to which serum ferritin levels reflect inflammation may reflect the total body iron stores. To further complicate this understanding, there are studies demonstrating that serum ferritin is not the most reliable marker for total body iron stores, especially when there are other complicating factors such as liver or kidney damage [12]. Put together, it seems that clinically, serum ferritin may be used as a marker for total body iron stores in the healthy individual, however, in a disease setting serum ferritin may be more indicative of the underlying pathophysiology such as organ damage or infection.

Another important consideration is while serum ferritin may be used clinically to suggest inflammation, serum ferritin measurements are focused largely on the L-ferritin subunit and as such, remain a poor indicator of iron status of the patient in this inflammatory state [97], as described earlier it is H-ferritin that is mostly responsive to the inflammatory process. H-ferritin has been detected in serum [106] and has the potential to be much more dynamic and informative than L-ferritin. A critical question that has yet to be answered clinically is: Is the iron saturation of serum ferritin in any given individual more informative to the total body iron stores than serum ferritin levels itself? Currently, it is rather trivial to measure serum ferritin levels but to measure the iron contained within serum ferritin is considerably more difficult. One recent study has looked at ferritin secretion from macrophages and determined that iron saturation of the ferritin was about a third as saturated as liver ferritin [24]. This is important as many consider serum ferritin to be iron-free or iron-poor, but the reality is that it contains a significant amount of iron. Thus, ferritin saturation may be the better measure of total body iron stores rather than the serum ferritin molecules themselves.

In addition to the utility of serum ferritin clinically, intracellular ferritin has also been implicated in the host response to microbial infection. Recent evidence demonstrates that H-ferritin confers tolerance to malaria and sepsis during infection by limiting reactive oxygen species (ROS) and overall oxidative stress. For example, Gozzelino et al. shows evidence that the activity of H-ferritin confers a metabolic adaptation to *Plasmodium* infection [107]. This activity is through the chelation ability of H-ferritin to limit labile iron from activating the pro-apoptotic c-Jun N-terminal kinase (JNK). Furthermore, the authors found that JNK activity inhibits H-ferritin expression and causes increased susceptibility of malaria coupled with tissue damage and oxidative stress. To extend this study, Weis et al. also looked at this metabolic adaptation in sepsis, a devastating syndrome resulting from a maladaptive host response to infection [108]. Much in the same way as Gozzelino et al., Weis and colleagues demonstrated a disease tolerance to sepsis that was facilitated by H-ferritin. Importantly, activity of H-ferritin to sequester cytosolic iron was critical for the setup of disease tolerance. Weis et al. showed that H-ferritin iron chelation prevents iron-driven oxidative inhibition of the glucose-6-phosphatase to sustain glucose production via liver gluconeogenesis. Another recent study that demonstrates the importance of H-ferritin in response to microbial infection was by Reddy et al. [109]. In this study, the authors infected H-ferritin knockout mice or wild-type mice with *Mycobacterium tuberculosis*, demonstrating that knocking out H-ferritin specifically in myeloid cell populations decreased survival after infection, increased the overall inflammatory response, and increased the total bacterial loads. These studies highlight the general importance of ferritin in the inflammatory response as well as for normal host iron homeostasis.

In contrast, ferritin has also been shown to have a role as an anti-inflammatory molecule. Ferritin in serum reportedly binds to high molecular weight kininogen (HK) [110]. Normally, HK is a co-factor in the intrinsic coagulation pathway; HK cleavage by the serine protease kallikrein leads to release of bradykinin and two-chain high molecular weight kininogen [111]. This particular pathway has large implications in the progression of a number of inflammatory diseases such as asthma [112], inflammatory bowel disease [113], and rheumatoid disorders [114,115]. Ferritin binding to HK serves as an anti-inflammatory signaling pathway, as the direct interaction of ferritin with HK prevents HK cleavage and a concomitant reduction in bradykinin release [102]. This overall interaction diminishes the total inflammatory response. In a similar paradigm, Fan and colleagues demonstrated that L-ferritin can play an important anti-inflammatory role in lipopolysaccharide (LPS)-stimulated macrophages [101]. In this study, Fan et al. show that overexpression of L-ferritin in macrophages can inhibit LPS-mediated transcription of TNF-α and IL-1β, both critical pro-inflammatory cytokines. Conversely, they showed that L-ferritin is significantly downregulated after LPS stimulation. From this study, the authors conclude that L-ferritin has an underappreciated role in the anti-inflammatory resolution cascade. Importantly, both of these studies are direct evidence of ferritin playing an anti-inflammatory role.

6. Ferritin as a Disease Biomarker

While the amount of iron has been shown to increase throughout the body with age [116–118], abnormal iron homeostasis can lead to devastating diseases. Typically, a concomitant increase in ferritin levels are paired with increased iron levels [119], attempting to ensure safe handling of this increase in iron. However, a failure of ferritin levels to concomitantly increase with iron may impact normal physiology and induce pathology as a result of iron-mediated induction of oxidative stress. This role for ferritin and a mishandling of systemic iron has been shown to be implicated in a number of diseases such as Still's disease, hemophagocytic syndrome, and sideroblastic anemia—implications of serum ferritin in these diseases and others have been critically reviewed in numerous other reviews [12,104,106]. Similarly, serum ferritin as a bioindicator for cancer has been extensively reviewed as well [120,121]. Here we will focus specifically on neurological disorders and the impact that ferritin has on diagnosis as a biomarker for disease or progression. One interesting new development has been proposed in Friedreich's Ataxia where the authors discuss the hypothesis that the mitochondrial protein frataxin may oligomerize like ferritin and perform functions redundant with mitochondrial ferritin, acting as another iron storage molecule [122]. Loss of frataxin and this iron storage property may result in Friedreich's Ataxia and subsequent neurodegeneration.

6.1. *Neuroferritinopathy*

Neuroferritinopathy (NF), an autosomal dominant disease resulting from mutations in L-ferritin, is classified as belonging to a group of movement disorders known as Neurodegeneration with Brain Iron Accumulation (NBIA). This disease is an extrapyramidal syndrome typically characterized by excessive iron accumulation in the basal ganglia. NF was originally characterized as a disease arising from an additional adenine at c.460 of exon 4 in the L-ferritin gene, but other mutations around the same region were quickly identified as contributing to disease pathology [123]. These mutations cause a frameshift in the C-terminus of the L-ferritin subunit resulting in reduced or ablated iron storage and subsequent iron-mediated damage, as this mutation creates a larger than normal pore [123]. In 2010, Barbeito et al. showed that fibroblasts from NF patients have higher levels of H- and L-ferritin as well as increased levels of total iron stores [124]. Furthermore, Maccarinelli and colleagues showed in 2014 that mice with the same L-ferritin mutation had a progressive impairment in motor coordination and a propensity to accumulate iron within post-natal hippocampal neurons [125]. Interestingly, this mutation in NF patients is present in all cells, but there is no evidence for iron mismanagement or dyshomeostasis by the rest of the body. It is currently unclear whether brain cells are simply more sensitive to iron-dependent toxicity or if there is a separate function for L-ferritin within the brain parenchyma. It is likely that the high oxygen and glucose consumption of the brain leads to an increase in iron utilization and therefore ROS/oxidative stress. Without functional L-ferritin, brain cells are rendered unable to survive this oxidative damage.

6.2. *Parkinson's Disease*

One of the most prominent neurodegenerative diseases with marked neurodegeneration as well as substantial iron accumulation in the substantia nigra pars compacta (SNpc) is Parkinson's disease (PD). In general, there is agreement that iron accumulation in the SNpc increases with age, but the additional increase in iron in the SNpc as a result of PD depends heavily on the stage and progression of PD [126]. With regard to ferritin in PD, there are a number of conflicting reports regarding the expression of ferritin within the SNpc; biochemical studies have shown both increased [126] and decreased [127] levels of ferritin within the SNpc in PD. In the 1-methyl-4-phenyl-1,2,3,6-tetrahydropyridine (MPTP) model of PD, H-ferritin overexpression in neurons is protective against disease progression [128]. Although there seems to be altered iron management specifically within the SNpc, cerebrospinal fluid (CSF) levels of ferritin and serum ferritin levels were not significantly different between PD and non-PD patients [127]. In contrast however, there is a recent study detailing how serum ferritin may serve as a potential biomarker for diagnosis in PD [129]. In this study, the authors found an increased level of serum ferritin in PD patients when compared to non-PD patients. Unfortunately, the sample size of the patient cohort used in this study was relatively small (40 healthy vs. 40 PD patients) and was limited to a cross-sectional analysis. Furthermore, there is a lack of consensus about the reliability of using serum ferritin as an indicator of brain iron status or even, as previously discussed, systemic iron status. Another consideration in the utilization of serum/CSF ferritin as a biomarker in PD is that peripheral inflammation plays a large role in PD disease progression [130]. As such, serum/CSF ferritin levels will likely be altered as a result and may not be informative of brain iron status.

6.3. *Restless Legs Syndrome*

In Restless Legs Syndrome (RLS), a disorder characterized by an irresistible urge to move the limbs and unpleasant sensations in the legs, a well-established neurobiological abnormality is low brain iron despite normal peripheral iron levels [131]. However, RLS is about five times more prevalent in iron deficient populations [132,133]. It is clear that ferritin levels are significantly impacted by and are important in RLS pathology, but it is not yet known how ferritin may specifically contribute to disease progression or disease symptoms. We have previously shown that Tf, TfR, and H-ferritin levels are decreased in the endothelial cells of RLS patients, indicating iron mismanagement at the level of the BBB, suggesting decreased brain iron acquisition in RLS brains [134]. Furthermore, studies have also demonstrated a decrease in H-ferritin and iron levels specifically in the SNpc of RLS brains compared to controls [135]. Currently, serum ferritin is used to guide treatment, but we have discussed the concerns regarding the utility of serum ferritin both as a measure of total body iron stores and serum ferritin levels are of no value in predicting response to treatment. Lammers et al. studied serum ferritin, bodily iron, and RLS, finding no association between early-onset RLS and longitudinal measures of iron stores [136]. Similarly, while serum ferritin is currently used clinically to guide treatment, it has been shown that serum ferritin levels have no predictive value in the response to treatment [131]. This is an important consideration as it underlines the fact that serum ferritin levels are not necessarily predictive of brain ferritin levels or total brain iron status.

6.4. *Amyotrophic Lateral Sclerosis*

Amyotrophic Lateral Sclerosis (ALS), a progressive and devastating disease, is characterized by loss of motor neurons in the cortex, brainstem, and spinal cord. While ALS is a relatively common disease, the exact mechanisms for this neurodegeneration is currently unknown, with a number of factors such as oxidative stress, excitotoxic stimulation, and genetic factors all implicated to play a role. It has long been known that in the ALS iron homeostasis is disrupted; there is higher iron in the CSF and spinal cord of ALS patients [137]. While there are a large number of studies that demonstrate elevated levels of serum ferritin in ALS [137–139], there is not yet a consensus regarding whether serum ferritin is predictive [139–141] or unrelated [137,138] to disease progression and survival rates.

7. Conclusions

Classically, ferritin has been described as a critical iron storage protein whose dual roles as both an antioxidant and an iron sink were essential to cellular survival. The importance of ferritin can directly be seen in knockout mouse models; both H and L homozygous knockout mice are embryonic lethal [128,142]. While not disputing the importance of these intracellular roles, it is clear that ferritin has highly dynamic and novel functions outside of the cells. Recent evidence has demonstrated the ability of ferritin to participate in iron delivery, delivery of macro/micromolecules, and as a potential biomarker in many neurologic diseases. Though serum ferritin is largely comprised of the L subunit, iron levels in ferritin remain much higher than transferrin; there is significant potential for serum ferritin to deliver anywhere between 10 to 100 times higher iron than transferrin [35]. Furthermore, while it is clear that ferritin can deliver iron to various organs throughout the body, it is still unclear as to why the body needs multiple iron delivery routes, especially with such drastic differences in amount of iron delivered. Besides iron, the delivery of ferritin-encapsulated macro- and micromolecules has important implications in the treatment and diagnoses of various disorders. While serum ferritin has been implicated in a number of diseases, the exact role and mechanism for serum ferritin in these disorders has not yet been fully characterized. There is a large volume of literature dedicated to exploring ferritin biology, but a number of questions and topics remain to be explored regarding ferritin delivery, downstream fate, role of ferritin in many diseases, and the utility of ferritin clinically.

Author Contributions: B.C. and J.R.C. were responsible for writing, editing, and overseeing all final drafts of the review.

References

1. Laufberger, V. Sur la cristallisation de la ferritine. *Bull. Soc. Chim. Biol.* **1937**, *19*, 1575–1582. (In French)
2. Bradley, J.M.; Le Brun, N.E.; Moore, G.R. Ferritins: Furnishing proteins with iron. *J. Biol. Inorg. Chem.* **2016**, *21*, 13–28. [CrossRef] [PubMed]

3. Arosio, P.; Levi, S. Ferritin, Iron Homeostasis, and Oxidative Damage. *Free Radic. Biol. Med.* **2002**, *33*, 457–463. [CrossRef]
4. Arosio, P.; Ingrassia, R.; Cavadini, P. Ferritins: A family of molecules for iron storage, antioxidation and more. *Biochim. Biophys. Acta Gen. Subj.* **2009**, *1790*, 589–599. [CrossRef] [PubMed]
5. Arosio, P.; Elia, L.; Poli, M. Ferritin, cellular iron storage and regulation. *IUBMB Life* **2017**, *69*, 414–422. [CrossRef] [PubMed]
6. Wang, Z.; Gao, H.; Zhang, Y.; Liu, G.; Niu, G.; Chen, X. Functional ferritin nanoparticles for biomedical applications. *Front. Chem. Sci. Eng.* **2017**, *11*, 633–646. [CrossRef] [PubMed]
7. Corsi, B.; Cozzi, A.; Arosio, P.; Drysdale, J.; Santambrogio, P.; Campanella, A.; Biasiotto, G.; Albertini, A.; Levi, S. Human mitochondrial ferritin expressed in HeLa cells incorporates iron and affects cellular iron metabolism. *J. Biol. Chem.* **2002**, *277*, 22430–22437. [CrossRef] [PubMed]
8. Waldo, G.S.; Wright, E.; Whang, Z.H.; Briat, J.F.; Theil, E.C.; Sayers, D.E. Formation of the ferritin iron mineral occurs in plastids. *Plant Physiol.* **1995**, *109*, 797–802. [CrossRef] [PubMed]
9. Surguladze, N.; Thompson, K.M.; Beard, J.L.; Connor, J.R.; Fried, M.G. Interactions and Reactions of Ferritin with DNA. *J. Biol. Chem.* **2004**, *279*, 14694–14702. [CrossRef] [PubMed]
10. Surguladze, N.; Patton, S.; Cozzi, A.; Fried, M.G.; Connor, J.R. Characterization of nuclear ferritin and mechanism of translocation. *Biochem. J.* **2005**, *388*, 731–740. [CrossRef] [PubMed]
11. Alkhateeb, A.A.; Connor, J.R. Nuclear ferritin: A new role for ferritin in cell biology. *Biochim. Biophys. Acta Gen. Subj.* **2010**, *1800*, 793–797. [CrossRef] [PubMed]
12. Knovich, M.A.; Storey, J.A.; Coffman, L.G.; Torti, S.V.; Torti, F.M. Ferritin for the clinician. *Blood Rev.* **2009**, *23*, 95–104. [CrossRef] [PubMed]
13. Kuiper, M.A.; Mulder, C.; van Kamp, G.J.; Scheltens, P.; Wolters, E.C. Cerebrospinal fluid ferritin levels of patients with Parkinson's disease, Alzheimer's disease, and multiple system atrophy. *J. Neural Transm.* **1994**, *7*, 109–114. [CrossRef]
14. Liu, X.; Madhankumar, A.B.; Slagle-Webb, B.; Sheehan, J.M.; Surguladze, N.; Connor, J.R. Heavy chain ferritin siRNA delivered by cationic liposomes increases sensitivity of cancer cells to chemotherapeutic agents. *Cancer Res.* **2011**, *71*, 2240–2249. [CrossRef] [PubMed]
15. Yang, H.; Yang, M.; Guan, H.; Liu, Z.; Zhao, S.; Takeuchi, S.; Yanagisawa, D.; Tooyama, I. Mitochondrial ferritin in neurodegenerative diseases. *Neurosci. Res.* **2013**, *77*, 1–7. [CrossRef] [PubMed]
16. Algarín, C.; Peirano, P.; Garrido, M.; Pizarro, F.; Lozoff, B. Iron Deficiency Anemia in Infancy: Long-Lasting Effects on Auditory and Visual System Functioning. *Pediatr. Res.* **2003**, *53*, 217–223. [CrossRef] [PubMed]
17. Tomatsu, S.; Orii, K.O.; Fleming, R.E.; Holden, C.C.; Waheed, A.; Britton, R.S.; Gutierrez, M.A.; Velez-Castrillon, S.; Bacon, B.R.; Sly, W.S. Contribution of the H63D mutation in HFE to murine hereditary hemochromatosis. *Proc. Natl. Acad. Sci. USA* **2003**, *100*, 15788–15793. [CrossRef] [PubMed]
18. Nixon, A.M.; Neely, E.; Simpson, I.A.; Connor, J.R. The role of HFE genotype in macrophage phenotype. *J. Neuroinflamm.* **2018**, *15*, 30. [CrossRef] [PubMed]
19. Stephenson, E.; Nathoo, N.; Mahjoub, Y.; Dunn, J.F.; Yong, V.W. Iron in multiple sclerosis: Roles in neurodegeneration and repair. *Nat. Rev. Neurol.* **2014**, *10*, 459–468. [CrossRef] [PubMed]
20. Peters, D.G.; Connor, J.R.; Meadowcroft, M.D. The relationship between iron dyshomeostasis and amyloidogenesis in Alzheimer's disease: Two sides of the same coin. *Neurobiol. Dis.* **2015**, *81*, 49–65. [CrossRef] [PubMed]
21. Biasiotto, G.; Di Lorenzo, D.; Archetti, S.; Zanella, I. Iron and Neurodegeneration: Is Ferritinophagy the Link? *Mol. Neurobiol.* **2016**, *53*, 5542–5574. [CrossRef] [PubMed]
22. ten Kate, J.; Wolthuis, A.; Westerhuis, B.; van Deursen, C. The Iron Content of Serum Ferritin: Physiological Importance and Diagnostic Value. *Clin. Chem. Lab. Med.* **1997**, *35*, 53–56. [CrossRef]
23. Hearnshaw, S.; Thompson, N.P.; Mcgill, A. The epidemiology of hyperferritinaemia. *World J. Gastroenterol.* **2006**, *12*, 5866–5869. [CrossRef] [PubMed]
24. Cohen, L.A.; Gutierrez, L.; Weiss, A.; Leichtmann-Bardoogo, Y.; Zhang, D.L.; Crooks, D.R.; Sougrat, R.; Morgenstern, A.; Galy, B.; Hentze, M.W.; et al. Serum ferritin is derived primarily from macrophages through a nonclassical secretory pathway. *Blood* **2010**, *116*, 1574–1584. [CrossRef] [PubMed]
25. Connor, J.R.; Zhang, X.; Nixon, A.M.; Webb, B.; Perno, J.R. Comparative evaluation of nephrotoxicity and management by macrophages of intravenous pharmaceutical iron formulations. *PLoS ONE* **2015**, *10*, e0125272. [CrossRef] [PubMed]

26. Leimberg, M.J.; Prus, E.; Konijn, A.M.; Fibach, E. Macrophages function as a ferritin iron source for cultured human erythroid precursors. *J. Cell. Biochem.* **2008**, *103*, 1211–1218. [CrossRef] [PubMed]
27. Kidane, T.Z.; Sauble, E.; Linder, M.C. Release of iron from ferritin requires lysosomal activity. *Am. J. Physiol. Cell Physiol.* **2006**, *291*, C445–C455. [CrossRef] [PubMed]
28. Briley-Saebo, K.; Bjørnerud, A.; Grant, D.; Ahlstrom, H.; Berg, T.; Kindberg, G.M. Hepatic cellular distribution and degradation of iron oxide nanoparticles following single intravenous injection in rats: Implications for magnetic resonance imaging. *Cell Tissue Res.* **2004**, *316*, 315–323. [CrossRef] [PubMed]
29. Blott, E.J.; Griffiths, G.M. Secretory lysosomes. *Nat. Rev. Mol. Cell Biol.* **2002**, *3*, 122–131. [CrossRef] [PubMed]
30. Truman-Rosentsvit, M.; Berenbaum, D.; Spektor, L.; Cohen, L.A.; Belizowsky-Moshe, S.; Lifshitz, L.; Ma, J.; Li, W.; Kesselman, E.; Abutbul-Ionita, I.; et al. Ferritin is secreted via 2 distinct nonclassical vesicular pathways. *Blood* **2018**, *131*, 342–352. [CrossRef] [PubMed]
31. Mrowczynski, O.D.; Madhankumar, A.B.; Slagle-Webb, B.; Lee, S.Y.; Zacharia, B.E.; Connor, J.R. HFE genotype affects exosome phenotype in cancer. *Biochim. Biophys. Acta Gen. Subj.* **2017**, *1861*, 1921–1928. [CrossRef] [PubMed]
32. Kimura, T.; Jia, J.; Kumar, S.; Won Choi, S.; Gu, Y.; Mudd, M.; Dupont, N.; Jiang, S.; Peters, R.; Farzam, F.; et al. Dedicated SNAREs and specialized TRIM cargo receptors mediate secretory autophagy. *EMBO J.* **2017**, *36*, 42–60. [CrossRef] [PubMed]
33. Fisher, J.; Devraj, K.; Ingram, J.; Slagle-Webb, B.; Madhankumar, A.B.; Liu, X.; Klinger, M.; Simpson, I.A.; Connor, J.R. Ferritin: A novel mechanism for delivery of iron to the brain and other organs. *Am J. Physiol. Cell Physiol.* **2007**, *293*, C641–C649. [CrossRef] [PubMed]
34. Chiou, B.; Neal, E.H.; Bowman, A.B.; Lippmann, E.S.; Simpson, I.A.; Connor, J.R. Endothelial cells are critical regulators of iron transport in a model of the human blood–brain barrier. *J. Cereb. Blood Flow Metab.* **2018**, in press. [CrossRef] [PubMed]
35. Chiou, B.; Neal, E.H.; Bowman, A.B.; Lippmann, E.S.; Simpson, I.A.; Connor, J.R. Pharmaceutical iron formulations do not cross a model of the human blood-brain barrier. *PLoS ONE* **2018**, *13*, e0198775. [CrossRef] [PubMed]
36. Simpson, I.A.; Ponnuru, P.; Klinger, M.E.; Myers, R.L.; Devraj, K.; Coe, C.L.; Lubach, G.R.; Carruthers, A.; Connor, J.R. A Novel Model for Brain Iron Uptake: Introducing the Concept of Regulation. *J. Cereb. Blood Flow Metab.* **2015**, *35*, 48–57. [CrossRef] [PubMed]
37. Duck, K.A.; Connor, J.R. Iron uptake and transport across physiological barriers. *BioMetals* **2016**, *29*, 573–591. [CrossRef] [PubMed]
38. Duck, K.A.; Simpson, I.A.; Connor, J.R. Regulatory mechanisms for iron transport across the blood-brain barrier. *Biochem. Biophys. Res. Commun.* **2017**, *494*, 70–75. [CrossRef] [PubMed]
39. Todorich, B.; Zhang, X.; Connor, J.R. H-ferritin is the major source of iron for oligodendrocytes. *Glia* **2011**, *59*, 927–935. [CrossRef] [PubMed]
40. Adams, P.C.; Chau, L.A. Uptake of ferritin by isolated rat hepatocytes. Effect of metabolic inhibitors and iron. *Clin. Investig. Med. Médecine Clin. Exp.* **1993**, *16*, 15–21.
41. Blight, G.D.; Morgan, E.H. Ferritin and iron uptake by reticulocytes. *Br. J. Haematol.* **1983**, *55*, 59–71. [CrossRef] [PubMed]
42. Moss, D.; Powell, L.W.; Arosio, P.; Halliday, J.W. Characterization of the ferritin receptors of human T lymphoid (MOLT-4) cells. *J. Lab. Clin. Med.* **1992**, *119*, 273–279. [PubMed]
43. Sakamoto, S.; Kawabata, H.; Masuda, T.; Uchiyama, T.; Mizumoto, C.; Ohmori, K.; Koeffler, H.P.; Kadowaki, N.; Takaori-Kondo, A. H-Ferritin is Preferentially Incorporated by Human Erythroid Cells through Transferrin Receptor 1 in a Threshold-Dependent Manner. *PLoS ONE* **2015**, *10*, e0139915. [CrossRef] [PubMed]
44. Gelvan, D.; Fibach, E.; Meyron-Holtz, E.G.; Konijn, A.M. Ferritin uptake by human erythroid precursors is a regulated iron uptake pathway. *Blood* **1996**, *88*, 3200–3207. [PubMed]
45. Beard, J.L.; Connor, J.R. Iron status and neural functioning. *Annu. Rev. Nutr.* **2003**, *23*, 41–58. [CrossRef] [PubMed]
46. Hulet, S.; Heyliger, S.; Powers, S.; Connor, J. Oligodendrocyte progenitor cells internalize ferritin via clathrin-dependent receptor mediated endocytosis. *J. Neurosci. Res.* **2000**, *61*, 52–60. [CrossRef]
47. Li, J.Y.; Paragas, N.; Ned, R.M.; Qiu, A.; Viltard, M.; Leete, T.; Drexler, I.R.; Chen, X.; Sanna-Cherchi, S.;

Mohammed, F.; et al. Scara5 is a Ferritin Receptor Mediating Non-Transferrin Iron Delivery. *Dev. Cell* **2009**, *16*, 35–46. [CrossRef] [PubMed]

48. Chen, T.T.; Li, L.; Chung, D.H.; Allen, C.D.C.; Torti, S.V.; Torti, F.M.; Cyster, J.G.; Chen, C.Y.; Brodsky, F.M.; Niemi, E.C.; et al. TIM-2 is expressed on B cells and in liver and kidney and is a receptor for H-ferritin endocytosis. *J. Exp. Med.* **2005**, *202*, 955–965. [CrossRef] [PubMed]
49. Todorich, B.; Zhang, X.; Slagle-Webb, B.; Seaman, W.E.; Connor, J.R. Tim-2 is the receptor for H-ferritin on oligodendrocytes. *J. Neurochem.* **2008**, *107*, 1495–1505. [CrossRef] [PubMed]
50. Han, J.; Seaman, W.E.; Di, X.; Wang, W.; Willingham, M.; Torti, F.M.; Torti, S.V. Iron uptake mediated by binding of H-ferritin to the TIM-2 receptor in mouse cells. *PLoS ONE* **2011**, *6*, e23800. [CrossRef] [PubMed]
51. Chiou, B.; Lucassen, E.; Sather, M.; Kallianpur, A.; Connor, J. Semaphorin4A and H-ferritin utilize Tim-1 on human oligodendrocytes: A novel neuro-immune axis. *Glia* **2018**, *66*, 1317–1330. [CrossRef] [PubMed]
52. Li, R.; Luo, C.; Mines, M.; Zhang, J.; Fan, G.H. Chemokine CXCL12 Induces Binding of Ferritin Heavy Chain to the Chemokine Receptor CXCR4, Alters CXCR4 Signaling, and Induces Phosphorylation and Nuclear Translocation of Ferritin Heavy Chain. *J. Biol. Chem.* **2006**, *281*, 37616–37627. [CrossRef] [PubMed]
53. Li, L.; Fang, C.J.; Ryan, J.C.; Niemi, E.C.; Lebrón, J.A.; Björkman, P.J.; Arase, H.; Torti, F.M.; Torti, S.V.; Nakamura, M.C.; et al. Binding and uptake of H-ferritin are mediated by human transferrin receptor-1. *Proc. Natl. Acad. Sci. USA* **2010**, *107*, 3505–3510. [CrossRef] [PubMed]
54. Hulet, S.; Powers, S.; Connor, J. Distribution of transferrin and ferritin binding in normal and multiple sclerotic human brains. *J. Neurol. Sci.* **1999**, *165*, 48–55. [CrossRef]
55. Akinc, A.; Battaglia, G. Exploiting Endocytosis for Nanomedicines. *Cold Spring Harb. Perspect. Biol.* **2013**, *5*, a016980. [CrossRef] [PubMed]
56. Das, A.; Nag, S.; Mason, A.B.; Barroso, M.M. Endosome–mitochondria interactions are modulated by iron release from transferrin. *J. Cell Biol.* **2016**, *214*, 831–845. [CrossRef] [PubMed]
57. Mancias, J.D.; Wang, X.; Gygi, S.P.; Harper, J.W.; Kimmelman, A.C. Quantitative proteomics identifies NCOA4 as the cargo receptor mediating ferritinophagy. *Nature* **2014**, *509*, 105–109. [CrossRef] [PubMed]
58. Mancias, J.D.; Vaites, L.P.; Nissim, S.; Biancur, D.E.; Kim, A.J.; Wang, X.; Liu, Y.; Goessling, W.; Kimmelman, A.C.; Harper, J.W. Ferritinophagy via NCOA4 is required for erythropoiesis and is regulated by iron dependent HERC2-mediated proteolysis. *Elife* **2015**, *4*, e10308. [CrossRef] [PubMed]
59. Mehlhase, J.; Sandig, G.; Pantopoulos, K.; Grune, T. Oxidation-induced ferritin turnover in microglial cells: Role of proteasome. *Free Radic. Biol. Med.* **2005**, *38*, 276–285. [CrossRef] [PubMed]
60. Linder, M.C. Mobilization of stored iron in mammals: A review. *Nutrients* **2013**, *5*, 4022–4050. [CrossRef] [PubMed]
61. Zhang, Y.; Mikhael, M.; Xu, D.; Li, Y.; Soe-Lin, S.; Ning, B.; Li, W.; Nie, G.; Zhao, Y.; Ponka, P. Lysosomal Proteolysis Is the Primary Degradation Pathway for Cytosolic Ferritin and Cytosolic Ferritin Degradation Is Necessary for Iron Exit. *Antioxid. Redox Signal.* **2010**, *13*, 999–1009. [CrossRef] [PubMed]
62. Kim, M.; Rho, Y.; Jin, K.S.; Ahn, B.; Jung, S.; Kim, H.; Ree, M. pH-Dependent Structures of Ferritin and Apoferritin in Solution: Disassembly and Reassembly. *Biomacromolecules* **2011**, *12*, 1629–1640. [CrossRef] [PubMed]
63. Ghinea, N.; Hasu, M. Charge effect on binding, uptake and transport of ferritin through fenestrated endothelium. *J. Submicrosc. Cytol.* **1986**, *18*, 647–659. [PubMed]
64. Mazzucchelli, S.; Truffi, M.; Baccarini, F.; Beretta, M.; Sorrentino, L.; Bellini, M.; Rizzuto, M.A.; Ottria, R.; Ravelli, A.; Ciuffreda, P.; et al. H-Ferritin-nanocaged olaparib: A promising choice for both BRCA-mutated and sporadic triple negative breast cancer. *Sci. Rep.* **2017**, *7*, 7505. [CrossRef] [PubMed]
65. Mazzucchelli, S.; Bellini, M.; Fiandra, L.; Truffi, M.; Rizzuto, M.A.; Sorrentino, L.; Longhi, E.; Nebuloni, M.; Prosperi, D.; Corsi, F. Nanometronomic treatment of 4T1 breast cancer with nanocaged doxorubicin prevents drug resistance and circumvents cardiotoxicity. *Oncotarget* **2016**, *8*, 8383–8396. [CrossRef] [PubMed]
66. Liang, M.; Fan, K.; Zhou, M.; Duan, D.; Zheng, J.; Yang, D.; Feng, J.; Yan, X. H-ferritin-nanocaged doxorubicin nanoparticles specifically target and kill tumors with a single-dose injection. *Proc. Natl. Acad. Sci. USA* **2014**, *111*, 14900–14905. [CrossRef] [PubMed]
67. Kwon, C.; Kang, Y.J.; Jeon, S.; Jung, S.; Hong, S.Y.; Kang, S. Development of Protein-Cage-Based Delivery Nanoplatforms by Polyvalently Displaying β-Cyclodextrins on the Surface of Ferritins Through Copper(I)-Catalyzed Azide/Alkyne Cycloaddition. *Macromol. Biosci.* **2012**, *12*, 1452–1458. [CrossRef] [PubMed]

68. Luo, Y.; Wang, X.; Du, D.; Lin, Y. Hyaluronic acid-conjugated apoferritin nanocages for lung cancer targeted drug delivery. *Biomater. Sci.* **2015**, *3*, 1386–1394. [CrossRef] [PubMed]
69. Truffi, M.; Fiandra, L.; Sorrentino, L.; Monieri, M.; Corsi, F.; Mazzucchelli, S. Ferritin nanocages: A biological platform for drug delivery, imaging and theranostics in cancer. *Pharmacol. Res.* **2016**, *107*, 57–65. [CrossRef] [PubMed]
70. Li, L.; Muñoz-Culla, M.; Carmona, U.; Lopez, M.P.; Yang, F.; Trigueros, C.; Otaegui, D.; Zhang, L.; Knez, M. Ferritin-mediated siRNA delivery and gene silencing in human tumor and primary cells. *Biomaterials* **2016**, *98*, 143–151. [CrossRef] [PubMed]
71. Li, X.; Qiu, L.; Zhu, P.; Tao, X.; Imanaka, T.; Zhao, J.; Huang, Y.; Tu, Y.; Cao, X. Epidermal Growth Factor-Ferritin H-Chain Protein Nanoparticles for Tumor Active Targeting. *Small* **2012**, *8*, 2505–2514. [CrossRef] [PubMed]
72. Conti, L.; Lanzardo, S.; Ruiu, R.; Cadenazzi, M.; Cavallo, F.; Aime, S.; Crich, S.G. L-Ferritin targets breast cancer stem cells and delivers therapeutic and imaging agents. *Oncotarget* **2016**, *7*, 66713–66727. [CrossRef] [PubMed]
73. Alkhateeb, A.A.; Han, B.; Connor, J.R. Ferritin stimulates breast cancer cells through an iron-independent mechanism and is localized within tumor-associated macrophages. *Breast Cancer Res. Treat.* **2013**, *137*, 733–744. [CrossRef] [PubMed]
74. Uchida, M.; Flenniken, M.L.; Allen, M.; Willits, D.A.; Crowley, B.E.; Brumfield, S.; Willis, A.F.; Jackiw, L.; Jutila, M.; Young, M.J.; et al. Targeting of cancer cells with ferrimagnetic ferritin cage nanoparticles. *J. Am. Chem. Soc.* **2006**, *128*, 16626–16633. [CrossRef] [PubMed]
75. Chen, Z.; Zhai, M.; Xie, X.; Zhang, Y.; Ma, S.; Li, Z.; Yu, F.; Zhao, B.; Zhang, M.; Yang, Y.; et al. Apoferritin Nanocage for Brain Targeted Doxorubicin Delivery. *Mol. Pharm.* **2017**, *14*, 3087–3097. [CrossRef] [PubMed]
76. Wu, T.; Li, Y.; Liu, B.; Zhang, S.; Wu, L.; Zhu, X.; Chen, Q. Expression of Ferritin Light Chain (FTL) is Elevated in Glioblastoma, and FTL Silencing Inhibits Glioblastoma Cell Proliferation via the GADD45/JNK Pathway. *PLoS ONE* **2016**, *11*, e0149361. [CrossRef] [PubMed]
77. Kanekiyo, M.; Wei, C.J.; Yassine, H.M.; McTamney, P.M.; Boyington, J.C.; Whittle, J.R.R.; Rao, S.S.; Kong, W.P.; Wang, L.; Nabel, G.J. Self-assembling influenza nanoparticle vaccines elicit broadly neutralizing H1N1 antibodies. *Nature* **2013**, *499*, 102–106. [CrossRef] [PubMed]
78. Kanekiyo, M.; Bu, W.; Joyce, M.G.; Meng, G.; Whittle, J.R.R.; Baxa, U.; Yamamoto, T.; Narpala, S.; Todd, J.-P.; Rao, S.S.; et al. Rational Design of an Epstein-Barr Virus Vaccine Targeting the Receptor-Binding Site. *Cell* **2015**, *162*, 1090–1100. [CrossRef] [PubMed]
79. Han, J.-A.; Kang, Y.J.; Shin, C.; Ra, J.S.; Shin, H.H.; Hong, S.Y.; Do, Y.; Kang, S. Ferritin protein cage nanoparticles as versatile antigen delivery nanoplatforms for dendritic cell (DC)-based vaccine development. *Nanomedicine* **2014**, *10*, 561–569. [CrossRef] [PubMed]
80. Puttick, S.; Bell, C.; Dowson, N.; Rose, S.; Fay, M. PET, MRI, and simultaneous PET/MRI in the development of diagnostic and therapeutic strategies for glioma. *Drug Discov. Today* **2015**, *20*, 306–317. [CrossRef] [PubMed]
81. Dubois, J.; Dehaene-Lambertz, G.; Kulikova, S.; Poupon, C.; Hüppi, P.S.; Hertz-Pannier, L. The early development of brain white matter: A review of imaging studies in fetuses, newborns and infants. *Neuroscience* **2014**, *276*, 48–71. [CrossRef] [PubMed]
82. Benders, M.J.N.L.; Kersbergen, K.J.; de Vries, L.S. Neuroimaging of White Matter Injury, Intraventricular and Cerebellar Hemorrhage. *Clin. Perinatol.* **2014**, *41*, 69–82. [CrossRef] [PubMed]
83. Essig, M.; Shiroishi, M.S.; Nguyen, T.B.; Saake, M.; Provenzale, J.M.; Enterline, D.; Anzalone, N.; Dörfler, A.; Rovira, À.; Wintermark, M.; et al. Perfusion MRI: The Five Most Frequently Asked Technical Questions. *Am. J. Roentgenol.* **2013**, *200*, 24–34. [CrossRef] [PubMed]
84. Bhogal, P.; Uff, C.; Makalanda, H.L.D. Vessel wall MRI and intracranial aneurysms. *J. Neurointerv. Surg.* **2016**, *8*, 1160–1162. [CrossRef] [PubMed]
85. He, D.; Marles-Wright, J. Ferritin family proteins and their use in bionanotechnology. *New Biotechnol.* **2015**, *32*, 651–657. [CrossRef] [PubMed]
86. Cutrin, J.C.; Crich, S.G.; Burghelea, D.; Dastrù, W.; Aime, S. Curcumin/Gd Loaded Apoferritin: A Novel "Theranostic" Agent To Prevent Hepatocellular Damage in Toxic Induced Acute Hepatitis. *Mol. Pharm.* **2013**, *10*, 2079–2085. [CrossRef] [PubMed]

87. Geninatti Crich, S.; Cadenazzi, M.; Lanzardo, S.; Conti, L.; Ruiu, R.; Alberti, D.; Cavallo, F.; Cutrin, J.C.; Aime, S. Targeting ferritin receptors for the selective delivery of imaging and therapeutic agents to breast cancer cells. *Nanoscale* **2015**, *7*, 6527–6533. [CrossRef] [PubMed]
88. Sevcenco, A.-M.; Paravidino, M.; Vrouwenvelder, J.S.; Wolterbeek, H.T.; van Loosdrecht, M.C.M.; Hagen, W.R. Phosphate and arsenate removal efficiency by thermostable ferritin enzyme from Pyrococcus furiosus using radioisotopes. *Water Res.* **2015**, *76*, 181–186. [CrossRef] [PubMed]
89. Muckenthaler, M.U.; Galy, B.; Hentze, M.W. Systemic Iron Homeostasis and the Iron-Responsive Element/Iron-Regulatory Protein (IRE/IRP) Regulatory Network. *Annu. Rev. Nutr.* **2008**, *28*, 197–213. [CrossRef] [PubMed]
90. Kwak, E.L.; Larochelle, D.A.; Beaumont, C.; Torti, S.V.; Torti, F.M. Role for NF-κB in the Regulation of Ferritin H by Tumor Necrosis Factor-α. *J. Biol. Chem.* **1995**, *270*, 15285–15293. [CrossRef] [PubMed]
91. Peyssonnaux, C.; Zinkernagel, A.S.; Schuepbach, R.A.; Rankin, E.; Vaulont, S.; Haase, V.H.; Nizet, V.; Johnson, R.S. Regulation of iron homeostasis by the hypoxia-inducible transcription factors (HIFs). *J. Clin. Investig.* **2007**, *117*, 1926–1932. [CrossRef] [PubMed]
92. Hoesel, B.; Schmid, J.A. The complexity of NF-κB signaling in inflammation and cancer. *Mol. Cancer* **2013**, *12*, 86. [CrossRef] [PubMed]
93. Xue, Y.; Yun, D.; Esmon, A.; Zou, P.; Zuo, S.; Yu, Y.; He, F.; Yang, P.; Chen, X. Proteomic Dissection of Agonist-Specific TLR-Mediated Inflammatory Responses on Macrophages at Subcellular Resolution. *J. Proteome Res.* **2008**, *7*, 3180–3193. [CrossRef] [PubMed]
94. Miller, L.L.; Miller, S.C.; Torti, S.V.; Tsuji, Y.; Torti, F.M. Iron-independent induction of ferritin H chain by tumor necrosis factor. *Proc. Natl. Acad. Sci. USA* **1991**, *88*, 4946–4950. [CrossRef] [PubMed]
95. Lissoni, P.; Cazzaniga, M.; Ardizzoia, A.; Rossini, F.; Fiorelli, G.; Tancini, G.; Pittalis, S.; Barni, S. Cytokine regulation of iron metabolism: Effect of low-dose interleukin-2 subcutaneous therapy on ferritin, transferrin and iron blood concentrations in cancer patients. *J. Biol. Regul. Homeost. Agents* **1993**, *7*, 31–33. [PubMed]
96. Gray, C.P.; Franco, A.V.; Arosio, P.; Hersey, P. Immunosuppressive effects of melanoma-derived heavy-chain ferritin are dependent on stimulation of IL-10 production. *Int. J. Cancer* **2001**, *92*, 843–850. [CrossRef] [PubMed]
97. Dignass, A.; Farrag, K.; Stein, J. Limitations of Serum Ferritin in Diagnosing Iron Deficiency in Inflammatory Conditions. *Int. J. Chronic Dis.* **2018**, *2018*, 9394060. [CrossRef] [PubMed]
98. Ruscitti, P.; Cipriani, P.; Di Benedetto, P.; Liakouli, V.; Berardicurti, O.; Carubbi, F.; Ciccia, F.; Guggino, G.; Triolo, G.; Giacomelli, R. H-ferritin and proinflammatory cytokines are increased in the bone marrow of patients affected by macrophage activation syndrome. *Clin. Exp. Immunol.* **2018**, *191*, 220–228. [CrossRef] [PubMed]
99. Kell, D.B.; Pretorius, E. Serum ferritin is an important inflammatory disease marker, as it is mainly a leakage product from damaged cells. *Metallomics* **2014**, *6*, 748. [CrossRef] [PubMed]
100. Gomes, A.; Moreira, A.; Mesquita, G.; Gomes, M. Modulation of Iron Metabolism in Response to Infection: Twists for All Tastes. *Pharmaceuticals* **2018**, *11*, 84. [CrossRef] [PubMed]
101. Fan, Y.; Zhang, J.; Cai, L.; Wang, S.; Liu, C.; Zhang, Y.; You, L.; Fu, Y.; Shi, Z.; Yin, Z.; et al. The effect of anti-inflammatory properties of ferritin light chain on lipopolysaccharide-induced inflammatory response in murine macrophages. *Biochim. Biophys. Acta Mol. Cell Res.* **2014**, *1843*, 2775–2783. [CrossRef] [PubMed]
102. Parthasarathy, N.; Torti, S.V.; Torti, F.M. Ferritin binds to light chain of human H-kininogen and inhibits kallikrein-mediated bradykinin release. *Biochem. J.* **2002**, *365*, 279–286. [CrossRef] [PubMed]
103. Cohen-Solal, A.; Leclercq, C.; Deray, G.; Lasocki, S.; Zambrowski, J.J.; Mebazaa, A.; de Groote, P.; Damy, T.; Galinier, M. Iron deficiency: an emerging therapeutic target in heart failure. *Heart* **2014**, *100*, 1414–1420. [CrossRef] [PubMed]
104. Wang, W.; Knovich, M.A.; Coffman, L.G.; Torti, F.M.; Torti, S. V Serum ferritin: Past, present and future. *Biochim. Biophys. Acta* **2010**, *1800*, 760–769. [CrossRef] [PubMed]
105. Ueda, N.; Takasawa, K. Impact of Inflammation on Ferritin, Hepcidin and the Management of Iron Deficiency Anemia in Chronic Kidney Disease. *Nutrients* **2018**, *10*, 1173. [CrossRef] [PubMed]
106. Recalcati, S.; Invernizzi, P.; Arosio, P.; Cairo, G. New functions for an iron storage protein: The role of ferritin in immunity and autoimmunity. *J. Autoimmun.* **2008**, *30*, 84–89. [CrossRef] [PubMed]

107. Gozzelino, R.; Andrade, B.B.; Larsen, R.; Luz, N.F.; Vanoaica, L.; Seixas, E.; Coutinho, A.; Cardoso, S.; Rebelo, S.; Poli, M.; et al. Metabolic Adaptation to Tissue Iron Overload Confers Tolerance to Malaria. *Cell Host Microbe* **2012**, *12*, 693–704. [CrossRef] [PubMed]
108. Weis, S.; Carlos, A.R.; Moita, M.R.; Singh, S.; Blankenhaus, B.; Cardoso, S.; Larsen, R.; Rebelo, S.; Schäuble, S.; Del Barrio, L.; et al. Metabolic Adaptation Establishes Disease Tolerance to Sepsis. *Cell* **2017**, *169*, 1263–1275. [CrossRef] [PubMed]
109. Reddy, V.P.; Chinta, K.C.; Saini, V.; Glasgow, J.N.; Hull, T.D.; Traylor, A.; Rey-Stolle, F.; Soares, M.P.; Madansein, R.; Rahman, M.A.; et al. Ferritin H Deficiency in Myeloid Compartments Dysregulates Host Energy Metabolism and Increases Susceptibility to Mycobacterium tuberculosis Infection. *Front. Immunol.* **2018**, *9*, 860. [CrossRef] [PubMed]
110. Torti, S.V.; Torti, F.M. Human H-kininogen is a ferritin-binding protein. *J. Biol. Chem.* **1998**, *273*, 13630–13635. [CrossRef] [PubMed]
111. Kaplan, A.P. The Bradykinin-Forming Cascade: A Historical Perspective. In *Chemical Immunology and Allergy*; Karger: Basel, Switzerland, 2014; Volume 100, pp. 205–213.
112. Barnes, P.J. Bradykinin and asthma. *Thorax* **1992**, *47*, 979–983. [CrossRef] [PubMed]
113. Stadnicki, A. Intestinal tissue kallikrein-kinin system in inflammatory bowel disease. *Inflamm. Bowel Dis.* **2011**, *17*, 645–654. [CrossRef] [PubMed]
114. Sharma, J.N. Involvement of the kinin-forming system in the physiopathology of rheumatoid inflammation. *Agents Actions* **1992**, *38*, 343–361. [PubMed]
115. Sharma, J.N.; Buchanan, W.W. Pathogenic responses of bradykinin system in chronic inflammatory rheumatoid disease. *Exp. Toxicol. Pathol.* **1994**, *46*, 421–433. [CrossRef]
116. Cook, C.I.; Yu, B.P. Iron accumulation in aging: Modulation by dietary restriction. *Mech. Ageing Dev.* **1998**, *102*, 1–13. [CrossRef]
117. Hagemeier, J.; Geurts, J.J.; Zivadinov, R. Brain iron accumulation in aging and neurodegenerative disorders. *Expert Rev. Neurother.* **2012**, *12*, 1467–1480. [CrossRef] [PubMed]
118. Pirpamer, L.; Hofer, E.; Gesierich, B.; De Guio, F.; Freudenberger, P.; Seiler, S.; Duering, M.; Jouvent, E.; Duchesnay, E.; Dichgans, M.; et al. Determinants of iron accumulation in the normal aging brain. *Neurobiol. Aging* **2016**, *43*, 149–155. [CrossRef] [PubMed]
119. Connor, J.R.; Snyder, B.S.; Arosio, P.; Loeffler, D.A.; LeWitt, P. A Quantitative Analysis of Isoferritins in Select Regions of Aged, Parkinsonian, and Alzheimer's Diseased Brains. *J. Neurochem.* **1995**, *65*, 717–724. [CrossRef] [PubMed]
120. Fonseca-Nunes, A.; Jakszyn, P.; Agudo, A. Iron and Cancer Risk-A Systematic Review and Meta-analysis of the Epidemiological Evidence. *Cancer Epidemiol. Biomarkers Prev.* **2014**, *23*, 12–31. [CrossRef] [PubMed]
121. Alkhateeb, A.A.; Connor, J.R. The significance of ferritin in cancer: Anti-oxidation, inflammation and tumorigenesis. *Biochim. Biophys. Acta Rev. Cancer* **2013**, *1836*, 245–254. [CrossRef] [PubMed]
122. Alsina, D.; Purroy, R.; Ros, J.; Tamarit, J. Iron in Friedreich Ataxia: A Central Role in the Pathophysiology or an Epiphenomenon? *Pharmaceuticals* **2018**, *11*, 89. [CrossRef] [PubMed]
123. Levi, S.; Rovida, E. Neuroferritinopathy: From ferritin structure modification to pathogenetic mechanism. *Neurobiol. Dis.* **2015**, *81*, 134–143. [CrossRef] [PubMed]
124. Barbeito, A.G.; Levade, T.; Delisle, M.B.; Ghetti, B.; Vidal, R. Abnormal iron metabolism in fibroblasts from a patient with the neurodegenerative disease hereditary ferritinopathy. *Mol. Neurodegener.* **2010**, *5*, 50. [CrossRef] [PubMed]
125. Maccarinelli, F.; Pagani, A.; Cozzi, A.; Codazzi, F.; Di Giacomo, G.; Capoccia, S.; Rapino, S.; Finazzi, D.; Politi, L.S.; Cirulli, F.; et al. A novel neuroferritinopathy mouse model (FTL 498InsTC) shows progressive brain iron dysregulation, morphological signs of early neurodegeneration and motor coordination deficits. *Neurobiol. Dis.* **2015**, *81*, 119–133. [CrossRef] [PubMed]
126. Riederer, P.; Sofic, E.; Rausch, W.D.; Schmidt, B.; Reynolds, G.P.; Jellinger, K.; Youdim, M.B.H. Transition Metals, Ferritin, Glutathione, and Ascorbic Acid in Parkinsonian Brains. *J. Neurochem.* **1989**, *52*, 515–520. [CrossRef] [PubMed]
127. Dexter, D.T.; Carayon, A.; Vidailhet, M.; Ruberg, M.; Agid, F.; Agid, Y.; Lees, A.J.; Wells, F.R.; Jenner, P.; Marsden, C.D. Decreased Ferritin Levels in Brain in Parkinson's Disease. *J. Neurochem.* **1990**, *55*, 16–20. [CrossRef] [PubMed]

128. Thompson, K.; Menzies, S.; Muckenthaler, M.; Torti, F.M.; Wood, T.; Torti, S.V.; Hentze, M.W.; Beard, J.; Connor, J. Mouse brains deficient in H-ferritin have normal iron concentration but a protein profile of iron deficiency and increased evidence of oxidative stress. *J. Neurosci. Res.* **2003**, *71*, 46–63. [CrossRef] [PubMed]
129. Hemmati-Dinarvand, M.; Taher-Aghdam, A.A.; Mota, A.; Zununi Vahed, S.; Samadi, N. Dysregulation of serum NADPH oxidase1 and ferritin levels provides insights into diagnosis of Parkinson's disease. *Clin. Biochem.* **2017**, *50*, 1087–1092. [CrossRef] [PubMed]
130. Kozina, E.; Sadasivan, S.; Jiao, Y.; Dou, Y.; Ma, Z.; Tan, H.; Kodali, K.; Shaw, T.; Peng, J.; Smeyne, R.J. Mutant LRRK2 mediates peripheral and central immune responses leading to neurodegeneration in vivo. *Brain* **2018**, *141*, 1753–1769. [CrossRef] [PubMed]
131. Connor, J.R.; Patton, S.M.; Oexle, K.; Allen, R.P. Iron and restless legs syndrome: Treatment, genetics and pathophysiology. *Sleep Med.* **2017**, *31*, 61–70. [CrossRef] [PubMed]
132. Allen, R.P.; Auerbach, S.; Bahrain, H.; Auerbach, M.; Earley, C.J. The prevalence and impact of restless legs syndrome on patients with iron deficiency anemia. *Am. J. Hematol.* **2013**, *88*, 261–264. [CrossRef] [PubMed]
133. Akyol, A.; Kiylioglu, N.; Kadikoylu, G.; Bolaman, A.Z.; Ozgel, N. Iron deficiency anemia and restless legs syndrome: Is there an electrophysiological abnormality? *Clin. Neurol. Neurosurg.* **2003**, *106*, 23–27. [CrossRef] [PubMed]
134. Connor, J.R.; Ponnuru, P.; Wang, X.-S.; Patton, S.M.; Allen, R.P.; Earley, C.J.; Leader, G.M. Profile of altered brain iron acquisition in restless legs syndrome. *Brain* **2011**, *134*, 959–968. [CrossRef] [PubMed]
135. Connor, J.R.; Boyer, P.J.; Menzies, S.L.; Dellinger, B.; Allen, R.P.; Ondo, W.G.; Earley, C.J. Neuropathological examination suggests impaired brain iron acquisition in restless legs syndrome. *Neurology* **2003**, *61*, 304–309. [CrossRef] [PubMed]
136. Lammers, N.; Curry-Hyde, A.; Smith, A.J.; Eastwood, P.R.; Straker, L.M.; Champion, D.; McArdle, N. Are serum ferritin and transferrin saturation risk markers for restless legs syndrome in young adults? Longitudinal and cross-sectional data from the Western Australian Pregnancy Cohort (Raine) Study. *J. Sleep Res.* **2018**, e12741. [CrossRef] [PubMed]
137. Zheng, Y.; Gao, L.; Wang, D.; Zang, D. Elevated levels of ferritin in the cerebrospinal fluid of amyotrophic lateral sclerosis patients. *Acta Neurol. Scand.* **2017**, *136*, 145–150. [CrossRef] [PubMed]
138. Su, X.W.; Clardy, S.L.; Stephens, H.E.; Simmons, Z.; Connor, J.R. Serum ferritin is elevated in amyotrophic lateral sclerosis patients. *Amyotroph. Lateral Scler. Front. Degener.* **2015**, *16*, 102–107. [CrossRef] [PubMed]
139. Nadjar, Y.; Gordon, P.; Corcia, P.; Bensimon, G.; Pieroni, L.; Meininger, V.; Salachas, F. Elevated Serum Ferritin Is Associated with Reduced Survival in Amyotrophic Lateral Sclerosis. *PLoS ONE* **2012**, *7*, e45034. [CrossRef] [PubMed]
140. Yu, J.; Wang, N.; Qi, F.; Wang, X.; Zhu, Q.; Lu, Y.; Zhang, H.; Che, F.; Li, W. Serum ferritin is a candidate biomarker of disease aggravation in amyotrophic lateral sclerosis. *Biomed. Rep.* **2018**, *9*, 333–338. [CrossRef] [PubMed]
141. Hu, X.; Yang, Y.; Su, J.; Yao, C. Meta-analysis of the relationship between amyotrophic lateral sclerosis and susceptibility to serum ferritin level elevation. *Neurosciences* **2016**, *21*, 120–125. [CrossRef] [PubMed]
142. Li, W.; Garringer, H.J.; Goodwin, C.B.; Richine, B.; Acton, A.; VanDuyn, N.; Muhoberac, B.B.; Irimia-Dominguez, J.; Chan, R.J.; Peacock, M.; et al. Systemic and cerebral iron homeostasis in ferritin knock-out Mice. *PLoS ONE* **2015**, *10*, e0117435. [CrossRef] [PubMed]

3

Reductive Mobilization of Iron from Intact Ferritin: Mechanisms and Physiological Implication

Fadi Bou-Abdallah [1,*], John J. Paliakkara [1], Galina Melman [2] and Artem Melman [2,*]

1 Department of Chemistry, State University of New York at Potsdam, Potsdam, NY 13676, USA; paliakjj199@potsdam.edu

2 Department of Chemistry & Biomolecular Science, Clarkson University, Potsdam, NY 13699, USA gmelman@clarkson.edu

* Correspondence: bouabdf@potsdam.edu (F.B.-A.); amelman@clarkson.edu (A.M.);

Abstract: Ferritins are highly conserved supramolecular protein nanostructures composed of two different subunit types, H (heavy) and L (light). The two subunits co-assemble into a 24-subunit heteropolymer, with tissue specific distributions, to form shell-like protein structures within which thousands of iron atoms are stored as a soluble inorganic ferric iron core. In-vitro (or in cell free systems), the mechanisms of iron(II) oxidation and formation of the mineral core have been extensively investigated, although it is still unclear how iron is loaded into the protein in-vivo. In contrast, there is a wide spread belief that the major pathway of iron mobilization from ferritin involves a lysosomal proteolytic degradation of ferritin, and the dissolution of the iron mineral core. However, it is still unclear whether other auxiliary iron mobilization mechanisms, involving physiological reducing agents and/or cellular reductases, contribute to the release of iron from ferritin. In vitro iron mobilization from ferritin can be achieved using different reducing agents, capable of easily reducing the ferritin iron core, to produce soluble ferrous ions that are subsequently chelated by strong iron(II)-chelating agents. Here, we review our current understanding of iron mobilization from ferritin by various reducing agents, and report on recent results from our laboratory, in support of a mechanism that involves a one-electron transfer through the protein shell to the iron mineral core. The physiological significance of the iron reductive mobilization from ferritin by the non-enzymatic FMN/NAD(P)H system is also discussed.

Keywords: ferritin; iron mobilization; chaotropes; flavin nucleotide; electron transfer; kinetics

1. Introduction

Iron is an essential element required for virtually all living organisms and is involved in numerous biological reactions including respiration, oxygen transport, electron transfer, oxidative metabolism, deoxyribonucleotide synthesis, and gene regulation [1,2]. Due to the wide range of redox potentials of Fe^{3+}/Fe^{2+} metal complexes (from approximately −500 to +600 mV), iron cations are indispensable cofactors for numerous enzymes catalyzing oxidation–reduction reactions [3–5]. Almost all iron cations in living cells are tightly bound to metalloproteins, leaving less than one percent as "labile iron pool" in the cytosol. The pool contains "free" or loosely bound iron cations predominantly in the reduced Fe^{2+} form. The labile iron pool serves as the main source of iron for the synthesis of iron proteins. However, the presence of labile ferrous ions constitutes a considerable problem for all aerobic organisms, due to their involvement in Fenton reaction in the presence of hydrogen peroxide, an inevitable byproduct of cellular respiration. The resultant hydroxyl radicals react rapidly with cellular biopolymers, including proteins, lipids, and nucleic acids, resulting in their oxidation and loss of functionality. In living cells iron(III) cations produced via Fenton reaction can be rapidly reduced back to iron(II) cations, leading to a continuous cycle of hydroxyl radicals (HO•) production. To avoid this dangerous cycle of hydroxyl radicals formation, the concentration of labile iron is regulated by a strict control of the rates of iron uptake and mobilization in iron transport and storage proteins. While cellular iron trafficking is suggested to occur via iron chaperons [6], the reported affinity of such chaperones to iron cations is relatively low, suggesting an easy iron exchange mechanism with the labile iron pool.

The most efficient way to protect cells from the toxic effect of elevated levels of labile iron cations is ferritin, a ubiquitous and well-characterized iron storage and detoxification protein. A single ferritin molecule is capable of sequestering up to thousands of iron atoms, in the form of insoluble inorganic ferrihydrite core [7–10]. In bacteria, plants, fish, and amphibians, ferritins are generally homopolymers composed of H-type subunits, while in animals, ferritin is a heteropolymer, typically consisting of 24 subunits of two types, H and L (Figure 1) [10,11]. The resultant protein nanocage, separating the inner cavity of ferritin from the outside environment is remarkably stable in the pH range of 3–9, and temperatures up to 80 °C. Small molecules and various cations have been shown to enter the ferritin interior through eight narrow hydrophilic three-fold channels, and possibly through six hydrophobic four-fold channels as well [10]. The natural Fe^{2+} cations rapidly diffuse through the ferritin shell, where it is oxidized to insoluble iron(III) cations to form the inorganic ferrihydrite core. In mammals, the H-subunit is responsible for the rapid oxidation of Fe(II) to Fe(III) by molecular oxygen (or by hydrogen peroxide) at a dinuclear center, while the L-subunit helps iron clearance from the center in support of iron nucleation and mineralization [12–15]. Ferritin composed exclusively of L-subunits is still capable of oxidizing iron(II) cations, although at a much lower rate.

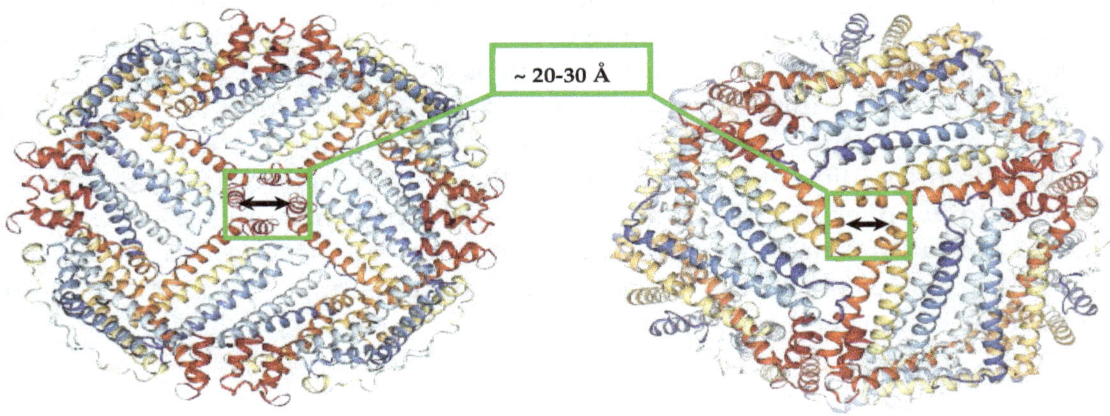

Figure 1. Ferritin molecule (PDB 1R03) with highlighted hydrophobic four-fold (**left**), and hydrophilic three-fold channels (**right**), that allow the transport of small molecules and ions to the inner cavity.

Bacteria can express at least four types of ferritin-like proteins with iron storage capability, two of which (FtnA and FtnB) are structurally similar to conventional ferritins, in term of subunit arrangement and the formation of nanocages (i.e., composed of 24 identical H-like subunits) [16]. The third type, bacterioferritin (Bfr), contains up to 12 protoporphyrin IX heme groups sandwiched between two-fold symmetry-related subunits, where they are bound covalently to methionine groups. The fourth ferritin type is called Dps (or DNA-binding protein from starved cells), contains 12 identical subunits, and thus has half the size of typical ferritins [17,18]. All ferritin types (except FtnB) possess rapid ferroxidase activity, and form ferrihydrite iron cores similar to conventional ferritins [19,20]. In bacteria, iron release from ferritin occurs through reduction of the inorganic iron core by bacterioferritin associated ferredoxin (Bfd) [19,20]. Transfer of electron from Bfd to the iron hydroxide core is mediated by bacterioferritin-bound heme molecules, most likely through electron transfer mechanisms [21]. However, very little is known about how the mechanisms of oxidative storage and reductive mobilization of iron are regulated in bacteria.

2. Brief Overview of Iron Reductive Mobilization from Intact Ferritin

While iron uptake and oxidation in conventional ferritin is relatively well understood, the mechanism of iron mobilization is rather controversial [22–26]. It is well established that the major pathway of iron mobilization from ferritin is based on proteolytic degradation, which involves transport of ferritin molecules into the lysosomes, followed by dissolution of the exposed iron hydroxide core [22,27,28]. The half-life of ferritin circulation in eukaryotic cells is about 19–24 h, under conditions of iron deficiency, but is much longer in iron-abundant environments [29], suggesting a tightly regulated cellular iron mobilization, although the exact mechanism remains unclear. We still do not know if proteolytic degradation of ferritin is the only mechanism by which iron is released from the protein, and whether other auxiliary iron mobilization mechanisms for the immediate access of cells to iron exist. Multiple reports on the reductive mobilization of iron cations from intact ferritin appeared in the literature, demonstrating the easy reduction of the iron core by a variety of one electron reducing agents, including flavin mononucleotide [30,31], ascorbate [32,33], sodium dithionite [34] and superoxide [35,36]. The rate of reduction is strongly dependent on the reduction potential of the electron donor [30]. In contrast, while two electron reductants, such as NADH [23] and glutathione [31], possess strongly negative reduction potentials, they generally reduce ferritin very slowly. One notable exception is thioglycolic acid [37], which reacts much more rapidly with the ferritin iron core, and is commonly used in the preparation of iron-free apoferritin. It has been shown that FtnA ferritin, from Pseudomonas aeruginosa, undergoes reductive mobilization of iron(III) by treatment with NADPH in the presence of ferredoxin-NADP$^+$ reductase and 2,2′-bipyridine; however, the physiological relevance of this process is not clear, even for anaerobic conditions [19,38].

The reduction of ferritin iron by these reducing agents, produces soluble Fe(II) cations that exit the ferritin internal cavity, through the eight hydrophilic three-fold channels, and join the cellular labile iron pool (Figure 2). The newly formed Fe(II) cations can be easily re-oxidized to Fe(III) , through the catalytic activity of the ferritin's ferroxidase centers. The rate of ferrous ions re-oxidation is very high [39,40], and their concentration is likely very low, and difficult to observe. This difficulty in detecting reduced iron(II) cations, can be resolved by the addition of iron(II) specific chelate ligands, such as 1,1′-bipyridine, phenanthroline, or ferrozine. The presence of excess chelators prevents the re-oxidation of iron(II) cations, and provides straightforward spectrophotometric detection of the resultant Fe(II)-chelate complexes, which typically have high (~10^3–10^4 $M^{-1}cm^{-1}$) absorbance metal-to-ligand-charge-transfer (MLCT) bands [41].

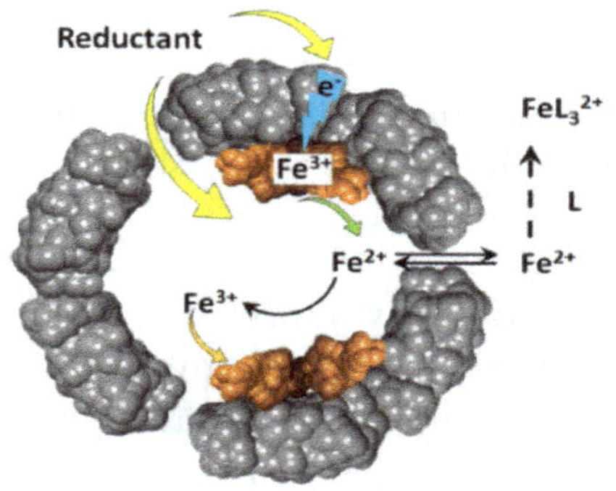

Figure 2. Schematic depiction of the oxidative deposition and reductive mobilization of iron in ferritin.

Amongst the most potent ferritin reducing agents in cell free systems are reduced flavins, including FMNH2 and FADH2 [31]. Reduced flavins can be prepared by chemical reduction of flavins, under oxygen-free conditions [31], or by in-situ reduction of NADH or NADPH. The latter reaction can be catalyzed by NAD(P)H:flavin oxidoreductase [30], or can proceed without enzymatic catalysis at higher concentrations of flavins and NADH [42]. Because a significant concentration (several mM) of flavins is commonly found in the cytosol of living cells, reduced flavins are possible candidates for the hypothetical reductive mobilization of iron cations from intact ferritins [30,31], although the physiological relevance of this mechanism is far from being obvious. Free reduced flavins, such as FMNH2 and FADH2, that are not protein-bound, are rapidly oxidized by molecular oxygen [43]. While FMN can be reduced back to FMNH2 by cellular NAD(P)H:flavin oxidoreductases [30], the rate constants for the re-oxidation of reduced flavins by molecular oxygen are very high [43], suggesting that the stationary concentrations of reduced flavins is extremely low. Unfortunately, there have been multiple studies on the reduction of ferritin iron by NADH without any consideration of the amount of dissolved oxygen present in solutions.

3. Iron Mobilization by the FMN-NADH System

To clarify the influence of each player on the reductive mobilization of iron from intact ferritins, we studied the kinetics of iron reduction by the FMN-NADH system, using horse spleen ferritin (HosF), and recombinant human heteropolymer apoferritin (~21H- and 3L-subunits, referred to as HuHLF), under a tight control of O_2 concentration [23]. In both cases (Figure 3), the iron release kinetics showed a biphasic behavior. The initial lag phase was followed by a second phase featuring a rapid iron release kinetic. The initial lag phase exhibited a small increase in absorption at 530 nm, indicating a slow iron release process. The second phase is characterized by a dramatic increase in the iron release rates, which depend on the concentrations of FMN and NADH, but not on the concentration of ferritin. The linear increase in the rates of iron mobilization suggests that the generation of FMNH2 by the FMN-NADH system, is the rate-limiting step under these conditions. Notably, the gradual decrease in the rates of iron mobilization from ferritin (as observed towards the end of the reactions in Figure 3 (right), is due to the depletion of the iron(III) hydroxide core, such as the reduction of the ferritin iron core becomes the rate limiting step [23].

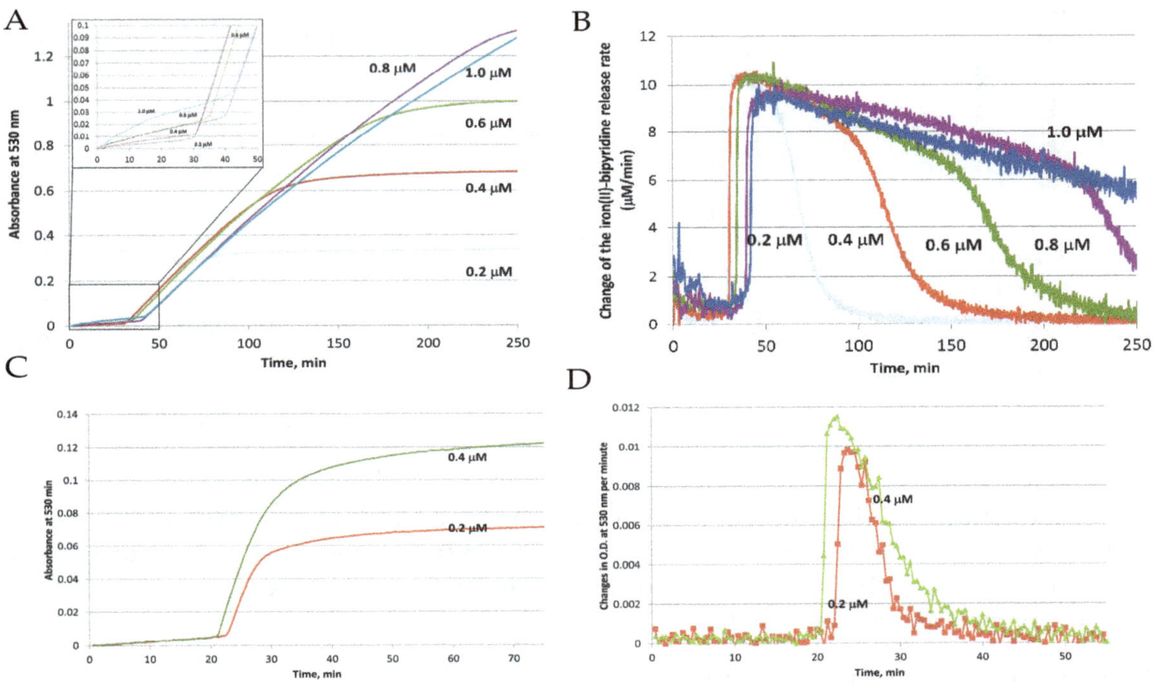

Figure 3. Reductive mobilization of iron from HosF containing 2250 Fe/shell. Conditions: 0.2–1 µM ferritin, 2 mM NADH, 200 µM FMN, 2 mM 2,2′-bipyridine, 2650 U/mL catalase, at pH 7.0 and 22 °C. (**A**) Absorbance change of $[Fe(bipy)_3]^{2+}$ as a function of time. (**B**) Change of the iron(II)–bipyridine release rate versus time for different concentrations of HosF. (**C**,**D**) Reductive mobilization of iron from human recombinant heteropolymer ferritin (0.2 and 0.4 µM) loaded with 500 Fe/protein, in the presence of 2 mM NADH, 200 µM FMN, 2 mM 2,2′-bipyridine, 2650 U/mL catalase, at pH 7.0 and 28 °C. (**C**) Absorbance change of $[Fe(bipy)_3]^{2+}$ as a function of time. (**D**) Change of the iron(II)–bipyridine release rate versus time, for different concentrations of heteropolymer ferritin. Reprinted with permission from Ref. [23].

The significant release of iron from ferritin does not occur until essentially all the dissolved oxygen has been depleted, as observed in Figure 3 (left). The duration of the lag phase depends on the concentration of dissolved oxygen, as well as the concentrations of NADH and FMN, but not on the concentration of ferritin. This indicates that most of the FMNH2, produced from the reaction between FMN and NADH, is re-oxidized back to FMN by dissolved molecular oxygen, without an appreciable release of iron. This re-oxidation reaction is very fast, even at a low concentration of dissolved oxygen, which can be expected, since the rate of FMNH2 oxidation by oxygen is much faster than that of iron reduction [43].

To further determine the effect of oxygen on the amount and rate of iron release from ferritin, the experiments were repeated, while simultaneously monitoring the concentration of molecular oxygen by a MI 730 Clark oxygen microelectrode [23]. As shown in Figure 4, the concentration of dissolved oxygen decreases sharply during the induction period (lag period), without any noticeable iron release. Only when oxygen concentration reaches a level of ~5 μM, that iron reduction and chelation by bipyridine is observed [23]. Because oxygen concentration in this experiment is well below typical normoxic conditions, the results presented in Figure 4 suggest that free reduced flavins are unlikely to serve as ferritin-reducing agents, in normally oxygenated cells. Significantly, under these conditions, the rates of iron mobilization from ferritin would be too low, even in the absence of inevitable re-oxidation of newly formed iron(II) cations. It is also highly improbable that the rates of iron mobilization are strongly dependent on cells oxygenation level, which is known to vary widely under different circumstances.

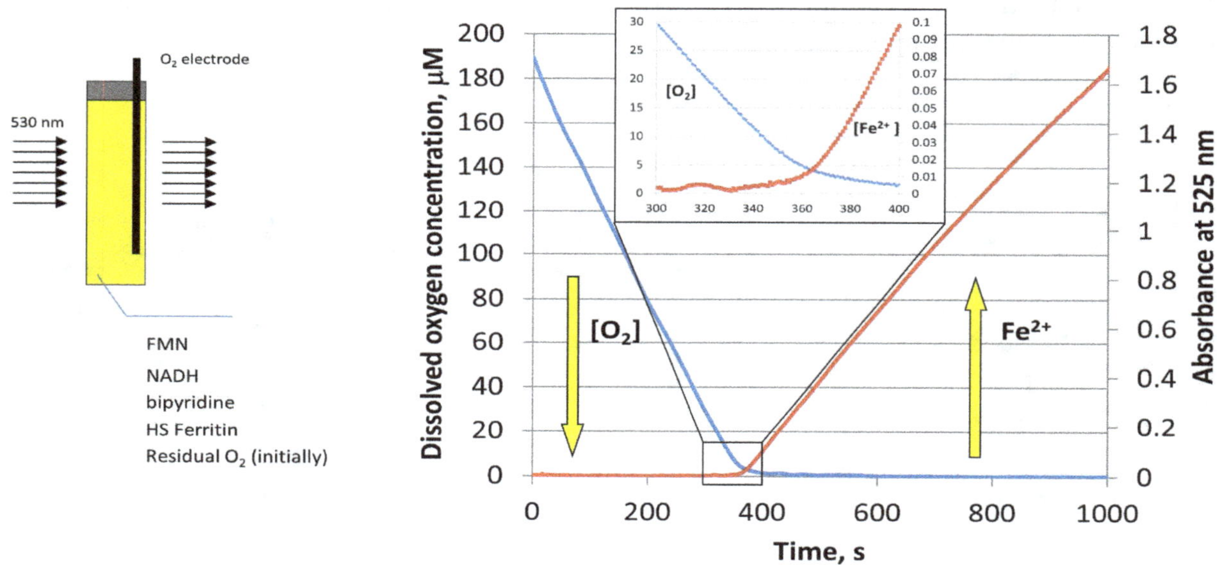

Figure 4. Schematic of the simultaneous monitoring of the dissolved oxygen concentration (blue curve), and light absorption of Fe(II)–bipyridine complex at 530 nm (red curve), during the reductive release of iron from HosF (0.6 μM), in the presence of 2 mM NADH, 2 mM FMN, and 2 mM 2,2′-bipyridine. Reprinted with permission from Ref. [23].

4. Iron Mobilization by Reduced Flavins

Reduction of ferritin iron cores by reduced flavins (and other reductants) has been the subject of intense investigation [23,25,26,30,31,44–46]. Iron reduction can proceed through two possible mechanisms that involve either a passive diffusion of reducing agents across the ferritin's shell [30], or the transfer of electrons through specific pathways along the protein shell [46] (Figure 5). Literature evidence in support of the diffusion mechanism is based on two experiments, the first of which employed agarose-bound FMNH2, produced by a reaction of agarose-bound FMN with NADH [30]. The inability of agarose-immobilized FMNH2 to induce reductive mobilization of iron cations from horse spleen ferritin [31], was considered as proof of the inability of FMNH2 to diffuse to the protein's interior, and that ferritin iron reduction reactions can only proceed through FMNH2 diffusion into ferritin. The problem with this experiment is that it failed to account for possible changes in the reactivity of reduced flavins caused by agarose binding. Alternatively, derivatization of agarose by FMN may occur at the surface of the agarose grains, but also inside the agarose beads, which may not be available for ferritin diffusion and subsequent iron reduction [31].

The second piece of evidence is the observation of increased rates of iron reductive mobilization in the presence of chaotropes, or specific peptide molecules in solution [42,47,48]. It was shown that the presence of 1 M urea resulted in a dramatic (more than five-fold) increase in the rates of iron reduction in ferritin, by the FMN-NADH system, in the presence of 2,2′-bipyridine [42]. The data were interpreted as a weakening of the ferritin inter-subunits interactions, which resulted in an enlarged diameter of the three-fold or four-fold axes, thus facilitating the diffusion of FMNH2 molecules into the ferritin interior. Furthermore, certain short peptide sequences (i.e., HSNTYYFPKGG) were shown to exhibit more than three-fold increased iron release rates from ferritin [48]. These later results, however, cannot be easily interpreted, given that the rates of iron reduction in ferritin by the non-enzymatic FMN-NADH system are limited by the rate of FMNH2 production [23], and not by the rate of iron reduction. Additionally, these experiments did not disclose the initial amount of dissolved oxygen in solution, or the possibility of oxygen diffusion inside the reaction cell, which, as reported above, dramatically alters the amount, and rates of iron release from ferritin.

Evidence for electron transfer reactions across the protein shell are based on the rapid oxidation of iron(II) cations inside the ferritin cavity, under anaerobic conditions, by large electron acceptors, such as plastocyanin, cytochrome c, or stellavyanin [26,46,49]. Because of the large size of these proteins, and their inability to diffuse across the protein shell, iron oxidation reactions can only be explained by electron transfer, from iron(II) cations to these electron acceptors. In further support of this mechanism, iron oxidation and deposition reactions were also observed in L-subunit ferritins, which lack ferroxidase centers, and therefore ferroxidase activity [49]. Such a long range electron transport across the 2 nm protein shell, can be facilitated by the redox activity of the protein shell [46].

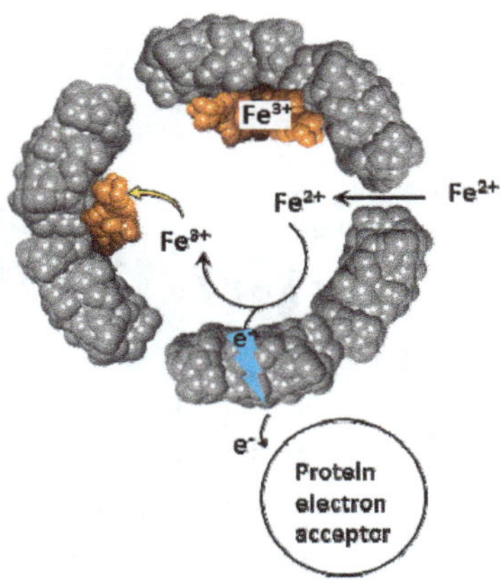

Figure 5. Schematic of Fe^{2+} cations diffusion and electron transfer across the ferritin shell, followed by Fe^{2+} oxidation and deposition.

To further understand the iron reductive mobilization from ferritin, and differentiate between the two mechanisms (diffusion vs. electron transfer), more data is needed, using different types of ferritin (i.e., heteropolymer horse spleen ferritin (HosF), homopolymer human H-chain or L-chain ferritin (HuHF or HuLF), and heteropolymer human H/L ferritin (HuHLF)). Recent experiments from our laboratory [25], using the FMN-NADH system (or reduced flavin FMNH2), were performed with HosF and HuHF, under controlled concentration of oxygen. In contrast to literature reports, our data showed no (or insignificant) difference in the reaction rates, in the presence of 0–2 M urea, guanidine chloride, or Triton X100 (Figure 6), suggesting that the kinetics of iron release from ferritin by flavins are independent on the type, or amount of chaotropes present. Additional experiments performed under strict anaerobic conditions, using solutions of $FMNH_2$ prepared by catalytic hydrogenation with Adams catalyst, revealed much faster reduction reactions, with no effect from chaotropes on the rates of the iron mobilization reactions [25].

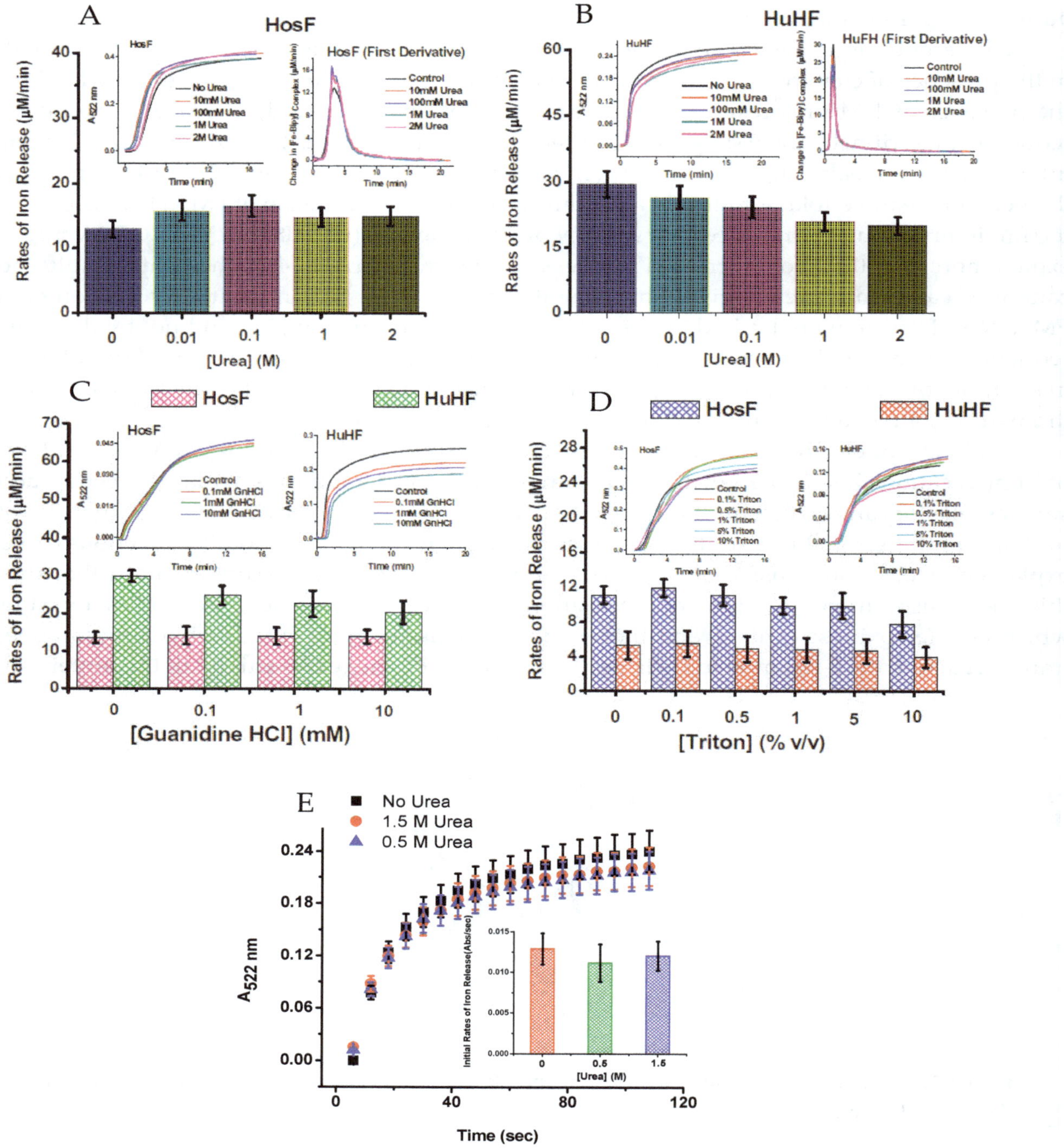

Figure 6. Rates of iron release from HosF and HuHF by the FMN-NADH system (**A–D**), and by $FMNH_2$ (**E**), in the absence or presence of different concentrations of chaotropes. In both experiments, the presence of urea does not affect the rates of iron mobilization. Reprinted with permission from Ref. [25].

The above results suggest that the earlier studies may have been inaccurately interpreted, and that the diffusion mechanism should be revisited. If FMNH2 is able to diffuse into the ferritin interior and reduce the iron(III) hydroxide core, then the produced FMN should be able to diffuse out of ferritin. Notably, the diffusion of various molecules of similar size to FMN, including cisplatin [50], curcumin [51], or anthocyanin [52] is known to be extremely slow, suggesting that diffusion of FMNH2 is unlikely to be responsible for the observed fast rates of iron reduction. To further explore the origin of these discrepancies, we carried out an experiment to unambiguously demonstrate that, neither FMN, nor FMNH2, both of which possess virtually identical steric size, can diffuse through the ferritin shell [25]. All of the aforementioned molecules, including FMN, can be trapped inside the inner cavity of ferritin, by first denaturing the protein down to its individual subunits at pH 2, followed by their re-assembly at neutral pH, and dialysis [50–53]. The resulting ferritin-FMN entrapped molecules, were found to be stable for days, without any sign of diffusing out. These results clearly indicate that the ferritin channels are too small for FMN (or FMNH2) diffusion, implying that electron transfer is most likely the pathway by which ferritin iron core is reduced by flavins. Given the thickness of the protein shell (~2 nm), it is reasonable to assume that these electron transfer processes are not arbitrary, but rather a conserved evolutionary feature of ferritin, accompanied by specific protein structural arrangements. Interestingly, recent reports demonstrated the importance of electron transfer reactions, carried by three aromatic residues surrounding the diiron center of *E. coli* bacterial ferritin in the formation of the iron mineral core [54,55].

We propose that these electron transfer pathways might be physiologically important processes for iron reductive mobilization from ferritin. However, as discussed above, FMNH2 is an unlikely electron donor candidate in cells. Protein-bound reduced flavins are more stable complexes in the presence of oxygen, and could serve as potential reducing agents, similarly to the ferredoxin-bacterioferritin complex [19,21], but this is purely speculative at the moment and requires further investigation. Some exogenous one-electron reducing agents, with less negative reduction potential than FMNH2, were reported to reduce ferritin iron cores in the presence of oxygen [56]; however, these measurements were conducted without the continuous monitoring of oxygen concentration in solution, and require further clarification.

5. Iron Mobilization by Other Reducing Agents

It has been reported that ascorbate and glutathione are capable of mobilizing iron(II) cations from ferritin [31]. While the rates of iron reduction were substantially lower than with reduced flavins, the high intracellular concentration (several mM) of the reduced forms of ascorbate and glutathione, could be sufficient for significant mobilization of iron from cellular ferritin, under physiological conditions. Surprisingly, under anaerobic conditions, iron core reduction by ascorbate and glutathione in horse spleen ferritin comes to a complete stop only after ~17–18% of the total iron has been reduced, in direct contrast with reduced flavins and dithionite, where complete iron mobilization was observed. The sudden halt of iron mobilization cannot be the result of a thermodynamic equilibrium, since the reduction potential of both ascorbate and glutathione is much more negative than that of iron(III). Damaged horse spleen ferritin molecules that cannot protect the inorganic iron core from reducing agents, is one possible explanation for this partial iron mobilization. If this were true, then iron(III) cations in undamaged ferritin can NOT be reduced by ascorbate and glutathione under anaerobic conditions, at least in the absence of other agents. In that regard, it is interesting to compare the iron reducing ability of glutathione, with that of thiolactic acid, which is known to induce complete iron mobilization from ferritin. This clear difference in outcome can be rationalized by the small size of thiolactate molecules, and their ability to easily diffuse through ferritin channels, in contrast to glutathione. Under anaerobic conditions, iron mobilization from ferritin by ascorbate is extremely slow, but the presence of oxygen, iron, or copper cations causes a dramatic increase in the rates of iron reduction [57,58]. This effect can be ascribed to the formation of different redox species, most likely free radical species [59].

Superoxide anion radicals were also reported to induce reductive mobilization of iron from ferritin [35,36]. Because superoxide anions are continuously produced by mitochondria, as a byproduct of oxidative phosphorylation, its tiny size would allow its fast diffusion into the ferritin interior, and the subsequent reduction of the inorganic iron core. However, the physiological importance of this process is questionable, since the stationary concentration of superoxide anions is very low (10^{-10} M), due to the presence of cellular superoxide dismutases [60].

Other compounds reported to induce reductive mobilization of iron from ferritin, include polyphenols [61,62], which are abundant in certain foods. While too large to diffuse inside ferritin, they have the ability to donate one electron, and thus reduce the iron core through electron transfer, but more studies are needed to confirm these electron transfer reactions. The challenges of these studies is that these reactions are often accompanied by the auto-oxidation of polyphenol compounds at neutral pH, giving rise to colored products that absorb light at the same wavelength as iron(II)-(bipy)$_3$ complexes, and other commonly used Fe(II)-complexes [63].

6. Iron Mobilization by Specific Iron(III) Chelating Agents

Iron is a typical "hard" metal capable of binding to a variety of "hard" chelate ligands, including catechols, carboxylates, phosphates, and hydroxamates. Several endogenous chelate ligands of that type, that exist in millimolar concentration in cells, include citrate and ATP [64]. Several other chelate ligands (i.e., DFO, DFX, and BHT; Figure 7), with very high affinity to iron(III) cations have been developed for the treatment of iron overload diseases, such as beta-thalassemia [1,65]. While citrate or EDTA are unable to significantly mobilize iron from ferritin, simple hydroxamates, such as acetyl- or benzoylhydroxamic acid (Figure 7), are able of slowly mobilizing iron from ferritin, presumably because their small size allow them to diffuse across the ferritin shell, and remove iron cations [66].

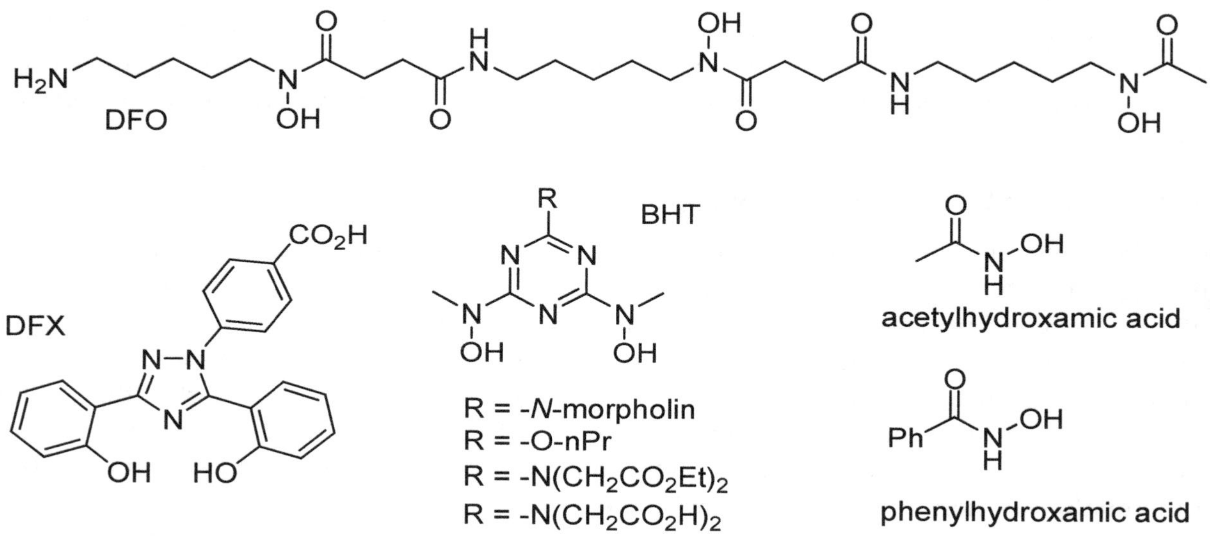

Figure 7. Structures of specific iron(III) chelators.

Surprisingly, relatively high rates of iron(III) mobilization were observed with large molecules, such as DFO and BHT [24]. These molecules, and their respective 1:1 or 2:1 iron(III) complexes, have molecular sizes too large to diffuse through ferritin channels. The mechanism and the iron release kinetics by these molecules are rather complicated, and strongly depend on the concentration of dissolved oxygen, and the presence of antioxidants, such as mannitol, urea, and superoxide dismutase [24]. Nonetheless, we have proposed a plausible mechanism that is mediated by superoxide anion radicals, which can readily diffuse into the ferritin interior to reduce the iron core, allowing the reduced and soluble iron(II) cations to exit out of ferritin, and be chelated by DFO or BHT ligands [24]. Because of the highly negative reduction potential of the Fe(II)-DFO, and the Fe(II)-BHT complexes (below −0.4 V vs. hydrogen electrode), they act as powerful electron donors capable of reducing dissolved molecular oxygen, thus replenishing superoxide anions (Figure 8). This theoretical cyclic process requires only a catalytic amount of superoxide anions, since they are regenerated after oxidation of the released iron(II) cations to iron(III). However, superoxide anions are unstable species, and can undergo disproportionation. One possible source for the regeneration of superoxide anions is iron(II) hydroxides, embedded within the iron(III) hydroxide core forming a magnetite phase [67]. Reduction of magnetite by one superoxide anion can produce two iron(II) cations, instead of one iron(II) cation in the case of a ferrihydrite phase (composed of only iron(III) hydroxides), thus continuously "breeding" superoxide anions.

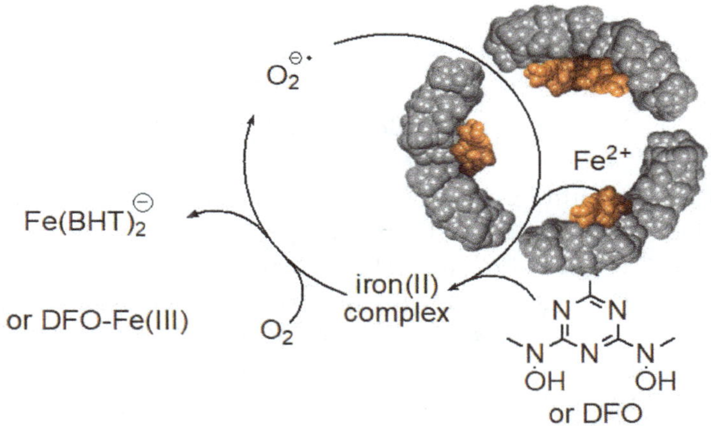

Figure 8. Superoxide mediated mobilization of iron(III) cations from the ferritin iron core by BHT (or DFO) chelators.

This unusual iron reduction mechanism is highly specific for exogenous chelators, possessing very high affinity to iron(III) cations, and is unlikely to be physiologically relevant for cells not exposed to these ligands. Endogenous iron(III) specific ligands with strong affinity for iron(III) (i.e., at least equal to that of pyrophosphate with a log $\beta = 22.2$), including nucleic acids [68] and nucleotide triphosphates, should be considered, although their ability to reach the inner cavity of ferritin is unknown. Smaller ions having lower affinity to iron(III) cations, such as phosphate, lactate, glutamate, or citrate may represent a better option that could assist with the dissolution of the inorganic iron core, similarly to that observed with acetohydroxamate [66]. In this latter case, iron(III) cations, complexed with these small chelates, are released from the interior cavity of ferritin, which upon exiting the ferritin shell encounter the stronger chelate agents (i.e., nucleotide triphosphate), followed by complexation and reduction to iron(II). Such process could constitute a futile cycle for the release of small amounts of iron cations, to help maintain the labile iron pool, under conditions that do not require large spikes in iron protein synthesis.

7. Conclusions and Perspective

Under anaerobic conditions, the reductive mobilization of iron from ferritin, in cell free systems, proceeds via electron transfer reactions across the protein shell. This process is likely to be physiologically relevant in anaerobic bacteria, where ferredoxin serves as the electron source, but its relevance under aerobic conditions is unknown. Reduced flavins are one-electron reducing agents that react much more rapidly with molecular oxygen than with the ferritin iron core, and are unlikely relevant iron reducing agents in oxygenated cells. Although some phenazine derivatives have been described as more efficient electron transfer mediators that facilitate the mobilization of iron from ferritin, even in the presence of dissolved oxygen [68], the exact mechanism of this electron mediation process is unclear. Additionally, the efficiency of these mediators in the presence of different concentration of molecular oxygen, and the relevance of this mechanism in vivo, remains to be determined. Nonetheless, this potential chemoselectivity for ferritin iron core reduction vs. oxygen reduction, is an attractive possibility that could support an auxiliary iron mobilization mechanism, in addition to ferritin proteolytic degradation. Other endogenous compounds including oxidoreductases are also worth exploring as potential ferritin-reducing agents.

Author Contributions: Conceptualization, F.B.-A. and A.M.; Methodology, F.B.-A. and A.M.; Software, F.B.-A., A.M., J.J.P. and G.M.; Validation, F.B.-A., A.M., J.J.P. and G.M.; Formal Analysis, F.B.-A., A.M., J.J.P. and G.M.; Investigation, F.B.-A., A.M., J.J.P. and G.M.; Resources, F.B.-A. and A.M.; Data Curation, F.B.-A., A.M., J.J.P. and G.M.; Writing-Original Draft Preparation, F.B.-A. and A.M.; Writing-Review & Editing, F.B.-A., A.M., J.J.P. and G.M.; Visualization, F.B.-A., A.M., J.J.P. and G.M.; Supervision, F.B.-A. and A.M.; Project Administration, F.B.-A. and A.M.; Funding Acquisition, F.B.-A. and A.M.

References

1. Britton, R.S.; Leicester, K.L.; Bacon, B.R. Iron toxicity and chelation therapy. *Int. J. Hematol.* **2002**, *76*, 219–228. [CrossRef] [PubMed]
2. Theil, E.C.; Goss, D.J. Living with Iron (and Oxygen): Questions and Answers about Iron Homeostasis. *Chem. Rev.* **2009**, *109*, 4568–4579. [CrossRef] [PubMed]
3. Cammack, R. Iron-Sulfur Clusters in Enzymes-Themes and Variations. *Adv. Inorg. Chem.* **1992**, *38*, 281–322.
4. Shaik, S.; Hirao, H.; Kumar, D. Reactivity of high-valent iron-oxo species in enzymes and synthetic reagents: A tale of many states. *Acc. Chem. Res.* **2007**, *40*, 532–542. [CrossRef] [PubMed]
5. Bruijnincx, P.C.A.; van Koten, G.; Gebbink, R. Mononuclear non-heme iron enzymes with the 2-His-1-carboxylate facial triad: Recent developments in enzymology and modeling studies. *Chem. Soc. Rev.* **2008**, *37*, 2716–2744. [CrossRef] [PubMed]
6. Shi, H.F.; Bencze, K.Z.; Stemmler, T.L.; Philpott, C.C. A cytosolic iron chaperone that delivers iron to ferritin. *Science* **2008**, *320*, 1207–1210. [CrossRef] [PubMed]
7. Bou-Abdallah, F. The iron redox and hydrolysis chemistry of the ferritins. *BBA-Gen. Subj.* **2010**, *1800*, 719–731. [CrossRef] [PubMed]
8. Harrison, P.M.; Arosio, P. The ferritins: Molecular properties, iron storage function and cellular regulation. *BBA-Bioenerg.* **1996**, *1275*, 161–203. [CrossRef]
9. Chasteen, N.D. Ferritin. Uptake, storage, and release of iron. *Met. Ions Biol. Syst.* **1998**, *35*, 479–514. [PubMed]
10. Arosio, P.; Ingrassia, R.; Cavadini, P. Ferritins: A family of molecules for iron storage, antioxidation and more. *BBA-Gen. Subj.* **2009**, *1790*, 589–599. [CrossRef] [PubMed]
11. Mehlenbacher, M.; Poli, M.; Arosio, P.; Santambrogio, P.; Levi, S.; Chasteen, N.D.; Bou-Abdallah, F. Iron oxidation and core formation in recombinant heteropolymeric human ferritins. *Biochemistry* **2017**, *56*, 3900–3912. [CrossRef] [PubMed]
12. Zhao, G.; Bou-Abdallah, F.; Arosio, P.; Levi, S.; Janus-Chandler, C.; Chasteen, N.D. Multiple pathways for mineral core formation in mammalian apoferritin. The role of hydrogen peroxide. *Biochemistry* **2003**, *42*, 3142–3150. [CrossRef] [PubMed]
13. Bou-Abdallah, F.; Yang, H.; Awomolo, A.; Cooper, B.; Woodhall, M.R.; Andrews, S.C.; Chasteen, N.D. Functionality of the three-site ferroxidase center of *Escherichia coli* bacterial ferritin (EcFtnA). *Biochemistry* **2014**, *53*, 483–495. [CrossRef] [PubMed]
14. Bou-Abdallah, F.; Zhao, G.; Biasiotto, G.; Poli, M.; Arosio, P.; Chasteen, N.D. Facilitated diffusion of iron(II) and dioxygen substrates into human H-chain ferritin. A fluorescence and absorbance study employing the ferroxidase center substitution Y34W. *J. Am. Chem. Soc.* **2008**, *130*, 17801–17811. [CrossRef] [PubMed]
15. Theil, E.C. Ferritin: The protein nanocage and iron biomineral in health and in disease. *Inorg. Chem.* **2013**, *52*, 12223–12233. [CrossRef] [PubMed]
16. Honarmand Ebrahimi, K.; Hagedoorn, P.-L.; Hagen, W.R. Unity in the *Biochemistry* of the iron-storage proteins ferritin and bacterioferritin. *Chem. Rev.* **2014**, *115*, 295–326. [CrossRef] [PubMed]
17. Haikarainen, T.; Papageorgiou, A.C. Dps-like proteins: Structural and functional insights into a versatile protein family. *Cell. Mol. Life Sci.* **2010**, *67*, 341–351. [CrossRef] [PubMed]
18. Zeth, K. Dps biomineralizing proteins: Multifunctional architects of nature. *Biochem. J.* **2012**, *445*, 297–311. [CrossRef] [PubMed]
19. Rivera, M. Bacterioferritin: Structure, Dynamics, and Protein-Protein Interactions at Play in Iron Storage and Mobilization. *Acc. Chem. Res.* **2017** *50*, 331–340. [CrossRef] [PubMed]
20. Eshelman, K.; Yao, H.; Hewage, A.N.D. P.; Deay, J.J.; Chandler, J.R.; Rivera, M. Inhibiting the BfrB: Bfd interaction in Pseudomonas aeruginosa causes irreversible iron accumulation in bacterioferritin and iron deficiency in the bacterial cytosol. *Metallomics* **2017** *9*, 646–659. [CrossRef] [PubMed]

21. Weeratunga, S.K.; Gee, C.E.; Lovell, S.; Zeng, Y.; Woodin, C.L.; Rivera, M. Binding of Pseudomonas aeruginosa apobacterioferritin-associated ferredoxin to bacterioferritin B promotes heme mediation of electron delivery and mobilization of core mineral iron. *Biochemistry* **2009**, *48*, 7420–7431. [CrossRef] [PubMed]
22. Linder, M.C. Mobilization of stored iron in mammals: A review. *Nutrients* **2013**, *5*, 4022–4050. [CrossRef] [PubMed]
23. Melman, G.; Bou-Abdallah, F.; Vane, E.; Maura, P.; Arosio, P.; Melman, A. Iron release from ferritin by flavin nucleotides. *BBA-Gen. Subj.* **2013**, *1830*, 4669–4674. [CrossRef] [PubMed]
24. Bou-Abdallah, F.; McNally, J.; Liu, X.X.; Melman, A. Oxygen catalyzed mobilization of iron from ferritin by iron(III) chelate ligands. *Chem. Commun.* **2011**, *47*, 731–733. [CrossRef] [PubMed]
25. Johnson, L.E.; Wilkinson, T.; Arosio, P.; Melman, A.; Bou-Abdallah, F. Effect of chaotropes on the kinetics of iron release from ferritin by flavin nucleotides. *BBA-Gen. Subj.* **2017**, *1861*, 3257–3262. [CrossRef] [PubMed]
26. Watt, R.K.; Hilton, R.J.; Graff, D.M. Oxido-reduction is not the only mechanism allowing ions to traverse the ferritin protein shell. *BBA-Gen. Subj.* **2010**, *1800*, 745–759. [CrossRef] [PubMed]
27. Kidane, T.Z.; Sauble, E.; Linder, M.C. Release of iron from ferritin requires lysosomal activity. *Am. J. Physiol. Cell Physiol.* **2006**, *291*, C445–C455. [CrossRef] [PubMed]
28. La, A.; Nguyen, T.; Tran, K.; Sauble, E.; Tu, D.; Gonzalez, A.; Kidane, T.Z.; Soriano, C.; Morgan, J.; Doan, M. Mobilization of iron from ferritin: New steps and details. *Metallomics* **2018**, *10*, 154–168. [CrossRef] [PubMed]
29. Truty, J.; Malpe, R.; Linder, M.C. Iron prevents ferritin turnover in hepatic cells. *J. Biol. Chem.* **2001**, *276*, 48775–48780. [CrossRef] [PubMed]
30. Jones, T.; Spencer, R.; Walsh, C. Mechanism and kinetics of iron release from ferritin by dihydroflavins and dihydroflavin analogs. *Biochemistry* **1978**, *17*, 4011–4017. [CrossRef] [PubMed]
31. Sirivech, S.; Frieden, E.; Osaki, S. The release of iron from horse spleen ferritin by reduced flavins. *Biochem. J.* **1974**, *143*, 311–315. [CrossRef] [PubMed]
32. Boyer, R.F.; Grabill, T.W.; Petrovich, R.M. Reductive release of ferritin iron: A kinetic assay. *Anal. Biochem.* **1988**, *174*, 17–22. [CrossRef]
33. Sakurai, K.; Nabeyama, A.; Fujimoto, Y. Ascorbate-mediated iron release from ferritin in the presence of alloxan. *Biometals* **2006**, *19*, 323–333. [CrossRef] [PubMed]
34. Funk, F.; Lenders, J.P.; Crichton, R.R.; Schneider, W. Reductive mobilisation of ferritin iron. *FEBS J.* **1985**, *152*, 167–172. [CrossRef]
35. Bolann, B.J.; Ulvik, R.J. Release of iron from ferritin by xanthine oxidase. Role of the superoxide radical. *Biochem. J.* **1987**, *243*, 55–59. [CrossRef] [PubMed]
36. Monteiro, H.P.; Winterbourn, C.C. The superoxide-dependent transfer of iron from ferritin to transferrin and lactoferrin. *Biochem. J.* **1988**, *256*, 923–928. [CrossRef] [PubMed]
37. Joo, M.S.; Tourillon, G.; Sayers, D.E.; Theil, E.C. Rapid reduction of iron in horse spleen ferritin by thioglycolic acid measured by dispersive X-ray absorption spectroscopy. *Biol. Met.* **1990**, *3*, 171–175. [CrossRef] [PubMed]
38. Yao, H.; Jepkorir, G.; Lovell, S.; Nama, P.V.; Weeratunga, S.; Battaile, K.P.; Rivera, M. Two Distinct Ferritin-like Molecules in Pseudomonas aeruginosa: The Product of the bfrA Gene Is a Bacterial Ferritin (FtnA) and Not a Bacterioferritin (Bfr). *Biochemistry* **2011**, *50*, 5236–5248. [CrossRef] [PubMed]
39. Orino, K.; Kamura, S.; Natsuhori, M.; Yamamoto, S.; Watanabe, K. Two pathways of iron uptake in bovine spleen apoferritin dependent on iron concentration. *Biometals* **2002**, *15*, 59–63. [CrossRef] [PubMed]
40. Sun, S.; Arosio, P.; Levi, S.; Chasteen, N.D. Ferroxidase kinetics of human liver apoferritin, recombinant H-chain apoferritin, and site-directed mutants. *Biochemistry* **1993**, *32*, 9362–9369. [CrossRef] [PubMed]
41. Haas, K.L.; Franz, K.J. Application of metal coordination chemistry to explore and manipulate cell biology. *Chem. Rev.* **2009**, *109*, 4921–4960. [CrossRef] [PubMed]
42. Liu, X.; Jin, W.; Theil, E.C. Opening protein pores with chaotropes enhances Fe reduction and chelation of Fe from the ferritin biomineral. *Proc. Natl. Acad. Sci. USA* **2003**, *100*, 3653–3658. [CrossRef] [PubMed]
43. Gibson, Q.H.; Hastings, J.W. The oxidation of reduced flavin mononucleotide by molecular oxygen. *Biochem. J.* **1962**, *83*, 368–377. [CrossRef] [PubMed]
44. Topham, R.; Goger, M.; Pearce, K.; Schultz, P. The mobilization of ferritin iron by liver cytosol. A comparison of xanthine and NADH as reducing substrates. *Biochem. J.* **1989**, *261*, 137–143. [CrossRef] [PubMed]
45. Theil, E.C.; Tosha, T.; Behera, R.K. Solving Biology's Iron Chemistry Problem with Ferritin Protein Nanocages. *Acc. Chem. Res.* **2016**, *49*, 784–791. [CrossRef] [PubMed]

46. Watt, G.D.; Jacobs, D.; Frankel, R.B. Redox reactivity of bacterial and mammalian ferritin: Is reductant entry into the ferritin interior a necessary step for iron release? *Proc. Natl. Acad. Sci. USA* **1988**, *85*, 7457–7461. [CrossRef] [PubMed]
47. Theil, E.C.; Liu, X.S.; Tosha, T. Gated pores in the ferritin protein nanocage. *Inorg. Chim. Acta* **2008**, *361*, 868–874. [CrossRef] [PubMed]
48. Liu, X.S.; Patterson, L.D.; Miller, M.J.; Theil, E.C. Peptides selected for the protein nanocage pores change the rate of iron recovery from the ferritin mineral. *J. Biol. Chem.* **2007**, *282*, 31821–31825. [CrossRef] [PubMed]
49. Carmona, U.; Li, L.; Zhang, L.; Knez, M. Ferritin light-chain subunits: Key elements for the electron transfer across the protein cage. *Chem. Commun.* **2014**, *50*, 15358–15361. [CrossRef] [PubMed]
50. Pontillo, N.; Pane, F.; Messori, L.; Amoresano, A.; Merlino, A. Cisplatin encapsulation within a ferritin nanocage: A high-resolution crystallographic study. *Chem. Commun.* **2016**, *52*, 4136–4139. [CrossRef] [PubMed]
51. Chen, L.; Bai, G.; Yang, S.; Yang, R.; Zhao, G.; Xu, C.; Leung, W. Encapsulation of curcumin in recombinant human H-chain ferritin increases its water-solubility and stability. *Food Res. Int.* **2014**, *62*, 1147–1153. [CrossRef]
52. Zhang, T.; Lv, C.; Chen, L.; Bai, G.; Zhao, G.; Xu, C. Encapsulation of anthocyanin molecules within a ferritin nanocage increases their stability and cell uptake efficiency. *Food Res. Int.* **2014**, *62*, 183–192. [CrossRef]
53. Chen, L.; Bai, G.; Yang, R.; Zang, J.; Zhou, T.; Zhao, G. Encapsulation of beta-carotene within ferritin nanocages greatly increases its water-solubility and thermal stability. *Food Chem.* **2014**, *149*, 307–312. [CrossRef] [PubMed]
54. Bradley, J.M.; Svistunenko, D.A.; Lawson, T.L.; Hemmings, A.M.; Moore, G.R.; Le Brun, N.E. Three Aromatic Residues are Required for Electron Transfer during Iron Mineralization in Bacterioferritin. *Angew. Chem. Int. Ed. Engl.* **2015**, *54*, 14763–14767. [CrossRef] [PubMed]
55. Bradley, J.M.; Svistunenko, D.A.; Moore, G.R.; Le Brun, N.E. Tyr25, Tyr58 and Trp133 of Escherichia coli bacterioferritin transfer electrons between iron in the central cavity and the ferroxidase centre. *Metallomics* **2017**, *9*, 1421–1428. [CrossRef] [PubMed]
56. Koochana, P.K.; Mohanty, A.; Das, S.; Subhadarshanee, B.; Satpati, S.; Dixit, A.; Sabat, S.C.; Behera, R.K. Releasing iron from ferritin protein nanocage by reductive method: The role of electron transfer mediator. *Biochim. Biophys. Acta Gen. Subj.* **2018**, *1862*, 1190–1198. [CrossRef] [PubMed]
57. Bienfait, H.F.; Van Den Briel, M.L. Rapid mobilization of ferritin iron by ascorbate in the presence of oxygen. *BBA-Gen. Subj.* **1980**, *631*, 507–510. [CrossRef]
58. Badu-Boateng, C.; Naftalin, R.J. Ascorbate and ferritin interactions: Consequences for iron release in vitro and in vivo and implications for inflammation. *Free Radic. Biol. Med.* **2018**, in press. [CrossRef] [PubMed]
59. Badu-Boateng, C.; Pardalaki, S.; Wolf, C.; Lajnef, S.; Peyrot, F.; Naftalin, R.J. Labile iron potentiates ascorbate-dependent reduction and mobilization of ferritin iron. *Free Radic. Biol. Med.* **2017**, *108*, 94–109. [CrossRef] [PubMed]
60. Gardner, P.R. Aconitase: Sensitive target and measure of superoxide. *Methods Enzymol.* **2002**, *349*, 9–23. [PubMed]
61. Hynes, M.J.; Coinceanainn, M.O. Investigation of the release of iron from ferritin by naturally occurring antioxidants. *J. Inorg. Biochem.* **2002**, *90*, 18–21. [CrossRef]
62. Ahmad, S.; Singh, V.; Rao, G.S. Release of iron from ferritin by 1, 2, 4-benzenetriol. *Chem. Biol. Interact.* **1995**, *96*, 103–111. [CrossRef]
63. Dangles, O.; Fargeix, G.; Dufour, C. One-electron oxidation of quercetin and quercetin derivatives in protic and non protic media. *J. Chem. Soc. Perkin Trans. 2* **1999**, 1387–1396. [CrossRef]
64. Bennett, B.D.; Kimball, E.H.; Gao, M.; Osterhout, R.; Van Dien, S.J.; Rabinowitz, J.D. Absolute metabolite concentrations and implied enzyme active site occupancy in *Escherichia coli*. *Nat. Chem. Biol.* **2009**, *5*, 593–599. [CrossRef] [PubMed]
65. Chaston, T.B.; Richardson, D.R. Iron Chelators for the treatment of iron overload disease: Relationship between structure, redox activity, and toxicity. *Am. J. Hematol.* **2003**, *73*, 200–210. [CrossRef] [PubMed]
66. Galvez, N.; Ruiz, B.; Cuesta, R.; Colacio, E.; Dominguez-Vera, J.M. Release of iron from ferritin by aceto-and benzohydroxamic acids. *Inorg. Chem.* **2005**, *44*, 2706–2709. [CrossRef] [PubMed]

67. Galvez, N.; Fernandez, B.; Sanchez, P.; Cuesta, R.; Ceolin, M.; Clemente-Leon, M.; Trasobares, S.; Lopez-Haro, M.; Calvino, J.J.; Stephan, O.; et al. Comparative structural and chemical studies of ferritin cores with gradual removal of their iron contents. *J. Am. Chem. Soc.* **2008**, *130*, 8062–8068. [CrossRef] [PubMed]
68. Netto, L.E.S.; Da Costa Ferreira, A.M.; Augusto, O. Iron(III) binding in DNA solutions: Complex formation and catalytic activity in the oxidation of hydrazine derivatives. *Chem. Biol. Interact.* **1991**, *79*, 1–14. [CrossRef]

4

Ferritin in Kidney and Vascular Related Diseases: Novel Roles for an Old Player

József Balla [1,2], György Balla [1,3] and Abolfazl Zarjou [4,5,*]

1 HAS-UD Vascular Biology and Myocardial Pathophysiology Research Group, Hungarian Academy of Sciences, H-4032 Debrecen, Hungary; balla@belklinika.com (J.B.); balla@med.unideb.hu (G.B.)
2 Division of Nephrology, Department of Medicine, Faculty of Medicine, University of Debrecen, H-4032 Debrecen, Hungary
3 Department of Pediatrics, Faculty of Medicine, University of Debrecen, H-4032 Debrecen, Hungary
4 Department of Medicine, University of Alabama at Birmingham, Birmingham, AL 35294, USA
5 Nephrology Research and Training Center, University of Alabama at Birmingham, Birmingham, AL 35294, USA
* Correspondence: azarjou@uabmc.edu

Abstract: Iron is at the forefront of a number of pivotal biological processes due to its ability to readily accept and donate electrons. However, this property may also catalyze the generation of free radicals with ensuing cellular and tissue toxicity. Accordingly, throughout evolution numerous pathways and proteins have evolved to minimize the potential hazardous effects of iron cations and yet allow for readily available iron cations in a wide variety of fundamental metabolic processes. One of the extensively studied proteins in the context of systemic and cellular iron metabolisms is ferritin. While clinicians utilize serum ferritin to monitor body iron stores and inflammation, it is important to note that the vast majority of ferritin is located intracellularly. Intracellular ferritin is made of two different subunits (heavy and light chain) and plays an imperative role as a safe iron depot. In the past couple of decades our understanding of ferritin biology has remarkably improved. Additionally, a significant body of evidence has emerged describing the significance of the kidney in iron trafficking and homeostasis. Here, we briefly discuss some of the most important findings that relate to the role of iron and ferritin heavy chain in the context of kidney-related diseases and, in particular, vascular calcification, which is a frequent complication of chronic kidney disease.

Keywords: iron; ferritin; acute kidney injury; chronic kidney disease; vascular calcification

1. The Superfamily of Ferritins

The ability of iron cations (the second most abundant element on earth) to change its valence serves as a unique and central capacity to contribute in multiple biological pathways, yet underscores its potential hazardous effects mainly by participating in Fenton's reaction [1,2].

$O_2^{\bullet-} + Fe^{3+} \leftarrow\rightarrow O_2 + Fe^{2+}$
$Fe^{2+} + H_2O_2 \rightarrow Fe^{3+} + HO^{\bullet} + OH^-$ (Fenton's reaction)
$O_2^{\bullet-} + H_2O_2 \leftarrow\rightarrow O_2 + HO^{\bullet} + OH^-$ (Haber–Weiss reaction)

The discovery of ferritin, a protein isolated from horse spleen, was a major step in our understanding of iron metabolism [3]. This discovery was followed by numerous studies that examined this multifaceted protein in various aspects of physiological and pathological conditions [4]. The highly conserved structure of ferritin and its universal expression among species further highlights the importance of this protein at the crossroads of multiple biological pathways that are mainly dictated by iron trafficking and homeostasis [4–6]. Ferritin is a globular protein made up of 24 subunits with a spherical hollow shell that allows for the safe storage of up to 4500 atoms of Fe^{3+}. These subunits are composed of heavy (FtH) and light (FtL) chains and their proportional contribution to the hollow spherical shell depends on the tissue and developmental stage of the organism [5,7]. For instance, while brain and heart ferritin is primarily composed of FtH chains, the liver and spleen mainly possess FtL [7]. One intriguing aspect of ferritin biology relates to serum ferritin that is predominantly composed of FtL chain, as evidenced by immunological cross reactivity with anti-ferritin L antibodies [8–10]. Serum ferritin is also relatively iron poor and its source was not completely understood until it was revealed by Cohen and colleagues that macrophages are the primary source of serum ferritin [11]. It must be noted that several investigators have reported that other cells, particularly hepatocytes, are also capable of secreting ferritin [12–14]. The study by Cohen et al. elegantly confirmed the light chain predominance of serum ferritin and its relatively low iron cations content, and provided evidence to support its secretion through the non-classical lysosomal secretory pathway [11]. More recently, another study reported that secretion of ferritin is mediated through two distinct non-classical pathways [15]. This study also examined the release of iron-rich ferritin and demonstrated that such secretion occurs via the multivesicular body-exosome pathway [15]. The release of iron-rich ferritin is particularly interesting as it may serve as an iron cargo predominantly in a paracrine fashion. The receptors, precise mode of uptake, and relevance of ferritin uptake by cells among species continues to be debated in the literature and future studies are needed to unequivocally describe the nature and significance of these processes.

Serum ferritin has long been used by clinicians to assess body iron stores in humans. However, it is also recognized that levels of serum ferritin rise in response to a number of clinical conditions particularly during inflammatory states and injury models, such as AKI [16–18]. Such elevation in response to inflammatory stimuli and the relatively iron-poor status of serum ferritin resulted in investigations to examine other potential roles in health and disease that were reviewed by Wang and colleagues [19]. More recently, an interesting pilot study examined the feasibility of measuring urinary ferritin (FtL) as a non-invasive diagnostic approach to assess neonates and young children for iron deficiency or iron overload [20]. This study was based on previous reports that confirmed the presence of urinary ferritin in healthy individuals [21,22] and, despite some limitations, found a correlation with paired serum ferritin. In contrast to FtL, the FtH subunit has crucial ferroxidase activity that converts Fe^{2+} to Fe^{3+}, facilitating its safe storage in the form of mineral ferrihydrite within the inner wall of the sphere [23,24]. Such functional properties have led to a significant amount of investigations into this field, leading to the discovery of seminal findings into the role of this superfamily of proteins in physiological processes and injury models [4,6,25,26].

The first description of a function for ferritin other than mere iron cation storage was reported by Balla and colleagues [27]. This seminal manuscript described an anti-oxidant role for ferritin in endothelial cells. In this study authors validated the cytotoxic properties of heme, but surprisingly found that briefly pulsing cells with heme remarkably increased their resistance against oxidant-mediated injury. While administration of apoferritin mimicked these beneficiary effects, a site-directed mutant form of FtH with subsequent loss of ferroxidase activity failed to recapitulate such protection against oxidative damage [27]. These findings generated significant interest in this field and were followed by additional pivotal findings. For instance, while ferritin was traditionally regarded as a cytosolic protein, others demonstrated its localization in other subcellular compartments, such as mitochondria [28,29] and the nucleus [30–32]. This review is intended to briefly discuss some of the aspects of ferritin in the context of kidney-related diseases and one of its major cardiovascular complications, namely vascular calcification.

2. Role of Iron and Ferritin in Acute Kidney Injury

Acute kidney injury (AKI) is a common clinical syndrome characterized by a sudden decrement in kidney function with ensuing derangements in multiple essential physiological parameters, such as dysregulated volume and electrolyte homeostasis [33,34]. It is well documented that AKI increases morbidity and mortality, particularly among critically ill patients [33,35,36]. Moreover, AKI incidence is on the rise and patients who survive AKI have an increased risk for the development of chronic kidney disease (CKD) [37–39]. These detrimental clinical consequences have led to vigorous investigations to better understand the individual and overlapping pathways that are involved in the pathogenesis of AKI. Iron metabolism and trafficking has emerged as one such pathway. The kidney was not considered a major organ involved in the regulation of iron homeostasis, mainly because of the lack of evidence of its involvement in hereditary hemochromatosis and the assumption that transferrin bound iron cations are not filtered by the glomerulus. However, along with other recent breakthroughs in the field of iron metabolism, our understanding of the delicate and well-orchestrated iron regulatory machinery in the kidney has evolved thanks to a number of pivotal observations. For example, the urinary proteomic analysis of Fanconi syndrome, which is characterized by overall dysfunctional proximal tubules and poor reabsorption capacity, demonstrates significantly elevated levels of transferrin in the urine samples of subjects, confirming its filtration [40,41]. Transferrin can be reabsorbed in the tubules via transferrin receptor-1 or cubilin-mediated endocytosis [42,43]. The kidneys also express high levels of divalent metal transporter-1, which was first described by Gunshin et al. [44], and their importance in renal iron handling under physiological and pathological conditions was subsequently confirmed by other investigations [45–49]. Some other iron regulatory proteins that are expressed in kidneys include neutrophil gelatinase-associated lipocalin [50], ferroportin [51,52], as well as hepcidin [53]. Additionally, among other tissues, mouse kidney expresses the highest levels of iron regulatory protein-1 with important functions in renal iron cations handling [54]. It must also be noted that the proximal tubules, workhouse of nephrons, possess a significant amount of mitochondria that contain notable amounts of heme, which encloses iron cations in its porphyrin ring. Based on the aforementioned evidence, it is apparent that the kidneys, particularly proximal tubules, are heavily involved in iron trafficking under both physiological and pathological conditions, and are accordingly more susceptible to injury [55]. In fact, several lines of evidence suggest a role for iron cations-mediated kidney injury in both humans and animal models of kidney disease [56–59]. The participation of iron cations in Fenton's reaction and their ability to aggravate oxidative stress led to the hypothesis that their removal would prove beneficial in kidney injury. In support of this premise, multiple investigations demonstrated that the removal of iron cations via deferoxamine (DFO), a potent iron cations chelator, was protective against AKI. These studies utilized DFO in the setting of glycerol-induced rhabdomyolysis [60], hemoglobin- and myoglobin-induced AKI [61], gentamicin nephrotoxicity [62], and ischemia-reperfusion (I/R) [63]. Notably, these salutary effects were recapitulated by the administration of apotransferrin in a model of I/R-mediated AKI [64]. The evidence to suggest iron as a main culprit and mediator of AKI has also been demonstrated in human studies. Work by Leaf and colleagues focused on the association between catalytic iron cations, non-transferrin bound iron cations, and the course of AKI in patients undergoing cardiac surgery with cardiopulmonary bypass [65]. They reported that primary outcomes, defined as in-hospital death or need for renal replacement therapy, AKI, and other adverse events post-operatively, were directly associated with higher plasma catalytic iron cation levels on post-operative day one [65]. In another study, the same group examined such association in 121 critically ill patients admitted to medical or surgical intensive care units [66]. Similarly, higher plasma catalytic iron cation levels were associated with a greater risk of death/need for renal replacement therapy, AKI, and hospital mortality. Importantly, the authors stated that these associations are independent of age, estimated glomerular filtration rate, and number of packed red blood cell transfusions [66]. Others also evaluated the role of plasma catalytic iron cations in relation to contrast-induced nephropathy. Their results confirmed higher levels of catalytic iron cations were associated with a higher risk of contrast nephropathy, as well as higher rates of mortality [67]. Other studies have suggested a role for catalytic iron cations in the context of glomerulopathies and proteinuria. For instance, in a rat model of nephrotic syndrome, a significant increase in the levels of glomerular catalytic iron cations was observed [68]. Importantly, chelation of iron cations with DFO was associated with complete protection against proteinuria [68]. Another clinical study validated these findings, where deferiprone, an oral iron cation chelator, was used in diabetic and non-diabetic glomerular disease [69]. While this study was rather small and non-randomized, iron cation chelation demonstrated a marked reduction of proteinuria in both groups of patients with and without diabetic glomerular nephropathy.

The above-mentioned evidence led to further investigations to examine how the proximal tubular expression of ferritin may affect the course of AKI. The importance and non-redundant function of FtH and its ferroxidase activity was reported by Ferreira and colleagues [70]. They demonstrated that global deletion of FtH in mice leads to embryonic lethality between 3.5 and 9.5 days of development [70]. Therefore, to understand the role of proximal tubule FtH expression during AKI, we generated transgenic mice with conditional deletion of FtH in proximal tubules. This was achieved by crossing FtH$^{lox/lox}$ mice that were generated and characterized by Darshan and colleagues [71] with phosphoenolpyruvate carboxykinase (PEPCK)-Cre mice [72]. Targeted deletion of FtH in proximal tubules led to heightened rhabdomyolysis-induced AKI, as evidenced by the higher rate of mortality, serum creatinine, and the higher expression of cleaved caspase-3, a marker of apoptosis [18]. The protective nature of FtH expression in proximal tubules was further supported by a histological analysis that revealed a greater number of tubular casts, necrotic tubules, and more prominent loss of proximal tubule brush border in the absence of FtH expression. Notably, rhabdomyolysis is primarily a heme-mediated injury model, given the significant amount of heme present in myoglobin. Therefore, to investigate whether FtH may play a protective role in other models of AKI that are not predominantly heme driven, cisplatin nephrotoxicity was used. These results indicated that, irrespective of the model of injury, deletion of FtH led to worse renal function, as evidenced by serum creatinine. Furthermore, the overall architecture of the kidneys was less preserved in the absence of FtH [18]. These studies led to another interesting observation that FtH deletion was accompanied by markedly higher levels of heme oxygenase-1 (HO-1) expression. HO-1 is a well-characterized anti-oxidant enzyme that has been shown to have protective effects against a number insults and kidney injury models [73,74]. Aggravated AKI, despite such high levels of HO-1, indicates that beneficial effects of HO-1 are co-dependent on FtH expression and this premise is further supported in a model of rodent anti-thymocyte antigen-1-induced glomerulonephritis [75]. This study showed that inhibition of HO activity was accompanied with downregulation of FtH expression and enhanced mesangial cell death. Additionally, while induction of HO-1 in cultured rat mesangial cells augmented its resistance to oxidative stress, FtH knockdown by RNA interference caused loss of such protective influences. Also of note, this study demonstrated adjacent expression of HO-1 and FtH in inflammatory glomeruli of human lupus nephritis biopsies [75]. In another study, Hatcher and colleagues examined FtH overexpression in a model of ischemia-reperfusion-induced AKI [76]. Using a conditional tissue-specific doxycycline-inducible system, about 6.5-fold higher levels of FtH expression was shown in mouse kidneys. Following injury, the authors demonstrated that FtH overexpression was associated with lesser apoptosis and improved tubular viability [76]. It was concluded that FtH overexpression protects the kidney via limiting oxidative stress induced by I/R. Another line of evidence to support the role of FtH in protecting the kidney against injurious insults comes from a more recent study by Scindia and colleagues [77]. In this study, the authors examined how modulation of iron homeostatic pathways via hepcidin alters the course of I/R-induced AKI. Hepcidin, a hormone produced primarily by hepatocytes [78], acts by directly binding to ferroportin, leading to its internalization and subsequent degradation in lysosomes [79]. This eventually leads to decreased iron cation absorption, as well as increased iron cation retention with subsequent upregulation of intracellular ferritin. It was demonstrated that hepcidin, given 24–48 h before I/R, mitigated kidney injury and reduced renal and systemic inflammation caused by I/R [77]. These effects were attributed to increased FtH expression in the kidney and the spleen. These overall beneficial properties were also corroborated in a model of hemoglobin-induced AKI, where hepcidin administration mitigated the upregulation of urinary kidney injury markers (neutrophil gelatinase-associated lipocalin and kidney injury molecule-1) and renal Interleukin-6 [80].

To further elaborate on the role of FtH and how its expression in different cells may contribute to the course of kidney damage, effects of FtH expression in myeloid cells were further investigated [81].

Using transgenic mice with conditional deletion of FtH in the proximal tubules or myeloid cells, it was found that myeloid FtH deficiency did not affect activation or accumulation of macrophages in the injured kidney compared with wild-type littermate controls. In contrast, a significant increase in the number of pro-inflammatory macrophages accompanied FtH deletion in proximal tubules in a model of unilateral ureteral obstruction (UUO). Moreover, while deletion of FtH in the myeloid compartment resulted in lesser fibrosis in a UUO model of kidney injury, the lack of FtH expression in proximal tubules exacerbated both inflammation and fibrosis [81]. These findings suggest a central role for FtH expression in various compartments that underscores its importance in the context of tubular-macrophage cross-talk during kidney injury. More recently, the effects of FtH expression in myeloid cells during sepsis and its clinical sequelae, including sepsis-induced AKI, were examined [82]. Results of this study demonstrated that the deletion of FtH in the myeloid compartment was associated with marked protection in two models of sepsis, namely cecal ligation puncture and lipopolysaccharide-induced endotoxemia. Deletion of FtH led to improved survival, reduced cytokine levels, and more preserved renal function. Mechanistic studies revealed that the protective effects were primarily mediated by the compensatory increase in circulating ferritin (FtL) in the absence of myeloid FtH [82]. It must be noted that the main circulatory form of ferritin is FtL and macrophages have been shown to be the primary source of serum ferritin [11]. Results also demonstrated that the protective effects of FtL during sepsis are attributed to its inhibitory actions against the activation of the NF-κB pathway. These findings not only provide a novel platform for future studies to better understand the pathogenesis of sepsis but also shed light on the immunomodulatory roles of circulating FtL.

3. Ferritin: A Potent Inhibitor of Osteoblastic Activity

Cardiovascular-related diseases remain the foremost cause of death in patients with CKD and those requiring renal replacement therapy [83–85]. About 10–15% of the U.S. population is estimated to have CKD and more than 450,000 Americans require dialysis resulting in a major burden of morbidity, mortality, and healthcare expenditure [86]. In this regard, vascular calcification (VC) is a common complication of CKD and is recognized as a portentous contributing factor to cardiovascular death in these patients [87–90]. The prevalence of VC is exceptionally high among patients with CKD and can be observed even in very young dialysis patients [91,92]. Two distinct patterns of VC have been described [93]. While intimal calcification occurs in atherosclerotic plaques, mineralization of the medial compartment is a common pathological finding in aging patients and patients with diabetes and advanced CKD [93,94]. The diffuse calcification that occurs in the medial layer of the vasculature is an important marker for all-cause mortality in patients undergoing dialysis [87,88,95]. There are several detrimental hemodynamic consequences of VC, including loss of arterial elasticity, increase in pulse wave velocity, development of left ventricular hypertrophy, and decrease in coronary artery perfusion, ensuing in myocardial ischemia and failure [95,96]. Following the description of VC as a tightly regulated cellular process where vascular smooth muscle cells (VSMC) transition into "osteoblast-like" cells, major research efforts have identified various pathways and mechanisms involved in the development and propagation of VC [97,98]. These proposed mechanisms include elastin degradation, apoptosis of VSMC, release of exosomes loaded with microRNAs, and extracellular vesicles that are rich in calcium and phosphate [99,100]. Nevertheless, multiple pivotal questions remain unanswered and currently no therapies exist for the treatment or prevention of VC. To better understand novel pathways that may be involved in the development and pathogenesis of VC, it was important to examine how derangements in iron metabolism may be contributing to the development of such detrimental pathological conditions. This principle was based on the fact that many patients with advanced CKD are also predisposed to iron-restricted erythropoiesis. Several factors lead to the development of anemia in patients with CKD and those requiring dialysis. These include decreased erythropoietin production, frequent diagnostic testing, blood loss during hemodialysis, and cannula puncture sites following hemodialysis, as well as a "functional iron deficiency state" [101–104]. This process, also known as anemia of chronic disease, is principally a result of the increased synthesis and secretion of hepcidin, which is a common paradigm of chronic inflammatory states such as CKD [105]. It must be noted that other cytokines have been demonstrated to have additional effects and further aggravate this state of functional iron deficiency [106]. Hepcidin leads to the internalization and degradation of ferroportin (membrane iron transporter) and the overall outcome is the decreased iron cation absorption from the small intestine along with the decreased egress of iron cations from the reticuloendothelial system [105]. Accordingly, while macrophages are loaded with iron cations, other cells within the body have a relatively lower iron cation content. It was therefore necessary to examine whether the repletion of iron cations and the subsequent upregulation of ferritin in VSMC mitigates the osteoblastic differentiation of these cells when exposed to high phosphate levels. Notably, increasing levels of serum phosphorus manifest during advanced stages of CKD and such hyperphosphatemia is a well-known risk factor for the development of VC [107–109]. Indeed, we found that the addition of hemin was able to significantly arrest the calcification and osteoblastic transition of VSMC [110].

To identify the mediator of such a salutary effect, we examined products of the HO/ferritin system that include biliverdin, bilirubin, carbon monoxide, and iron cations. It was demonstrated that iron administration inhibited calcium deposition and led to about a five-fold increment in intracellular ferritin levels. Subsequent studies using recombinant ferritin proteins confirmed the paramount role of ferritin upregulation in this inhibitory process. Using exogenous recombinant FtH, FtL, and a mutant form of FtH that lacks ferroxidase activity, we demonstrated the paramount role of FtH/ferroxidase activity in the abrogation of VSMC mineralization and osteoblastic transformation [110]. Importantly, the inhibitory role of FtH was not limited to the mere inhibition of hydroxyapatite deposition, but it also prevented the expression of the core binding factor alpha-1 (cbfa-1), a key transcription factor in osteogenesis [111].

Other studies have also suggested a potential inhibitory role for iron and iron-induced upregulation of ferritin in the context of VC. For example, Rajendran et al. used various detection methods to map the spatial distribution of the elements and quantify them simultaneously in atherosclerotic rabbit arteries [112]. They demonstrated that within atherosclerotic plaques, iron cations (likely sequestered within ferritin shell) and calcium exhibited a highly significant spatial inverse correlation. Moreover, an adenine-induced model of CKD in rats was employed to investigate the role of PA-21, an iron-based non-calcium phosphate binder in VC. They reported a higher degree of inhibition of VC when compared to another frequently used phosphate binder, calcium carbonate [113]. Furthermore, Seto et al. examined the role of iron loading on the progression of VC in an adenine diet-induced CKD rat model [114]. It was demonstrated that iron loading resulted in the suppression of VC and attributed these findings to the reduced expression of phosphate transporter (Pit-1) and cbfa-1. Others have also reported the inhibition of high phosphate-induced VC using ferric citrate and attributed these results to the suppression of apoptosis [115]. These results are interesting when taking into account a study that was published in 1995 and reported the inhibition of calcium deposition in bioprostethic valves when pre-treated with iron [116]. However, it is also noteworthy that some studies have failed to recapitulate the overall inhibitory effects of iron during VC [117].

Based on these findings, we hypothesized that osteoporosis induced by iron overload states, such as primary hemochromatosis [118,119], may be attributed to the increased expression of FtH in osteoblasts secondary to excessive iron accumulation. Indeed, investigating the mechanism(s) leading to decreased bone deposition in iron overload states, we were able to demonstrate the central role of FtH in this process [120]. We showed that the administration of apoferritin or recombinant FtH (both devoid of iron cations) markedly inhibited the mineralization and expression of osteoblastic specific genes, such as osteocalcin, alkaline phosphatase, and cbfa-1 [120]. Overall these results confirmed previous findings that increased iron cation levels mitigate calcification, but they also provided a novel mechanism for this process and identified FtH upregulation as a main inhibitory factor in this regard.

The potential hazardous effects of excessive iron cations are well recognized, and their optimal dosage and utilization frequency in CKD patients have been a major point of debate among nephrologists [121–123]. Accordingly, based on the aforementioned evidence, we sought to identify other approaches to upregulate FtH expression in VSMC without using excessive iron and examine how the pharmacological induction of ferritin may affect VC. To achieve this objective, we tested the effects of 3H-1,2-Dithiole-3-thione (D3T), a well-known cancer chemopreventive agent [124] and inducer of FtH expression [125], in a model of VSMC calcification. It was demonstrated that D3T inhibited osteoblastic transition of VSMC in a dose-dependent manner [126]. However, the central role of ferritin was further corroborated in experiments where the inhibitory effects of D3T on osteoblastic transition were arrested during FtH knockdown by RNA interference [126]. The overall effect of iron/D3T-induced FtH upregulation and inhibition of VSMC calcification is illustrated in Figure 1.

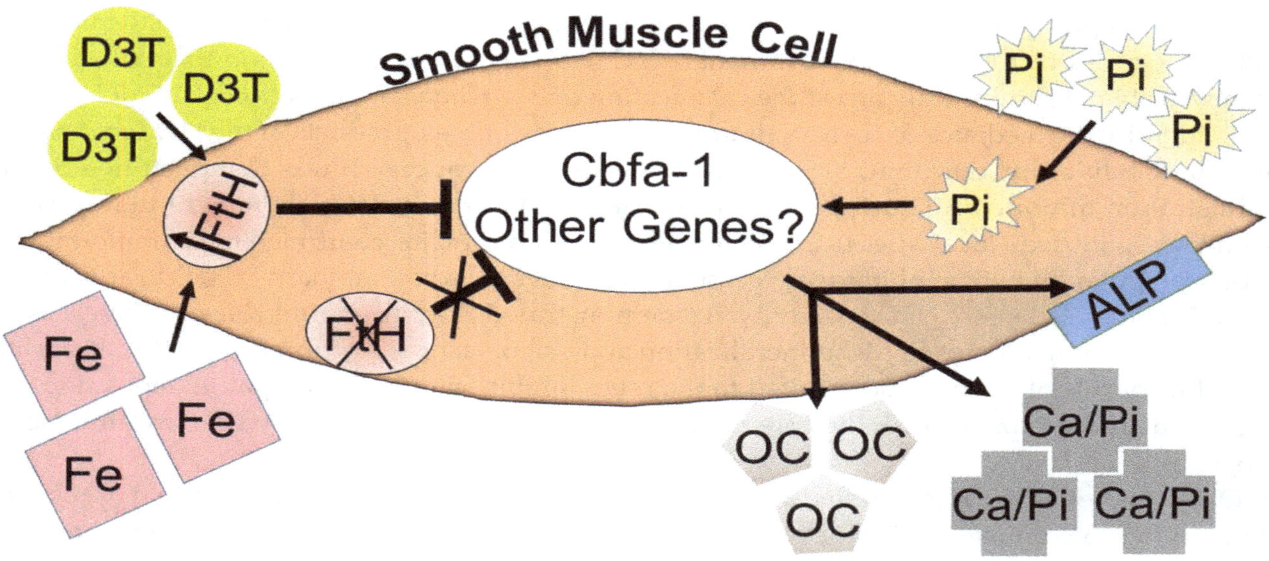

Figure 1. Overall schematic of the proposed mechanism of the inhibition of VSMC calcification via the upregulation of FtH. The figure depicts a vascular smooth muscle cell (VSMC) where elevated levels of Pi (phosphorus) induce the upregulation of cbfa-1 (core binding factor alpha-1), leading to the deposition of extracellular Ca/Pi (hydroxyapatite crystals) and the activation of osteoblastic genes, including OC (osteocalcin) and ALP (alkaline phosphatase). This process can be exacerbated by the deletion of FtH (ferritin heavy chain) or mitigated via D3T (3H-1,2-Dithiole-3-thione) and Fe (iron)-induced FtH upregulation. There may still be novel genes and pathways modulated by FtH expression that require further investigations.

More recently, similar inhibitory effects in mitigating the calcification of valvular tissues were demonstrated [127]. Valvular calcification and stenosis (particularly aortic valve) is a common finding in patients undergoing dialysis and the elderly population. In this study we showed that the induction of FtH was associated with the decreased osteoblastic activity of valvular interstitial cells. This inhibitory effect was attributed to the reduced nuclear accumulation of cbfa-1, and as a reciprocal effect, its enhancement of the nuclear localization of transcription factor Sox9 (SRY [sex-determining region Y]-box 9) [127]. These findings provide additional support to previous observations that identified reduced Sox9 function as a potential culprit of calcific valvular disease [128] and further corroborate the "anti-osteoblastic activity" of FtH. It must be emphasized that while a significant body of evidence is emerging to support the role of intracellular FtH expression as an inhibitory mechanism against calcification, additional targeted studies in animal models are required to unequivocally demonstrate and confirm these results.

It is also noteworthy that the implication and functional significance of iron and ferritin in the context of atherosclerosis and coronary artery disease continues to generate contradicting results and is heavily debated in the literature. While we do not elaborate further on these studies in this review, others have discussed these results in detail [129 134]

In conclusion, it is evident that ferritin and its role in both cellular and systemic iron homeostasis, as well as its participation in a number of pathways that are central to various pathological conditions, is increasingly recognized. Future studies and additional genetic manipulations (for instance, the targeted deletion of FtL or the over-expression of FtH) would be germane to pave the way for potential therapeutic targets utilizing this intriguing, ancient, and almost ubiquitous superfamily of proteins.

Author Contributions: Writing—original draft preparation: A.Z., G.B., and J.B.; writing—review and editing: A.Z., G.B., and J.B.; funding acquisition: A.Z. and J.B.

References

1. Haber, F.; Weiss, J. The Catalytic Decomposition of Hydrogen Peroxide by Iron Salts. *Proc. R. Soc. Lond. Ser. A Math. Phys. Sci.* **1934**, *147*, 332–351.
2. Fenton, H.J.H. LXXIII.—Oxidation of tartaric acid in presence of iron. *J. Chem. Soc. Trans.* **1894**, *65*, 899–910. [CrossRef]
3. Laufberger, V. Sur la cristallisation de la ferritine. *Bull. Soc. Chim. Biol.* **1937**, *19*, 1575–1582.
4. Arosio, P.; Ingrassia, R.; Cavadini, P. Ferritins: A family of molecules for iron storage, antioxidation and more. *Biochim. Biophys. Acta* **2009**, *1790*, 589–599. [CrossRef] [PubMed]
5. Arosio, P.; Levi, S. Cytosolic and mitochondrial ferritins in the regulation of cellular iron homeostasis and oxidative damage. *Biochim. Biophys. Acta* **2010**, *1800*, 783–792. [CrossRef]
6. Arosio, P.; Levi, S. Ferritin, iron homeostasis, and oxidative damage. *Free Radic. Biol. Med.* **2002**, *33*, 457–463. [CrossRef]
7. Harrison, P.M.; Arosio, P. The ferritins: Molecular properties, iron storage function and cellular regulation. *Biochim. Biophys. Acta* **1996**, *1275*, 161–203. [CrossRef]
8. Santambrogio, P.; Cozzi, A.; Levi, S.; Arosio, P. Human serum ferritin G-peptide is recognized by anti-L ferritin subunit antibodies and concanavalin-A. *Br. J. Haematol.* **1987**, *65*, 235–237. [CrossRef]
9. Cazzola, M.; Arosio, P.; Bellotti, V.; Bergamaschi, G.; Dezza, L.; Iacobello, C.; Ruggeri, G.; Zappone, E.; Albertini, A.; Ascari, E. Immunological reactivity of serum ferritin in patients with malignancy. *Tumori* **1985**, *71*, 547–554. [CrossRef]
10. Lukina, E.A.; Levina, A.A.; Mokeeva, R.A.; Tokarev Yu, N. The diagnostic significance of serum ferritin indices in patients with malignant and reactive histiocytosis. *Br. J. Haematol.* **1993**, *83*, 326–329. [CrossRef]
11. Cohen, L.A.; Gutierrez, L.; Weiss, A.; Leichtmann-Bardoogo, Y.; Zhang, D.L.; Crooks, D.R.; Sougrat, R.; Morgenstern, A.; Galy, B.; Hentze, M.W.; et al. Serum ferritin is derived primarily from macrophages through a nonclassical secretory pathway. *Blood* **2010**, *116*, 1574–1584. [CrossRef] [PubMed]
12. Ghosh, S.; Hevi, S.; Chuck, S.L. Regulated secretion of glycosylated human ferritin from hepatocytes. *Blood* **2004**, *103*, 2369–2376. [CrossRef]
13. Mack, U.; Cooksley, W.G.; Ferris, R.A.; Powell, L.W.; Halliday, J.W. Regulation of plasma ferritin by the isolated perfused rat liver. *Br. J. Haematol.* **1981**, *47*, 403–412. [CrossRef] [PubMed]
14. Tran, T.N.; Eubanks, S.K.; Schaffer, K.J.; Zhou, C.Y.; Linder, M.C. Secretion of ferritin by rat hepatoma cells and its regulation by inflammatory cytokines and iron. *Blood* **1997**, *90*, 4979–4986. [PubMed]
15. Truman-Rosentsvit, M.; Berenbaum, D.; Spektor, L.; Cohen, L.A.; Belizowsky-Moshe, S.; Lifshitz, L.; Ma, J.; Li, W.; Kesselman, E.; Abutbul-Ionita, I.; et al. Ferritin is secreted via 2 distinct nonclassical vesicular pathways. *Blood* **2018**, *131*, 342–352. [CrossRef] [PubMed]
16. Kalantar-Zadeh, K.; Kalantar-Zadeh, K.; Lee, G.H. The fascinating but deceptive ferritin: To measure it or not to measure it in chronic kidney disease? *Clin. J. Am. Soc. Nephrol.* **2006**, *1* (Suppl. 1), S9–S18. [CrossRef]
17. Zandman-Goddard, G.; Shoenfeld, Y. Ferritin in autoimmune diseases. *Autoimmun. Rev.* **2007**, *6*, 457–463. [CrossRef] [PubMed]
18. Zarjou, A.; Bolisetty, S.; Joseph, R.; Traylor, A.; Apostolov, E.O.; Arosio, P.; Balla, J.; Verlander, J.; Darshan, D.; Kuhn, L.C.; et al. Proximal tubule H-ferritin mediates iron trafficking in acute kidney injury. *J. Clin. Invest.* **2013**, *123*, 4423–4434. [CrossRef]
19. Wang, W.; Knovich, M.A.; Coffman, L.G.; Torti, F.M.; Torti, S.V. Serum ferritin: Past, present and future. *Biochim. Biophys. Acta* **2010** *1800*, 760–769. [CrossRef] [PubMed]

20. Bahr, T.M.; Christensen, R.D.; Ward, D.M.; Meng, F.; Jackson, L.K.; Doyle, K.; Christensen, D.R.; Harvey, A.G.; Yaish, H.M. Ferritin in serum and urine: A pilot study. *Blood Cells Mol. Dis.* **2019**, *76*, 59–62. [CrossRef] [PubMed]
21. Ishikawa, K.; Narita, O.; Saito, H.; Kato, K. Determination of ferritin in urine and in serum of normal adults with a sensitive enzyme immunoassay. *Clin. Chim. Acta* **1982**, *123*, 73–81. [CrossRef]
22. Gonzales, P.A.; Pisitkun, T.; Hoffert, J.D.; Tchapyjnikov, D.; Star, R.A.; Kleta, R.; Wang, N.S.; Knepper, M.A. Large-scale proteomics and phosphoproteomics of urinary exosomes. *J. Am. Soc. Nephrol.* **2009**, *20*, 363–379. [CrossRef] [PubMed]
23. Hentze, M.W.; Keim, S.; Papadopoulos, P.; O'Brien, S.; Modi, W.; Drysdale, J.; Leonard, W.J.; Harford, J.B.; Klausner, R.D. Cloning, characterization, expression, and chromosomal localization of a human ferritin heavy-chain gene. *Proc. Natl. Acad. Sci. USA* **1986**, *83*, 7226–7230. [CrossRef] [PubMed]
24. Lawson, D.M.; Treffry, A.; Artymiuk, P.J.; Harrison, P.M.; Yewdall, S.J.; Luzzago, A.; Cesareni, G.; Levi, S.; Arosio, P. Identification of the ferroxidase centre in ferritin. *FEBS Lett.* **1989**, *254*, 207–210. [CrossRef]
25. Arosio, P.; Elia, L.; Poli, M. Ferritin, cellular iron storage and regulation. *IUBMB Life* **2017**, *69*, 414–422. [CrossRef] [PubMed]
26. Watt, R.K. The many faces of the octahedral ferritin protein. *Biometals* **2011**, *24*, 489–500. [CrossRef]
27. Balla, G.; Jacob, H.S.; Balla, J.; Rosenberg, M.; Nath, K.; Apple, F.; Eaton, J.W.; Vercellotti, G.M. Ferritin: A cytoprotective antioxidant strategem of endothelium. *J. Biol. Chem.* **1992**, *267*, 18148–18153.
28. Levi, S.; Corsi, B.; Bosisio, M.; Invernizzi, R.; Volz, A.; Sanford, D.; Arosio, P.; Drysdale, J. A human mitochondrial ferritin encoded by an intronless gene. *J. Biol. Chem.* **2001**, *276*, 24437–24440. [CrossRef]
29. Drysdale, J.; Arosio, P.; Invernizzi, R.; Cazzola, M.; Volz, A.; Corsi, B.; Biasiotto, G.; Levi, S. Mitochondrial ferritin: A new player in iron metabolism. *Blood Cells Mol. Dis.* **2002**, *29*, 376–383. [CrossRef]
30. Cai, C.X.; Birk, D.E.; Linsenmayer, T.F. Nuclear ferritin protects DNA from UV damage in corneal epithelial cells. *Mol. Biol. Cell* **1998**, *9*, 1037–1051. [CrossRef]
31. Cai, C.; Ching, A.; Lagace, C.; Linsenmayer, T. Nuclear ferritin-mediated protection of corneal epithelial cells from oxidative damage to DNA. *Dev. Dyn.* **2008**, *237*, 2676–2683. [CrossRef] [PubMed]
32. Thompson, K.J.; Fried, M.G.; Ye, Z.; Boyer, P.; Connor, J.R. Regulation, mechanisms and proposed function of ferritin translocation to cell nuclei. *J. Cell Sci.* **2002**, *115*, 2165–2177. [PubMed]
33. Zarjou, A.; Sanders, P.W.; Mehta, R.L.; Agarwal, A. Enabling innovative translational research in acute kidney injury. *Clin. Transl. Sci.* **2012**, *5*, 93–101. [CrossRef] [PubMed]
34. Choudhury, D. Acute kidney injury: Current perspectives. *Postgrad. Med.* **2010**, *122*, 29–40. [CrossRef] [PubMed]
35. Maxwell, R.A.; Bell, C.M. Acute Kidney Injury in the Critically Ill. *Surg. Clin. N. Am.* **2017**, *97*, 1399–1418. [CrossRef] [PubMed]
36. Bevc, S.; Ekart, R.; Hojs, R. The assessment of acute kidney injury in critically ill patients. *Eur. J. Intern. Med.* **2017**, *45*, 54–58. [CrossRef] [PubMed]
37. Chawla, L.S.; Eggers, P.W.; Star, R.A.; Kimmel, P.L. Acute kidney injury and chronic kidney disease as interconnected syndromes. *N. Engl. J. Med.* **2014**, *371*, 58–66. [CrossRef]
38. Basile, D.P.; Donohoe, D.; Roethe, K.; Osborn, J.L. Renal ischemic injury results in permanent damage to peritubular capillaries and influences long-term function. *Am. J. Physiol. Ren. Physiol.* **2001**, *281*, F887–F899. [CrossRef]
39. Chawla, L.S.; Kimmel, P.L. Acute kidney injury and chronic kidney disease: An integrated clinical syndrome. *Kidney Int.* **2012**, *82*, 516–524. [CrossRef]
40. Cutillas, P.R.; Chalkley, R.J.; Hansen, K.C.; Cramer, R.; Norden, A.G.; Waterfield, M.D.; Burlingame, A.L.; Unwin, R.J. The urinary proteome in Fanconi syndrome implies specificity in the reabsorption of proteins by renal proximal tubule cells. *Am. J. Physiol. Ren. Physiol.* **2004**, *287*, F353–F364. [CrossRef]
41. Norden, A.G.; Lapsley, M.; Lee, P.J.; Pusey, C.D.; Scheinman, S.J.; Tam, F.W.; Thakker, R.V.; Unwin, R.J.; Wrong, O. Glomerular protein sieving and implications for renal failure in Fanconi syndrome. *Kidney Int.* **2001**, *60*, 1885–1892. [CrossRef] [PubMed]
42. Kozyraki, R.; Fyfe, J.; Verroust, P.J.; Jacobsen, C.; Dautry-Varsat, A.; Gburek, J.; Willnow, T.E.; Christensen, E.I.; Moestrup, S.K. Megalin-dependent cubilin-mediated endocytosis is a major pathway for the apical uptake of transferrin in polarized epithelia. *Proc. Natl. Acad. Sci. USA* **2001**, *98*, 12491–12496. [CrossRef] [PubMed]

43. Smith, C.P.; Lee, W.K.; Haley, M.; Poulsen, S.B.; Thevenod, F.; Fenton, R.A. Proximal tubule transferrin uptake is modulated by cellular iron and mediated by apical membrane megalin-cubilin complex and transferrin receptor 1. *J. Biol. Chem.* **2019**, *294*, 7025–7036. [CrossRef] [PubMed]
44. Gunshin, H.; Mackenzie, B.; Berger, U.V.; Gunshin, Y.; Romero, M.F.; Boron, W.F.; Nussberger, S.; Gollan, J.L.; Hediger, M.A. Cloning and characterization of a mammalian proton-coupled metal-ion transporter. *Nature* **1997**, *388*, 482–488. [CrossRef] [PubMed]
45. Tchernitchko, D.; Bourgeois, M.; Martin, M.E.; Beaumont, C. Expression of the two mRNA isoforms of the iron transporter Nramp2/DMTI in mice and function of the iron responsive element. *Biochem. J.* **2002**, *363*, 449–455. [CrossRef] [PubMed]
46. Abouhamed, M.; Gburek, J.; Liu, W.; Torchalski, B.; Wilhelm, A.; Wolff, N.A.; Christensen, E.I.; Thevenod, F.; Smith, C.P. Divalent metal transporter 1 in the kidney proximal tubule is expressed in late endosomes/lysosomal membranes: Implications for renal handling of protein-metal complexes. *Am. J. Physiol. Ren. Physiol.* **2006**, *290*, F1525–F1533. [CrossRef] [PubMed]
47. Wareing, M.; Ferguson, C.J.; Delannoy, M.; Cox, A.G.; McMahon, R.F.; Green, R.; Riccardi, D.; Smith, C.P. Altered dietary iron intake is a strong modulator of renal DMT1 expression. *Am. J. Physiol. Ren. Physiol.* **2003**, *285*, F1050–F1059. [CrossRef]
48. Ferguson, C.J.; Wareing, M.; Ward, D.T.; Green, R.; Smith, C.P.; Riccardi, D. Cellular localization of divalent metal transporter DMT-1 in rat kidney. *Am. J. Physiol. Ren. Physiol.* **2001**, *280*, F803–F814. [CrossRef]
49. Ferguson, C.J.; Wareing, M.; Delannoy, M.; Fenton, R.; McLarnon, S.J.; Ashton, N.; Cox, A.G.; McMahon, R.F.; Garrick, L.M.; Green, R.; et al. Iron handling and gene expression of the divalent metal transporter, DMT1, in the kidney of the anemic Belgrade (b) rat. *Kidney Int.* **2003**, *64*, 1755–1764. [CrossRef]
50. Mori, K.; Lee, H.T.; Rapoport, D.; Drexler, I.R.; Foster, K.; Yang, J.; Schmidt-Ott, K.M.; Chen, X.; Li, J.Y.; Weiss, S.; et al. Endocytic delivery of lipocalin-siderophore-iron complex rescues the kidney from ischemia-reperfusion injury. *J. Clin. Investig.* **2005**, *115*, 610–621. [CrossRef]
51. Donovan, A.; Brownlie, A.; Zhou, Y.; Shepard, J.; Pratt, S.J.; Moynihan, J.; Paw, B.H.; Drejer, A.; Barut, B.; Zapata, A.; et al. Positional cloning of zebrafish ferroportin1 identifies a conserved vertebrate iron exporter. *Nature* **2000**, *403*, 776–781. [CrossRef] [PubMed]
52. Wolff, N.A.; Liu, W.; Fenton, R.A.; Lee, W.K.; Thevenod, F.; Smith, C.P. Ferroportin 1 is expressed basolaterally in rat kidney proximal tubule cells and iron excess increases its membrane trafficking. *J. Cell Mol. Med.* **2011**, *15*, 209–219. [CrossRef] [PubMed]
53. Kulaksiz, H.; Theilig, F.; Bachmann, S.; Gehrke, S.G.; Rost, D.; Janetzko, A.; Cetin, Y.; Stremmel, W. The iron-regulatory peptide hormone hepcidin: Expression and cellular localization in the mammalian kidney. *J. Endocrinol.* **2005**, *184*, 361–370. [CrossRef] [PubMed]
54. Meyron-Holtz, E.G.; Ghosh, M.C.; Iwai, K.; LaVaute, T.; Brazzolotto, X.; Berger, U.V.; Land, W.; Ollivierre-Wilson, H.; Grinberg, A.; Love, P.; et al. Genetic ablations of iron regulatory proteins 1 and 2 reveal why iron regulatory protein 2 dominates iron homeostasis. *EMBO J.* **2004**, *23*, 386–395. [CrossRef] [PubMed]
55. Smith, C.P.; Thevenod, F. Iron transport and the kidney. *Biochim. Biophys. Acta* **2009**, *1790*, 724–730. [CrossRef] [PubMed]
56. Leaf, D.E.; Swinkels, D.W. Catalytic iron and acute kidney injury. *Am. J. Physiol. Ren. Physiol.* **2016**, *311*, F871–F876. [CrossRef] [PubMed]
57. Walker, V.J.; Agarwal, A. Targeting Iron Homeostasis in Acute Kidney Injury. *Semin. Nephrol.* **2016**, *36*, 62–70. [CrossRef] [PubMed]
58. Martines, A.M.; Masereeuw, R.; Tjalsma, H.; Hoenderop, J.G.; Wetzels, J.F.; Swinkels, D.W. Iron metabolism in the pathogenesis of iron-induced kidney injury. *Nat. Rev. Nephrol.* **2013**, *9*, 385–398. [CrossRef] [PubMed]
59. Swaminathan, S. Iron Homeostasis Pathways as Therapeutic Targets in Acute Kidney Injury. *Nephron* **2018**, *140*, 156–159. [CrossRef]
60. Shah, S.V.; Walker, P.D. Evidence suggesting a role for hydroxyl radical in glycerol-induced acute renal failure. *Am. J. Physiol.* **1988**, *255*, F438–F443. [CrossRef]
61. Paller, M.S. Hemoglobin- and myoglobin-induced acute renal failure in rats: Role of iron in nephrotoxicity. *Am. J. Physiol.* **1988**, *255*, F539–F544. [CrossRef] [PubMed]
62. Walker, P.D.; Shah, S.V. Evidence suggesting a role for hydroxyl radical in gentamicin-induced acute renal failure in rats. *J. Clin. Investig.* **1988**, *81*, 334–341. [CrossRef] [PubMed]

63. Paller, M.S.; Hedlund, B.E. Role of iron in postischemic renal injury in the rat. *Kidney Int.* **1988**, *34*, 474–480. [CrossRef] [PubMed]
64. De Vries, B.; Walter, S.J.; von Bonsdorff, L.; Wolfs, T.G.; van Heurn, L.W.; Parkkinen, J.; Buurman, W.A. Reduction of circulating redox-active iron by apotransferrin protects against renal ischemia-reperfusion injury. *Transplantation* **2004**, *77*, 669–675. [CrossRef] [PubMed]
65. Leaf, D.E.; Rajapurkar, M.; Lele, S.S.; Mukhopadhyay, B.; Rawn, J.D.; Frendl, G.; Waikar, S.S. Increased plasma catalytic iron in patients may mediate acute kidney injury and death following cardiac surgery. *Kidney Int.* **2015**, *87*, 1046–1054. [CrossRef]
66. Leaf, D.E.; Rajapurkar, M.; Lele, S.S.; Mukhopadhyay, B.; Waikar, S.S. Plasma catalytic iron, AKI, and death among critically ill patients. *Clin. J. Am. Soc. Nephrol.* **2014**, *9*, 1849–1856. [CrossRef]
67. Lele, S.S.; Mukhopadhyay, B.N.; Mardikar, M.M.; Patel, T.A.; Vasavada, A.K.; Banker, D.N.; Kapasi, K.D.; Chauhan, V.C.; Chawla, K.C.; Raju, S.R.; et al. Impact of catalytic iron on mortality in patients with acute coronary syndrome exposed to iodinated radiocontrast-The Iscom Study. *Am. Heart J.* **2013**, *165*, 744–751. [CrossRef]
68. Ueda, N.; Baliga, R.; Shah, S.V. Role of 'catalytic' iron in an animal model of minimal change nephrotic syndrome. *Kidney Int.* **1996**, *49*, 370–373. [CrossRef]
69. Rajapurkar, M.M.; Hegde, U.; Bhattacharya, A.; Alam, M.G.; Shah, S.V. Effect of deferiprone, an oral iron chelator, in diabetic and non-diabetic glomerular disease. *Toxicol. Mech. Methods* **2013**, *23*, 5–10. [CrossRef]
70. Ferreira, C.; Bucchini, D.; Martin, M.E.; Levi, S.; Arosio, P.; Grandchamp, B.; Beaumont, C. Early embryonic lethality of H ferritin gene deletion in mice. *J. Biol. Chem.* **2000**, *275*, 3021–3024. [CrossRef]
71. Darshan, D.; Vanoaica, L.; Richman, L.; Beermann, F.; Kuhn, L.C. Conditional deletion of ferritin H in mice induces loss of iron storage and liver damage. *Hepatology* **2009**, *50*, 852–860. [CrossRef] [PubMed]
72. Rankin, E.B.; Tomaszewski, J.E.; Haase, V.H. Renal cyst development in mice with conditional inactivation of the von Hippel-Lindau tumor suppressor. *Cancer Res.* **2006**, *66*, 2576–2583. [CrossRef] [PubMed]
73. Bolisetty, S.; Zarjou, A.; Agarwal, A. Heme Oxygenase 1 as a Therapeutic Target in Acute Kidney Injury. *Am. J. Kidney Dis.* **2017**, *69*, 531–545. [CrossRef] [PubMed]
74. Ayer, A.; Zarjou, A.; Agarwal, A.; Stocker, R. Heme Oxygenases in Cardiovascular Health and Disease. *Physiol. Rev.* **2016**, *96*, 1449–1508. [CrossRef] [PubMed]
75. Cheng, H.T.; Yen, C.J.; Chang, C.C.; Huang, K.T.; Chen, K.H.; Zhang, R.Y.; Lee, P.Y.; Miaw, S.C.; Huang, J.W.; Chiang, C.K.; et al. Ferritin heavy chain mediates the protective effect of heme oxygenase-1 against oxidative stress. *Biochim. Biophys. Acta* **2015**, *1850*, 2506–2517. [CrossRef] [PubMed]
76. Hatcher, H.C.; Tesfay, L.; Torti, S.V.; Torti, F.M. Cytoprotective Effect of Ferritin H in Renal Ischemia Reperfusion Injury. *PLoS ONE* **2015**, *10*, e0138505. [CrossRef] [PubMed]
77. Scindia, Y.; Dey, P.; Thirunagari, A.; Liping, H.; Rosin, D.L.; Floris, M.; Okusa, M.D.; Swaminathan, S. Hepcidin Mitigates Renal Ischemia-Reperfusion Injury by Modulating Systemic Iron Homeostasis. *J. Am. Soc. Nephrol.* **2015**, *26*, 2800–2814. [CrossRef]
78. Roetto, A.; Papanikolaou, G.; Politou, M.; Alberti, F.; Girelli, D.; Christakis, J.; Loukopoulos, D.; Camaschella, C. Mutant antimicrobial peptide hepcidin is associated with severe juvenile hemochromatosis. *Nat. Genet.* **2003**, *33*, 21–22. [CrossRef]
79. Girelli, D.; Nemeth, E.; Swinkels, D.W. Hepcidin in the diagnosis of iron disorders. *Blood* **2016**, *127*, 2809–2813. [CrossRef]
80. Van Swelm, R.P.; Wetzels, J.F.; Verweij, V.G.; Laarakkers, C.M.; Pertijs, J.C.; van der Wijst, J.; Thevenod, F.; Masereeuw, R.; Swinkels, D.W. Renal Handling of Circulating and Renal-Synthesized Hepcidin and Its Protective Effects against Hemoglobin-Mediated Kidney Injury. *J. Am. Soc. Nephrol.* **2016**, *27*, 2720–2732. [CrossRef]
81. Bolisetty, S.; Zarjou, A.; Hull, T.D.; Traylor, A.M.; Perianayagam, A.; Joseph, R.; Kamal, A.I.; Arosio, P.; Soares, M.P.; Jeney, V.; et al. Macrophage and epithelial cell H-ferritin expression regulates renal inflammation. *Kidney Int.* **2015**, *88*, 95–108. [CrossRef] [PubMed]
82. Zarjou, A.; Black, L.M.; McCullough, K.R.; Hull, T.D.; Esman, S.K.; Boddu, R.; Varambally, S.; Chandrashekar, D.S.; Feng, W.; Arosio, P.; et al. Ferritin Light Chain Confers Protection Against Sepsis-Induced Inflammation and Organ Injury. *Front. Immunol.* **2019**, *10*, 131. [CrossRef] [PubMed]

83. Schiffrin, E.L.; Lipman, M.L.; Mann, J.F. Chronic kidney disease: Effects on the cardiovascular system. *Circulation* **2007**, *116*, 85–97. [CrossRef] [PubMed]
84. Bloembergen, W.E. Cardiac disease in chronic uremia: Epidemiology. *Adv. Ren. Replace. Ther.* **1997**, *4*, 185–193. [CrossRef]
85. Herzog, C.A.; Asinger, R.W.; Berger, A.K.; Charytan, D.M.; Diez, J.; Hart, R.G.; Eckardt, K.U.; Kasiske, B.L.; McCullough, P.A.; Passman, R.S.; et al. Cardiovascular disease in chronic kidney disease. A clinical update from Kidney Disease: Improving Global Outcomes (KDIGO). *Kidney Int.* **2011**, *80*, 572–586. [CrossRef] [PubMed]
86. Norton, J.M.; Newman, E.P.; Romancito, G.; Mahooty, S.; Kuracina, T.; Narva, A.S. CE: Improving Outcomes for Patients with Chronic Kidney Disease: Part 1. *Am. J. Nurs.* **2017**, *117*, 22–32. [CrossRef] [PubMed]
87. Covic, A.; Kanbay, M.; Voroneanu, L.; Turgut, F.; Serban, D.N.; Serban, I.L.; Goldsmith, D.J. Vascular calcification in chronic kidney disease. *Clin. Sci. (Lond.)* **2010**, *119*, 111–121. [CrossRef] [PubMed]
88. McIntyre, C.W. The functional cardiovascular consequences of vascular calcification. *Semin. Dial.* **2007**, *20*, 122–128. [CrossRef]
89. London, G.M.; Marchais, S.J.; Guerin, A.P.; Metivier, F. Arteriosclerosis, vascular calcifications and cardiovascular disease in uremia. *Curr. Opin. Nephrol. Hypertens.* **2005**, *14*, 525–531. [CrossRef]
90. Gusbeth-Tatomir, P.; Covic, A. Causes and consequences of increased arterial stiffness in chronic kidney disease patients. *Kidney Blood Press Res.* **2007**, *30*, 97–107. [CrossRef]
91. Goodman, W.G.; Goldin, J.; Kuizon, B.D.; Yoon, C.; Gales, B.; Sider, D.; Wang, Y.; Chung, J.; Emerick, A.; Greaser, L.; et al. Coronary-artery calcification in young adults with end-stage renal disease who are undergoing dialysis. *N. Engl. J. Med.* **2000**, *342*, 1478–1483. [CrossRef] [PubMed]
92. Lumpaopong, A.; Mathew, A.V.; John, E.; Jelnin, V.; Benedetti, E.; Testa, G.; Oberholzer, J.; Sankary, H.; Ruiz, C. Early coronary calcification in children and young adults with end-stage renal disease. *Transplant. Proc.* **2007**, *39*, 37–39. [CrossRef]
93. Jono, S.; Shioi, A.; Ikari, Y.; Nishizawa, Y. Vascular calcification in chronic kidney disease. *J. Bone Miner. Metab.* **2006**, *24*, 176–181. [CrossRef]
94. Yamada, S.; Giachelli, C.M. Vascular calcification in CKD-MBD: Roles for phosphate, FGF23, and Klotho. *Bone* **2017**, *100*, 87–93. [CrossRef] [PubMed]
95. Mizobuchi, M.; Towler, D.; Slatopolsky, E. Vascular calcification: The killer of patients with chronic kidney disease. *J. Am. Soc. Nephrol.* **2009**, *20*, 1453–1464. [CrossRef] [PubMed]
96. Zhu, D.; Mackenzie, N.C.; Farquharson, C.; Macrae, V.E. Mechanisms and clinical consequences of vascular calcification. *Front. Endocrinol. (Lausanne)* **2012**, *3*, 95. [CrossRef] [PubMed]
97. El-Abbadi, M.; Giachelli, C.M. Mechanisms of vascular calcification. *Adv. Chronic Kidney Dis.* **2007**, *14*, 54–66. [CrossRef] [PubMed]
98. Shroff, R.C.; Shanahan, C.M. The vascular biology of calcification. *Semin. Dial.* **2007**, *20*, 103–109. [CrossRef]
99. McCarty, M.F.; DiNicolantonio, J.J. The molecular biology and pathophysiology of vascular calcification. *Postgrad. Med.* **2014**, *126*, 54–64. [CrossRef]
100. Liberman, M.; Marti, L.C. Vascular Calcification Regulation by Exosomes in the Vascular Wall. *Adv. Exp. Med. Biol.* **2017**, *998*, 151–160.
101. Zarychanski, R.; Houston, D.S. Anemia of chronic disease: A harmful disorder or an adaptive, beneficial response? *CMAJ* **2008**, *179*, 333–337. [CrossRef]
102. Webster, A.C.; Nagler, E.V.; Morton, R.L.; Masson, P. Chronic Kidney Disease. *Lancet* **2017**, *389*, 1238–1252. [CrossRef]
103. Panwar, B.; Gutierrez, O.M. Disorders of Iron Metabolism and Anemia in Chronic Kidney Disease. *Semin. Nephrol.* **2016**, *36*, 252–261. [CrossRef] [PubMed]
104. Babitt, J.L.; Lin, H.Y. Mechanisms of anemia in CKD. *J. Am. Soc. Nephrol.* **2012**, *23*, 1631–1634. [CrossRef] [PubMed]
105. Ueda, N.; Takasawa, K. Role of Hepcidin-25 in Chronic Kidney Disease: Anemia and Beyond. *Curr. Med. Chem.* **2017**, *24*, 1417–1452. [CrossRef] [PubMed]
106. Cassat, J.E.; Skaar, E.P. Iron in infection and immunity. *Cell Host Microbe* **2013**, *13*, 509–519. [CrossRef] [PubMed]
107. Fuery, M.A.; Liang, L.; Kaplan, F.S.; Mohler, E.R., 3rd. Vascular ossification: Pathology, mechanisms, and clinical implications. *Bone* **2018**, *109*, 28–34. [CrossRef] [PubMed]

108. Burke, S.K. Phosphate is a uremic toxin. *J. Ren. Nutr.* **2008**, *18*, 27–32. [CrossRef] [PubMed]
109. Block, G.A.; Klassen, P.S.; Lazarus, J.M.; Ofsthun, N.; Lowrie, E.G.; Chertow, G.M. Mineral metabolism, mortality, and morbidity in maintenance hemodialysis. *J. Am. Soc. Nephrol.* **2004**, *15*, 2208–2218. [CrossRef]
110. Zarjou, A.; Jeney, V.; Arosio, P.; Poli, M.; Antal-Szalmas, P.; Agarwal, A.; Balla, G.; Balla, J. Ferritin prevents calcification and osteoblastic differentiation of vascular smooth muscle cells. *J. Am. Soc. Nephrol.* **2009**, *20*, 1254–1263. [CrossRef]
111. Lian, J.B.; Stein, G.S. Runx2/Cbfa1: A multifunctional regulator of bone formation. *Curr. Pharm. Des.* **2003**, *9*, 2677–2685. [CrossRef] [PubMed]
112. Rajendran, R.; Minqin, R.; Ronald, J.A.; Rutt, B.K.; Halliwell, B.; Watt, F. Does iron inhibit calcification during atherosclerosis? *Free Radic. Biol. Med.* **2012**, *53*, 1675–1679. [CrossRef] [PubMed]
113. Phan, O.; Maillard, M.; Peregaux, C.; Mordasini, D.; Stehle, J.C.; Funk, F.; Burnier, M. PA21, a new iron-based noncalcium phosphate binder, prevents vascular calcification in chronic renal failure rats. *J. Pharmacol. Exp. Ther.* **2013**, *346*, 281–289. [CrossRef] [PubMed]
114. Seto, T.; Hamada, C.; Tomino, Y. Suppressive effects of iron overloading on vascular calcification in uremic rats. *J. Nephrol.* **2014**, *27*, 135–142. [CrossRef] [PubMed]
115. Ciceri, P.; Elli, F.; Braidotti, P.; Falleni, M.; Tosi, D.; Bulfamante, G.; Block, G.A.; Cozzolino, M. Iron citrate reduces high phosphate-induced vascular calcification by inhibiting apoptosis. *Atherosclerosis* **2016**, *254*, 93–101. [CrossRef] [PubMed]
116. Carpentier, S.M.; Carpentier, A.F.; Chen, L.; Shen, M.; Quintero, L.J.; Witzel, T.H. Calcium mitigation in bioprosthetic tissues by iron pretreatment: The challenge of iron leaching. *Ann. Thorac. Surg.* **1995**, *60*, S332–S338. [CrossRef]
117. Neven, E.; De Schutter, T.M.; Behets, G.J.; Gupta, A.; D'Haese, P.C. Iron and vascular calcification. Is there a link? *Nephrol. Dial. Transplant.* **2011**, *26*, 1137–1145. [CrossRef]
118. Balogh, E.; Paragh, G.; Jeney, V. Influence of Iron on Bone Homeostasis. *Pharmaceuticals (Basel)* **2018**, *11*, 107. [CrossRef]
119. Jeney, V. Clinical Impact and Cellular Mechanisms of Iron Overload-Associated Bone Loss. *Front. Pharmacol.* **2017**, *8*, 77. [CrossRef]
120. Zarjou, A.; Jeney, V.; Arosio, P.; Poli, M.; Zavaczki, E.; Balla, G.; Balla, J. Ferritin ferroxidase activity: A potent inhibitor of osteogenesis. *J. Bone Miner. Res.* **2010**, *25*, 164–172. [CrossRef]
121. Fishbane, S.; Mathew, A.; Vaziri, N.D. Iron toxicity: Relevance for dialysis patients. *Nephrol. Dial. Transplant.* **2014**, *29*, 255–259. [CrossRef] [PubMed]
122. Afzali, B.; Goldsmith, D.J. Intravenous iron therapy in renal failure: Friend and foe? *J. Nephrol.* **2004**, *17*, 487–495. [PubMed]
123. Brewster, U.C. Intravenous iron therapy in end-stage renal disease. *Semin. Dial.* **2006**, *19*, 285–290. [CrossRef] [PubMed]
124. Zhang, Y.; Munday, R. Dithiolethiones for cancer chemoprevention: Where do we stand? *Mol. Cancer Ther.* **2008**, *7*, 3470–3479. [CrossRef] [PubMed]
125. Pietsch, E.C.; Chan, J.Y.; Torti, F.M.; Torti, S.V. Nrf2 mediates the induction of ferritin H in response to xenobiotics and cancer chemopreventive dithiolethiones. *J. Biol. Chem.* **2003**, *278*, 2361–2369. [CrossRef]
126. Becs, G.; Zarjou, A.; Agarwal, A.; Kovacs, K.E.; Becs, A.; Nyitrai, M.; Balogh, E.; Banyai, E.; Eaton, J.W.; Arosio, P.; et al. Pharmacological induction of ferritin prevents osteoblastic transformation of smooth muscle cells. *J. Cell. Mol. Med.* **2016**, *20*, 217–230. [CrossRef] [PubMed]
127. Sikura, K.E.; Potor, L.; Szerafin, T.; Zarjou, A.; Agarwal, A.; Arosio, P.; Poli, M.; Hendrik, Z.; Mehes, G.; Oros, M.; et al. Potential Role of H-Ferritin in Mitigating Valvular Mineralization. *Arterioscler. Thromb. Vasc. Biol.* **2019**, *39*, 413–431. [CrossRef]
128. Peacock, J.D.; Levay, A.K.; Gillaspie, D.B.; Tao, G.; Lincoln, J. Reduced sox9 function promotes heart valve calcification phenotypes in vivo. *Circ. Res.* **2010**, *106*, 712–719. [CrossRef]
129. Kraml, P. The role of iron in the pathogenesis of atherosclerosis. *Physiol. Res.* **2017**, *66*, S55–S67.
130. Das De, S.; Krishna, S.; Jethwa, A. Iron status and its association with coronary heart disease: Systematic review and meta-analysis of prospective studies. *Atherosclerosis* **2015**, *238*, 296–303. [CrossRef]
131. Silvestre, O.M.; Goncalves, A.; Nadruz, W., Jr.; Claggett, B.; Couper, D.; Eckfeldt, J.H.; Pankow, J.S.; Anker, S.D.; Solomon, S.D. Ferritin levels and risk of heart failure-the Atherosclerosis Risk in Communities Study. *Eur. J. Heart Fail.* **2017**, *19*, 340–347. [CrossRef] [PubMed]

132. Galesloot, T.E.; Janss, L.L.; Burgess, S.; Kiemeney, L.A.; den Heijer, M.; de Graaf, J.; Holewijn, S.; Benyamin, B.; Whitfield, J.B.; Swinkels, D.W.; et al. Iron and hepcidin as risk factors in atherosclerosis: What do the genes say? *BMC Genet.* **2015**, *16*, 79. [CrossRef] [PubMed]
133. Lapice, E.; Masulli, M.; Vaccaro, O. Iron deficiency and cardiovascular disease: An updated review of the evidence. *Curr. Atheroscler. Rep.* **2013**, *15*, 358. [CrossRef] [PubMed]
134. Sullivan, J.L. Do hemochromatosis mutations protect against iron-mediated atherogenesis? *Circ. Cardiovasc. Genet.* **2009**, *2*, 652–657. [CrossRef] [PubMed]

5

Unraveling Hepcidin Plasma Protein Binding: Evidence from Peritoneal Equilibration Testing

Laura E. Diepeveen [1,*], Coby M. Laarakkers [1], Hilde P.E. Peters [2], Antonius E. van Herwaarden [1], Hans Groenewoud [3], Joanna IntHout [3], Jack F. Wetzels [4], Rachel P.L. van Swelm [1] and Dorine W. Swinkels [1]

1 Department of Laboratory Medicine, Radboud University Medical Center, 6525 Nijmegen, The Netherlands
2 Department of Nephrology, Isala Hospital, 8025 Zwolle, The Netherlands
3 Department of Health Evidence, Radboud University Medical Center, 6525 Nijmegen, The Netherlands
4 Department of Nephrology, Radboud University Medical Center, 6525 Nijmegen, The Netherlands
* Correspondence: Laura.Diepeveen@radboudumc.nl

Abstract: Peptide hormone hepcidin regulates systemic iron metabolism and has been described to be partially bound to α2-macroglobulin and albumin in blood. However, the reported degree of hepcidin protein binding varies between <3% and ≈89%. Since protein-binding may influence hormone function and quantification, better insight into the degree of hepcidin protein binding is essential to fully understand the biological behavior of hepcidin and interpretation of its measurement in patients. Here, we used peritoneal dialysis to assess human hepcidin protein binding in a functional human setting for the first time. We measured freely circulating solutes in blood and peritoneal fluid of 14 patients with end-stage renal disease undergoing a peritoneal equilibration test to establish a curve describing the relation between molecular weight and peritoneal clearance. Calculated binding percentages of total cortisol and testosterone confirmed our model. The protein-bound fraction of hepcidin was calculated to be 40% (±23%). We, therefore, conclude that a substantial proportion of hepcidin is freely circulating. Although a large inter-individual variation in hepcidin clearance, besides patient-specific peritoneal transport characteristics, may have affected the accuracy of the determined binding percentage, we describe an important step towards unraveling human hepcidin plasma protein binding in vivo including the caveats that need further research.

Keywords: iron homeostasis; hepcidin; protein binding; peritoneal dialysis

---

1. Introduction

The peptide hormone hepcidin, produced by hepatocytes, regulates iron entry into the circulation and iron distribution throughout the body by degradation of the cellular iron exporter ferroportin [1]. Hormones can circulate freely or partially bound to carrier proteins in the human body [2,3]. These carrier proteins allow transport of non-soluble hormones through the blood plasma, prevent excretion, and function as a reservoir thereby regulating hormone bioavailability. The free hormone hypothesis indicates that most hormones are not capable of exerting their physiological effect in a protein-bound form [2,4–6]. Hence, for partially bound hormones, such as thyroxine, testosterone, triiodothyronine, and cortisol, assays were designed to specifically quantify the bioactive free hormone concentration [5,7–9].

It is suggested that hepcidin in blood is partially bound to both α2-macroglobulin (α2M) and albumin [10]. However, there is large controversy on the subject since the reported plasma protein-bound fraction of hepcidin varies between <3% and ≈89% [10–12]. Consequently, it is uncertain to what degree currently available analytical assays quantify (only) bioactive hepcidin. Differences in extent of quantification of the freely circulating hepcidin relative to the protein bound compound between assays may influence interpretation and comparability of hepcidin measurement and hampers recent achievements on standardization of hepcidin assays [13]. Characterization of the measured analyte will add the final aspect to the metrological traceability chain of hepcidin, which describes an unbroken calibration hierarchy from a measurement result to a defined reference in SI units. Additionally, unraveling the protein binding properties of hepcidin will improve our understanding of its biology and will allow its correct quantification, which is essential in the assessment and interpretation of the pharmacokinetic and pharmacodynamic effects of hepcidin agonist or antagonist therapies [1,14]. To address these issues, we aimed to study the degree of hepcidin protein binding in a functional human setting for the first time, rather than using previously reported in vitro (research) techniques [10,11], mice in vivo studies [11], or human ex vivo serum analysis [12]. Especially since current in vitro techniques to assess free hormone concentrations in diagnostic medicine, such as equilibrium dialysis and ultrafiltration methods, have limitations amongst which are risk for leakage, non-specific absorption of the hormone leading to low reproducibility, and bias of results, osmotic effects or the Gibbs-Donnan effect [15].

To circumvent the limitations of in vitro studies, we aimed to unravel hepcidin plasma protein binding with a new approach using the principle of peritoneal dialysis (PD). PD is a treatment option for patients with end-stage renal disease (ESRD), in which the peritoneal cavity is filled with dialysis fluid. During a certain dwell time, plasma components are transported into the peritoneal cavity. Transport of molecules is mainly driven by diffusion and ultrafiltration and depends on peritoneal membrane characteristics [16]. To assess these individual characteristics, all patients treated with PD frequently undergo a standardized and highly reproducible peritoneal equilibration test (PET) [17–19]. During a four-hour dialysis exchange, the peritoneal membrane transport function of a patient treated with PD is characterized to classify them as either a high, low, or average transporter in order to optimize the dwell time [17]. These peritoneal equilibration rates reflect peritoneal clearance (PC) and can be calculated using the dialysate-to-plasma ratio (D/P ratio) for any given solute that is transported from the peritoneal capillary blood into dialysate fluid. The transport rate over the peritoneal membrane into the peritoneal cavity is largely size-selective and thus the PC is inversely related to the radius or molecular weight (MW) of a molecule, regardless of molecular properties such as charge or hydrophobicity [20–24]. Therefore, the transport rate of small molecules that are bound to large plasma proteins will be determined by the size of the complex. This has been verified using the protein-bound solute p-cresol (MW: 108 Da), since its PC was found to be similar to β2-microglobulin (MW: 11,815 Da) [25]. Although a high PC was expected based on the low MW of p-cresol, its clearance was much lower, confirming protein-binding.

In this study, we measured hepcidin, along with known freely circulating and protein-bound solutes, in blood and dialysate of patients with ESRD undergoing PET. We used this model to explore its suitability to quantify hormone binding, and therefore to unravel the extent of hepcidin binding in the circulation, by studying if the measured PC of hepcidin fits the curve describing the relation between MW and PC of free circulating solutes.

2. Results

In total, 14 patients with ESRD participated in this study. Mean age was 67 years, total creatinine clearance was between 56.4 and 129.5 L/week/1.73 m^2, and residual creatinine clearance was between 25.7 and 100.0 L/week/1.73 m^2 (Table 1). The start time of the PET after an overnight dwell was between 8:30 a.m. and noon. Four patients used prednisone (Table 1), which interferes with both total and free cortisol measurement due to metabolism into prednisolone. Therefore, cortisol measurements were not performed in these patients.

Table 1. Patient characteristics.

ID	Age (yrs)	Gender (M/F)	Underlying Disease	Use of Prednisone [1]	Creatinine Clearance (L/week/1.73 m^2) Total (residual)	Start Time PET (a.m.)
1	73	F	Primary amyloidosis	No	61.1 (32.3)	10:00
2	82	M	Renal vascular disease due to hypertension	No	56.4 (25.7)	09:30
3	55	F	Lupus erythematosus	1 × 7.5 mg	99.3 (73.7)	10:00
4	74	M	Renal vascular disease due to hypertension	No	68.2 (34.5)	08:30
5	72	M	IgA nephropathy	No	118.2 (69.6)	10:00
6	64	M	Renal vascular disease type unspecified	1 × 7.5 mg	70.5 (37.1)	12:00
7	66	M	Diabetes mellitus type 2	No	100.8 (63.9)	10:15
8	53	M	Chronic renal failure etiology unknown/uncertain	No	71.7 (43.2)	12:00
9	76	M	Renal vascular disease due to hypertension	No	114.0 (75.7)	12:00
10	72	M	Renal vascular disease type unspecified	No	128.6 (100.0)	10:00
11	55	F	IgA nephropathy	2 × 5 mg	122.6 (77.8)	11:30
12	61	F	Renal vascular disease type unspecified	1 × 5 mg	129.5 (96.7)	11:00
13	64	F	Diabetes mellitus type 2	No	101.8 (35.9)	09:30
14	77	M	Renal vascular disease due to hypertension	No	118.1 (73.1)	09:00

[1] Since use of prednisone was found to decrease the serum cortisol concentrations and interferes with measurement of both free and total cortisol, these measurements were not performed in patients using prednisone.

We measured and subsequently calculated the PC of free circulating solutes urea, creatinine, β2-microglobulin, albumin, and IgG (Table 2), and plotted the logarithmically transformed PC of each analyte against its MW for each patient. By applying a linear mixed model, we obtained a curve with a 95% prediction interval describing the relation between MW and PC of free circulating solutes (Figure 1, solid dots). We found the equation defining the curve to be:

$$\text{Log10 (PC)} = 4.5744 - 0.05063 * \sqrt[3]{\text{MW}}. \quad (1)$$

Table 2. Molecular weight, measured plasma, and dialysate concentrations (mean ± sd) and subsequent calculated peritoneal clearances (mean ± sd) for all solutes.

Solute	MW (Da)	[Plasma] t = 0 h Mean (sd)	[Dialysate] [1] t = 1 h Mean (sd)	Peritoneal Clearance (μL/min) t = 0–1 h Mean (sd)	N
Urea (mmol/L)	60.0	21.5 (6.6)	15.0 (6.1)	26,959.1 (6211.8)	14
Creatinine (μmol/L)	113.1	542.0 (172.6)	296.9 (119.9)	21,499.6 (5861.6)	14
Testosterone, total (nmol/L) [2]	288.0	8.6 (7.3)	0.1 (0.1)	507.7 (260.5)	13 [3]
Cortisol, total (nmol/L) [4]	362.5	229.1 (134.4)	8.4 (5.8)	1439.0 (490.8)	10 [5]
Cortisol, free (nmol/L)	362.5	12.7 (7.7)	8.4 (5.8)	25,030.8 (8123.9)	9 [5,6]
Hepcidin (nmol/L)	2789.4	10.6 (9.1)	1.2 (1.1)	4337.5 (1713.1)	13 [7]
β2-microglobulin (mg/L)	13,713.0	18.7 (5.0)	1.4 (0.9)	2804.0 (1587.8)	14
Albumin (g/L)	66437.0	32.1 (4.9)	0.2 (0.1)	242.3 (164.2)	14
IgG (mg/L)	150,000.0	7496.0 (1730.3)	23.1 (12.7)	129.3 (84.7)	14

[1] Average dialysate volumes were 2364 mL (range 1500-2250 mL). [2] Approximately 2% of the total plasma testosterone is circulating free in both men and women [9,26]; in men 44–65% of testosterone is bound to sex hormone binding globulin and 33–54% bound to albumin; in women 66–78% of testosterone is bound to sex hormone binding globulin (MW 90 kDa), and 20–32% to albumin (MW 66,437 Da) [9]. [3] One patient was excluded since dialysate concentrations of testosterone were below the LLOD. [4] Approximately 5% of the total plasma cortisol is circulating free, since 80–90% of cortisol is bound to corticosteroid binding globulin (MW 52 kDa) and 10–15% to albumin (MW 66,437 Da) [6]. [5] Patient 3, 6, 11, and 12 used prednisone, which interferes with cortisol measurement. The results of these patients were excluded. [6] For one patient material was insufficient to measure free cortisol. [7] One patient was excluded since both plasma and dialysate concentrations of hepcidin were below the LLOD.

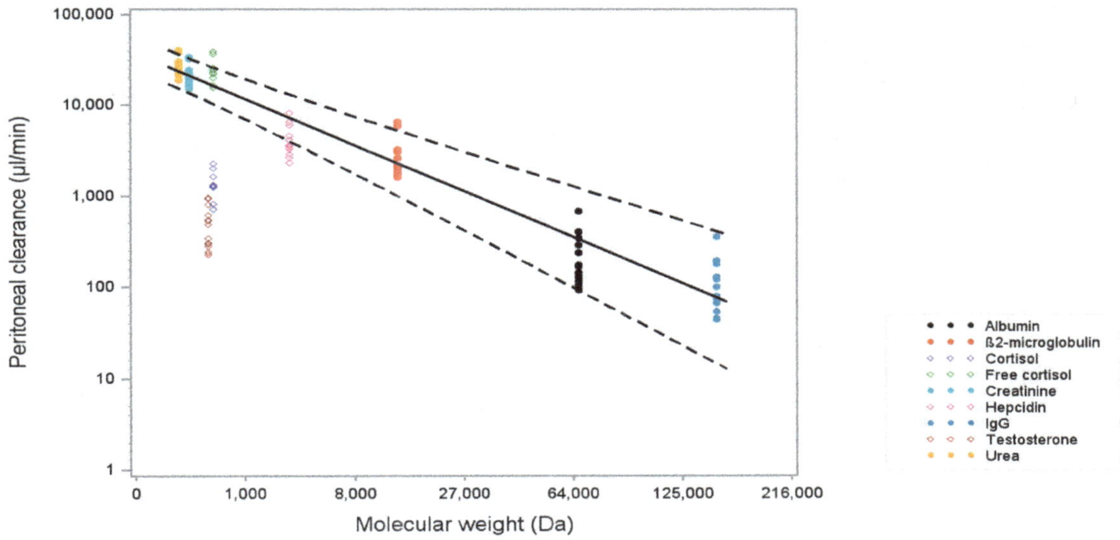

Figure 1. Peritoneal clearances (µL/min) as a function of molecular weight (Da). The logarithmically transformed peritoneal clearance (y-axis) of each specific analyte for each patient was plotted against the cube root of their molecular weight (x-axis). Based on the known free circulating analytes, i.e., urea, creatinine, β2-microglobulin, albumin, and IgG (solid dots), a curve was established describing the relation between clearance and molecular weight (solid line) with a 95% prediction interval (dashed lines). Hepcidin, free cortisol, total cortisol, and total testosterone measurements (open dots) were plotted in the figure thereafter.

We tested the validity of our model by measuring both total (i.e., free and protein-bound) and free cortisol and total testosterone. As expected, the PC measurements of total cortisol (Figure 1, open blue dots) and total testosterone (Figure 1, open brown dots) plotted against the MW of the unbound molecules were below the free solutes curve, confirming their predominantly bound status. Their binding percentages were calculated to be 91% (±3%) and 97% (±1.5%), respectively, corresponding to what is described in literature [6,9]. The mean of free cortisol PC measurements (Figure 1, open green dots) fell within the 95% confidence interval to the free solutes curve, confirming its unbound status.

We subsequently plotted the hepcidin PC measurements against the MW of hepcidin in the graph (Figure 1, open pink dots). Interestingly, the mean PC for hepcidin was found to lie below the established free solute curve. The calculated binding percentage is 40% (±23%), suggesting that hepcidin circulates in a more unbound than bound status, with a large inter-individual variability. Since several hepcidin PC measurements fell within the 95% confidence interval, we can exclude a predominantly protein-bound status of hepcidin, as we found for total cortisol and testosterone.

Last, we correlated the PC of all analytes with the PC of urea (Figure 2) to ensure that the variation in PC measurement of each analyte is solely caused by patient-specific transport characteristics. We have chosen urea for this since its PC measurements showed the lowest variation. We found a strong correlation between urea and creatinine (Spearman r = 0.9604, $p < 0.0001$), β2-microglobulin (Spearman r = 0.7890, $p = 0.0008$), free cortisol (Spearman r = 0.9333, $p = 0.0002$), total cortisol (Spearman r = 0.7697, $p = 0.0092$), and total testosterone (Spearman r = 0.6593, $p = 0.0142$). We observed a weaker correlation between urea and IgG (Spearman r = 0.5516, $p = 0.0408$) and urea and albumin (Spearman r = 0.5077, $p = 0.0638$). However, we did not find any correlation between urea and hepcidin (Spearman r = 0.2198, $p = 0.4706$). Further analysis showed that hepcidin does not correlate with any of the other analytes (Figure 3), except albumin (Spearman r = 0.6648, $p = 0.0132$). These results confirm a large inter-individual variation in hepcidin clearance, independent of peritoneal transport characteristics. Although this might influence the accuracy of the determined binding percentage, we conclude that a substantial proportion of hepcidin is freely circulating and exclude that circulating hepcidin is predominantly bound to plasma proteins.

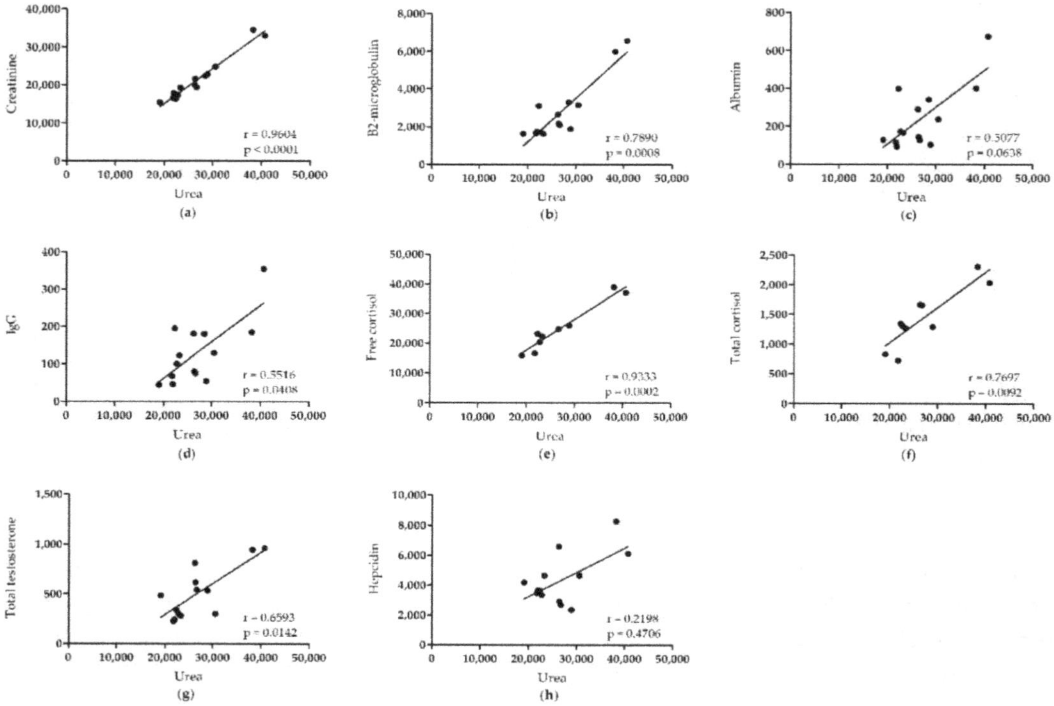

Figure 2. Correlations among the peritoneal clearance of urea with all analytes in patients with end-stage renal disease undergoing a peritoneal equilibration test. The peritoneal clearance of urea was correlated to the peritoneal clearance of (**a**) creatinine, (**b**) β2-microglobulin, (**c**) albumin, (**d**) IgG, (**e**) free cortisol, (**f**) total cortisol, (**g**) total testosterone, and (**h**) hepcidin. The strength of the correlation was measured using Spearman's correlation coefficient (r).

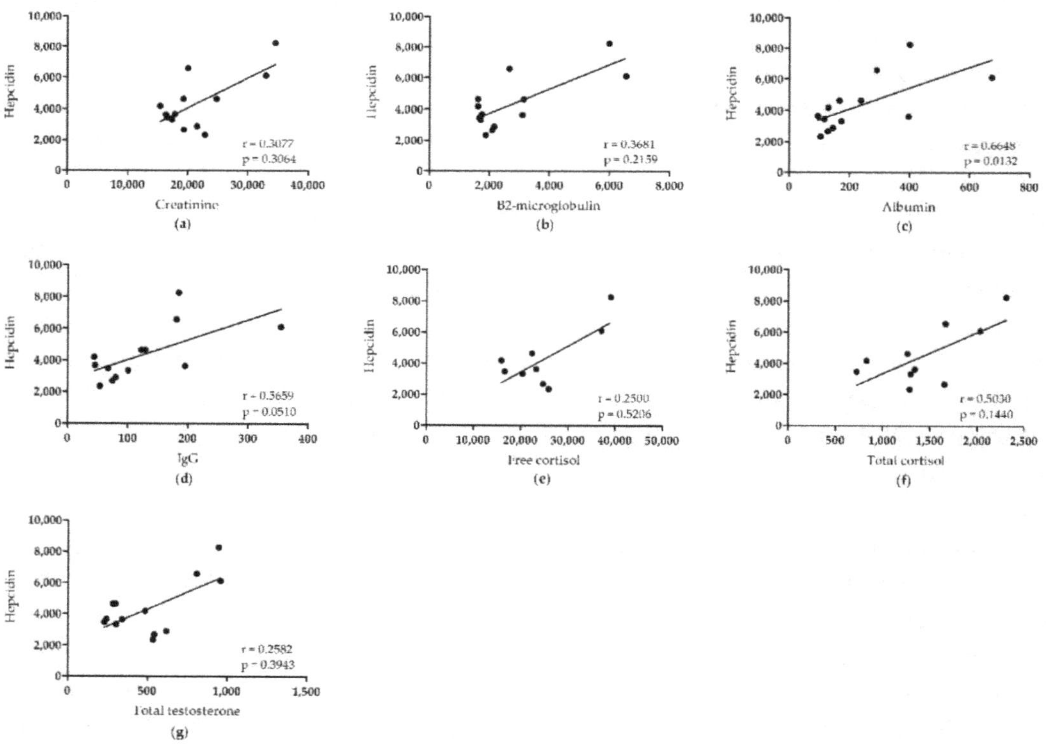

Figure 3. Correlations among the peritoneal clearance of hepcidin with all analytes in patients with end-stage renal disease undergoing a peritoneal equilibration test. The peritoneal clearance of hepcidin was correlated to the peritoneal clearance of (**a**) creatinine, (**b**) β2-microglobulin, (**c**) albumin, (**d**) IgG, (**e**) free cortisol, (**f**) total cortisol, and (**g**) total testosterone. The strength of the correlation was measured using Spearman's correlation coefficient (r).

3. Discussion

We applied the principle of PD to study the plasma protein binding of hepcidin in a functional human setting for the first time. To this end, we measured hepcidin along with known freely circulating and predominantly protein-bound solutes in blood and dialysate of patients with ESRD treated with PD undergoing PET. Our findings exclude that circulating hepcidin is predominantly bound to plasma proteins; however, the lack of correlation between hepcidin clearance and the clearance of the other analytes question the suitability of this model to determine an accurate binding percentage for this hormone.

Our finding that hepcidin is not predominantly bound is in line with other literature, in which a merely freely circulating hepcidin was observed using gel chromatography on human serum samples, followed by Liquid Chromatography-Mass Spectrometry (LC-MS/MS) [12]. In fact, other peptide hormones such as human growth hormone [27], insulin [28], and cardiac natriuretic hormones [29] circulate freely, since peptide hormones are often water-soluble and can, therefore, easily be transported via the cardiovascular system without requiring carrier proteins [30,31]. In addition, hepcidin is rapidly excreted by the kidneys, leading to a short half-life of only several hours [32–34]. Moreover, circulating hepcidin concentrations can change rapidly with subsequent effects on the circulating iron levels within 1–2 h [35,36]. Theoretically, this potential of a fast production [33,35,37] and quick turnover of hepcidin would preclude the need for protein binding [30].

Our observations differ from previous findings describing high hepcidin binding [10,11]. We believe this reported high binding percentage of ≈89% might be attributed to the excess of hepcidin (i.e., 100 times higher than physiological conditions) that was used in the experimental set-up, in combination with physiological α2M concentrations. This might have caused nonspecific binding of hepcidin, which the molecule is prone to due to its amphipathic character [38].

To the best of our knowledge, there are currently no established in vivo models to study protein binding and free drug or biomarker concentrations, which makes our explorative approach to study the functional protein binding of hormones unique. PET is regularly used as diagnostic test to characterize the functionality and transport properties of the peritoneal membrane in PD patients. Therefore, the strength of using PET is that dialysate sampling for research purposes provides human data with no additional burden for patients and it is a relatively simple, quick, and affordable method. Albeit we circumvent the disadvantages of in vitro techniques used to assess free hormone concentrations in diagnostic medicine, several limitations of our method were discovered during the study.

First, hepcidin did not correlate with urea or any of the other analytes, except albumin, suggesting that other variables besides patient-specific peritoneal transport characteristics may have affected hepcidin PC quantification. This raises the question if we can infer an accurate binding percentage for hepcidin, despite the fact that the validity of our model is confirmed by total cortisol and testosterone measurements and deduction of their binding percentages.

One of the possible explanations for the lack of correlation is the circadian rhythm of hepcidin, with plasma levels increasing during the day [39–43]. Due to practical concerns, blood and dialysate samples were not collected at the same time point, which could influence the determined hepcidin clearance differently for each patient. Nonetheless, in our previous study [43], the serum hepcidin median increased only by 2.5% between 11:00 and 13:30 amongst 24 participants. Therefore, the influence of hepcidins circadian rhythm seems unlikely since we used a time interval of only 1 h between blood and dialysate collection and PET start times were between 8:30 and noon. In addition, we did find a strong correlation between urea and both free and total cortisol, a hormone which also follows a circadian rhythm [44], suggesting the influence of a circadian rhythm is negligible.

Second, our study population suffers from ESRD and may therefore differ from healthy subjects, although there is no data to support the idea that peritoneal transport is affected by kidney function. It is described, however, that renal failure leads to the accumulation of uremic toxins in blood and tissues. These toxins can compete with other substrates for plasma protein binding to, for example, albumin [45]. As a result, the free fraction of a substrate of albumin will be increased. The strong correlation between hepcidin and albumin could imply binding of hepcidin to albumin and, therefore, the presence of uremic toxins might explain the observed inter-individual variability between hepcidin measurements. This might have led to an overestimation of the free fraction of hepcidin. However, testosterone and cortisol are also partially bound to albumin and we see no effect on their measurements. Therefore, interference of uremic toxins appears less likely. Nonetheless, we suggest our data should be validated and confirmed in healthy individuals or patients with a normal glomerular filtration rate.

Third, we cannot exclude our results are affected by production of hepcidin by mesothelial cells of the peritoneal membrane [46]. However, we feel that this is rather unlikely due to the high volume (2000 mL) new dialysate infused at t = 0 and the short dialysate time of 60 min.

Fourth, it is known that macromolecules may be removed from the peritoneal cavity by lymphatic absorption, which is independent of molecular size [47]. We observed a weak correlation between the small molecule urea and both macromolecules albumin and IgG. This might indicate that transport of these molecules is not solely dependent on permeability of the peritoneum, but also on lymphatic absorption, which would influence the established curve and could possibly introduce the observed inter-individual variation.

Last, clearance measurements of both hepcidin and albumin might be affected by their adherence to the dialysis bag, since both molecules possess nonspecific binding characteristics [38,48]. Due to their amphipathic character and suggested subsequent adherence to laboratory plastics, an extra factor of inter-individual variation is introduced, independent of patient specific peritoneal transport characteristics. This could explain the lack of correlation with other analytes. Regarding the assessment of hepcidins binding percentage, this would imply that the hepcidin concentration in dialysate, and therefore its clearance, might be underestimated and the free fraction would actually be higher.

Knowledge on the binding percentage of hepcidin is of great importance for correct quantification of the bioactive hormone, which in turn is key for both interpretation and standardization of hepcidin measurements in diagnostics of iron related disorders [1]. Characterization of hepcidin as measurand will add a key aspect to its metrological traceability chain that has recently been established, which is needed to obtain global uniform reference intervals and clinical decision limits for diagnostics [13]. Furthermore, correct analysis and interpretation of hepcidin measurement is essential in target assessment of clinical trials with hepcidin agonists and antagonists. These therapeutics are in development for treatment of several iron metabolism disorders such as hereditary hemochromatosis or anemia of inflammation [1,14]. A strong correlation has been observed between hepcidin-25 results of a wide variety of assays [13,49,50]. However, possible protein-binding could be an issue in correct hepcidin quantification when measuring target engagement of hepcidin antagonists that directly bind hepcidin in the circulation. These compounds display a high affinity for hepcidin and therefore specifically for the assessment of hepcidin antagonist efficiency, the remaining free, non-antagonist bound hepcidin should be quantified [51] rather than total hepcidin [52–54].

We can conclude that hepcidin is not predominantly bound and suggest that a substantial proportion is freely circulating, enabling direct and rapid bioactivity of the hormone. This is an important step towards unraveling human hepcidin plasma protein binding, although refinement of the model by inclusion of more patients and using more analytes with different MWs could help improve accuracy of our findings. Thereby, analytes with a high MW should preferably be excluded to circumvent influence of lymphatic absorption. Moreover, to definitively unravel hepcidin plasma protein binding, future studies must include studies on hepcidin production by mesothelial layer of the peritoneum and the prevention of nonspecific adherence of hepcidin in pre-analysis, which currently hampers (standard) dialysis techniques in diagnostic medicine.

4. Materials and Methods

4.1. Sample Collection

PET was performed according to the protocol of Isala hospital, Zwolle, The Netherlands. After an 10–12 h overnight dwell, a 2-Liter bag of 3.86% glucose solution (Baxter Healthcare Ltd., Newbury, UK) was instilled and allowed to dwell for 4 h [18]. Dialysate sampling was performed at 1 h of dwell time (t = 1 h), since peritoneal transport of solutes with a low MW (<200 Da) will decrease over a longer period of time due to saturation of the dialysate [22]. For sampling, all dialysate fluid was collected in a plastic (PVC) bag and mixed ex vivo before a sample was taken, to assure dialysate samples were representative for the fluid in the peritoneal cavity. Thereafter, the remaining dialysate was returned into the peritoneal cavity. Dialysate from 14 consecutive patients with ESRD who underwent PD was collected in tubes both with and without bovine serum albumin (1 g/50 mL, Sigma-Aldrich, Saint Louis, MO, USA), as for measurements of hepcidin and IgG, addition of albumin prevents adhesion to the tubes and subsequent loss. Blood samples were drawn prior to dialysis (t = 0 h) in both heparin plasma and serum tubes. All were centrifuged at 2000 g for 10 min. Blood and dialysate samples were aliquoted and immediately stored at −80 °C until measurement.

4.2. Laboratory Measurements

We measured total hepcidin concentrations (i.e., the sum of bound and unbound full length hepcidin-25), as well as freely circulating solutes urea, creatinine, β2-microglobulin, albumin, IgG, total testosterone (free and protein-bound), total cortisol (free and protein-bound), and free cortisol in blood and dialysate.

Analytical methods are described in Appendix A. All measurements were performed in freshly thawed aliquots within 8 months after collection.

4.3. Ethics

The study was approved by the Ethics Committee and the Board of Directors of Isala hospital, Zwolle, The Netherlands, and has been in accordance with the Helsinki Declaration. All patients signed informed consent prior to participation and all samples were blinded.

4.4. Calculations and Statistical Analysis

Measurement results for solutes below the lower limit of detection (LLOD) were excluded. We calculated PC (μL/min) for each analyte using the dialysate sample taken at t = 1 h and blood sample taken at t = 0 h of each analyte, using the patient-specific dialysate volume and a dialysis time of 60 min as:

$$\text{Peritoneal clearance } (\mu\text{L/min}) = [\text{Dialysate}]/[\text{Blood}] \times (\text{Volume dialysate})/(\text{Duration of dialysis}). \quad (2)$$

Logarithmic transformation was used for PC data before statistical analysis, as the data was not normally distributed. In addition, we used a cube root scaling for MW, since transport rates are related to size and thus radius (r), and considering volume as a three-dimensional characteristic of the radius (r^3). The curve describing the relation between MW and PC of all analytes was estimated with a linear mixed model using a random slope and random intercept. The expected PC of each analyte could be calculated using its MW and the equation of the curve. We calculated the binding percentage as:

$$\text{Binding percentage } (\%) = (1 - (\text{Measured PC})/(\text{Expected PC})) \times 100\%. \quad (3)$$

In this equation, the measured PC divided by the expected PC represents the free hormone fraction. The strength of a linear association between the clearances of two analytes was measured using Spearman's correlation coefficient.

All statistical analyses were performed with SAS software, version 9.4 (SAS Institute, Inc. Cary, NC, USA) and GraphPad Prism 5.03 (GraphPad Software Inc., La Jolla, CA, USA).

Author Contributions: Conceptualization, C.L.; H.P.; J.W. and D.S.; methodology, L.D.; C.L.; H.P.; J.W. and D.S.; software, H.G.; validation, A.H. and D.S.; formal analysis, H.G. and J.H.; investigation, L.D.; C.L. and H.P.; resources, C.L.; data curation, L.D.; writing—original draft preparation, L.D.; writing—review and editing, A.H.; R.S., J.W. and D.S.; visualization, H.G. and J.H.; supervision, D.S.; project administration, L.D.

Acknowledgments: We would like to thank the nurses of the dialysis department of Isala hospital for their help with collecting the samples during PET.

Appendix A

Laboratory Chemistry Measurements

Measurements of urea, creatinine, and IgG were performed on a Cobas C8000 random access analyzer (Roche Diagnostics, Basel, Switzerland). Albumin was measured by nephelometry on a BNII system (Siemens, München, Germany). β2-microglobulin was measured by a direct sandwich-ELISA, using two polyclonal rabbit anti-human β2-microglobulin antibodies, of which one was HRP labeled. The pH of all peritoneal dialysate samples was 7.5 allowing accurate measurements of β2-microglobulin.

Measurement of Hepcidin in Serum and Peritoneal Dialysate

Measurements of hepcidin were performed by a combination of weak cation exchange chromatography and time-of-flight mass spectrometry (WCX-TOF MS) using a stable hepcidin-25^{+40} isotope as internal standard for quantification [55]. This MS-based assay determines total hepcidin (i.e., the sum of bound and unbound fraction). Peptide spectra were generated on a Microflex LT matrix-enhanced laser desorption/ionisation TOF MS platform (Bruker Daltonics, Hamburg, Germany). Hepcidin concentrations were expressed as nmol/L. The lower limit of quantification of this method was 0.5 nM.

Measurement of Total Cortisol and Total Testosterone in Serum

Cortisol and testosterone were analyzed by Liquid Chromatography-Mass Spectrometry (LC-MS/MS) after protein precipitation and solid-phase extraction. Internal standard [$^2H_4$]-cortisol and [$^{13}C_3$]-testosterone (Isoscience, Ambler, PA, USA) was added to 100 μL serum. Subsequently, 300 μL acetonitrile with 0.1% formic acid was added for protein precipitation and 300 μL H_2O was added to 200 μL supernatant followed by solid phase extraction (Oasis HLB 1cc, Waters, Milford, MA, USA). The eluate (methanol:isopropanol 95:5) was dried under a stream of N_2 gas, reconstituted in methanol:water (3:7) and injected (10 μL) into an Agilent Technologies 1290 Infinity Ultra High Performance Liquid Chromatography (UHPLC)-system (Agilent Technologies, Agilent, Santa Clara, CA, USA) equipped with a BEH C18 (1.7 μm 2.1 × 50 mm) analytical column (Waters Corp.) at 60 °C. Mobile phase A (methanol:water 20:80 + 2 mM NH_4CH_3COO + 0.1% formic acid) and B (methanol:water 98:2 + 2 mM NH_4CH_3COO + 0.1% formic acid) were run in a gradient (0.4 mL/min). Start gradient 70:30 A:B for 2.5 min; then to 40:60 A:B in 3.5 min; followed by a gradient in 0.5 min to 2:98 to remain such for 0.5 min and thereafter to 70:30 A:B in 0.5 min and remain such for 0.5 min. Retention time was 1.41 min and 4.37 min for cortisol and testosterone, respectively. Total run time was 8 min. A 9-point calibration curve was used (cortisol and testosterone, Steraloids). An Agilent 6490 tandem mass spectrometer (Agilent Technologies, Agilent, Santa Clara, CA, USA) was operated in the electrospray positive ion mode, with a capillary voltage 3.5 kV, fragmentor voltage 380 V, sheath gas temperature 350 °C, and gas temperature 150 °C with N_2 collision gas. Two transitions (qualitative and quantitative) were monitored. Transitions (Q1 > Q3) were m/z 363.4 > 97.1 (34 V) and m/z 363.4 >

121.1 (25 V) for cortisol; m/z 367.4 > 97.1 (34 V) and m/z 367.4 > 121.1 (25 V) for [2H4]-cortisol. m/z 289.2 > 109.1 (30 kEV) and m/z 289.2 > 97.1 (30 kEV) for testosterone; m/z 292.3 > 112.1 (30 kEV) and m/z 292.3 > 100.1 (30 kEV) for 13C3-testosterone. Dwell time was 100 ms and 50 ms for cortisol and testosterone, respectively. The method was linear assessed by CLSI EP6 protocol [56]. For cortisol total CV is 3.6% at 300 nmol/L and 3.1% at 1080 nmol/L. For testosterone total CV is 6.0% at 0.9 nmol/L and 5.3% at 19 nmol/L.

Measurement of Free Cortisol in Serum by Equilibrium Dialysis—Liquid Chromatography Tandem Mass Spectrometry (LC-MS/MS)

Serum was dialyzed in a multi-cell equilibrium dialyzer using Teflon dialyzing cells consisting of two identical parts between which a flat membrane is fitted (Dianorm-Geräte). The dialysis cells are incubated in a water bath with constant agitation by a rotating apparatus and temperature during dialysis was maintained at 37 ± 0.5 °C, by constant monitoring with an immersion thermostatic system (Tinytag TGP-4020 logger and PB5001-1M5 sonde; Gemini data loggers). The dialysis membranes were prepared from Dianorm (Diachema dialysis membranes 10.14) with a cut-off of 5 kDa. Equilibrium dialysis was performed for 5 h with 180 µL serum against 180 µL HEPES buffer; while rotating the dialysis apparatus at 20 rpm. The HEPES buffer used for equilibrium dialysis was composed to reflect the electrolyte composition and pH of serum and contained in addition to 12.570 g/L N-(2-hydroxyethyl)piperazine-N′-(2-ethanesulfonic acid (HEPES), 5.353 g/L NaCl, 0.200 g/L KCl, 0.224 g/L KH_2PO_4, 0.275 g/L $MgSO_4{\cdot}7\,H_2O$, 0.300 g/L urea, 0.275 g/L $CaCl_2{\cdot}2\,H_2O$, 0.900 g/L NaOH, and 0.520 g/L NaN_3 (Merck, Darmstadt, Germany). The pH was adjusted with HCl to pH 7.40 (at 37 °C). The buffer was diluted by ultrapure water produced with a Milli Advantage A10 and 100 µL dialysate was subsequently used for total cortisol measurement by LC-MS/MS as described above.

Measurement of Total Cortisol and Total Testosterone in Peritoneal Dialysate

Testosterone and cortisol in peritoneal dialysate were analyzed by LC-MS/MS after solid-phase extraction. Sample preparation consisted of internal standard addition [13C3]-testosterone (Isoscience, Ambler, PA, USA) and [$^3H_4$]-cortisol (Isoscience) to 1000 µL dialysate and solid phase extraction (SPE) using Oasis® MCX 1cc cartridges (Waters Corp, Milford, MA, USA).

Columns were pre-equilibrated with 1 mL MeOH:IPA (95:5) and subsequently washed with 1 mL H_2O. After application of the sample, columns were washed with 1 mL H_2O:NH_4OH (95:5) and 1 mL MeOH:H_2O (20/80) + 2% HCOOH. The 300 µL eluate (MeOH) was dried under a stream of N_2 gas, reconstituted in MeOH:H_2O (30:70). A nine-point calibration series was used (using testosterone and cortisol both from Steraloids). Calibrators, quality controls, and samples (reconstituted in 100 µL) were injected (10 µL) into an Agilent Technologies 1290 Infinity VL UHPLC-system (Agilent Technologies, Santa Clara, USA), equipped with a BEH C18 (1.7 µm 2.1 X 50 mm) analytical column (Waters Corp., Milford, MA, USA) at 60 °C. Mobile phase A (MeOH/H_2O (20:80) + 2 mM NH_4CH_3COO + 0.1% HCOOH) and B (MeOH/H_2O (98:2) + 2 mM NH_4CH_3COO + 0.1% HCOOH) were run in a gradient (0.4 mL/min). The gradient program was as follows: Start gradient A:B (70:30) for 2.5 min; followed by a gradient in 2 min to A:B (60:40) and subsequent 2.5 min A:B (35:65). For column washing, a gradient 0.5 min A:B (98:2) was established to remain such for 0.5 min. The column was re-equilibrated to A:B (70:30) in 0.5 min and remained such for 0.5 min. Retention times were 1.5 min and 4.5 min for cortisol and testosterone, respectively. An Agilent 6490 tandem mass spectrometer (Agilent Technologies, Santa Clara, CA, USA) was operated in the electrospray positive ion mode. Operating conditions were as follows: Capillary voltage 3.5 kV, fragmentor voltage 380 V, sheath gas temperature 350 °C, and gas temperature 150 °C. The collision energy was optimized between 25 and 34 eV for all solutes and Nitrogen was used as collision gas. Two mass transitions were monitored for each analyte and the internal standards. The first transition was used for quantification, the second for confirmation. The transitions (Q1 > Q3) were m/z 289 > 97 and m/z 289 > 109 for testosterone; m/z 292 > 100 and m/z

292 > 112 for [13C3]-testosterone; m/z 363 > 121 and m/z 363 > 97 for cortisol; m/z 367 > 121 and m/z 367 > 97 for [3H4]-cortisol. Total run time was 9 min.

For both total and free cortisol PC calculations, we used total cortisol measurements in dialysate, since we assume that all cortisol present in dialysate after 1 h of dwell time is free considering the large MW of its main binding protein corticosteroid binding globulin (MW 52 kDa).

References

1. Girelli, D.; Nemeth, E.; Swinkels, D.W. Hepcidin in the diagnosis of iron disorders. *Blood* **2016**, *127*, 2809–2813. [CrossRef] [PubMed]
2. Ekins, R. Measurement of free hormones in blood. *Endocr. Rev.* **1990**, *11*, 5–46. [CrossRef] [PubMed]
3. Ekins, R. The free hormone hypothesis and measurement of free hormones. *Clin. Chem.* **1992**, *38*, 1289–1293.
4. Mendel, C.M. The free hormone hypothesis: A physiologically based mathematical model. *Endocr. Rev.* **1989**, *10*, 232–274. [CrossRef] [PubMed]
5. Faix, J.D. Principles and pitfalls of free hormone measurements. *Best Pract. Res. Clin. Endocrinol. Metab.* **2013**, *27*, 631–645. [CrossRef] [PubMed]
6. Bae, Y.J.; Kratzsch, J. Corticosteroid-binding globulin: Modulating mechanisms of bioavailability of cortisol and its clinical implications. *Best Pract. Res. Clin. Endocrinol. Metab.* **2015**, *29*, 761–772. [CrossRef]
7. Thienpont, L.M.; Van Uytfanghe, K.; Poppe, K.; Velkeniers, B. Determination of free thyroid hormones. *Best Pract. Res. Clin. Endocrinol. Metab.* **2013**, *27*, 689–700. [CrossRef]
8. Morley, J.E.; Patrick, P.; Perry, H.M. Evaluation of assays available to measure free testosterone. *Metabolism* **2002**, *51*, 554–559. [CrossRef]
9. Shea, J.; Wong, P.; Chen, Y. Free Testosterone: Clinical Utility and Important Analytical Aspects of Measurement. *Adv. Clin. Chem.* **2014**, *63*, 59–84.
10. Peslova, G.; Petrak, J.; Kuzelova, K.; Hrdy, I.; Halada, P.; Kuchel, P.W.; Soe-Lin, S.; Ponka, P.; Sutak, R.; Becker, E.; et al. Hepcidin, the hormone of iron metabolism, is bound specifically to alpha-2-macroglobulin in blood. *Blood* **2009**, *113*, 6225–6236. [CrossRef]
11. Huang, M.L.; Austin, C.J.; Sari, M.A.; Rahmanto, Y.S.; Ponka, P.; Vyoral, D.; Richardson, D.R. Hepcidin bound to alpha2-macroglobulin reduces ferroportin-1 expression and enhances its activity at reducing serum iron levels. *J. Biol. Chem.* **2013**, *288*, 25450–25465. [CrossRef] [PubMed]
12. Itkonen, O.; Stenman, U.H.; Parkkinen, J.; Soliymani, R.; Baumann, M.; Hamalainen, E. Binding of hepcidin to plasma proteins. *Clin. Chem.* **2012**, *58*, 1158–1160. [CrossRef] [PubMed]
13. Diepeveen, L.E.; Laarakkers, C.M.M.; Martos, G.; Pawlak, M.E.; Uguz, F.F.; Verberne, K.; van Swelm, R.P.L.; Klaver, S.; de Haan, A.F.J.; Pitts, K.R.; et al. Provisional standardization of hepcidin assays: Creating a traceability chain with a primary reference material, candidate reference method and a commutable secondary reference material. *Clin. Chem. Lab. Med.* **2019**, *57*, 864–872. [CrossRef] [PubMed]
14. Crielaard, B.J.; Lammers, T.; Rivella, S. Targeting iron metabolism in drug discovery and delivery. *Nat. Rev. Drug Discov.* **2017**, *16*, 400–423. [CrossRef] [PubMed]
15. Bowers, W.F.; Fulton, S.; Thompson, J. Ultrafiltration vs. equilibrium dialysis for determination of free fraction. *Clin. Pharmacokinet.* **1984**, *9* (Suppl. 1), 49–60. [CrossRef] [PubMed]
16. Khanna, R. Solute and Water Transport in Peritoneal Dialysis: A Case-Based Primer. *Am. J. Kidney Dis.* **2017**, *69*, 461–472. [CrossRef] [PubMed]
17. Twardowski, Z.J.; Nolph, K.D.; Khanna, R.; Prowant, B.F.; Ryan, L.P.; Moore, H.L.; Nielsen, M.P. Peritoneal equilibration test. *Perit. Dial. Bull.* **1987**, *7*, 138–147.
18. Ho-dac-Pannekeet, M.M.; Schouten, N.; Langendijk, M.J.; Hiralall, J.K.; de Waart, D.R.; Struijk, D.G.; Krediet, R.T. Peritoneal transport characteristics with glucose polymer based dialysate. *Kidney Int.* **1996**, *50*, 979–986. [CrossRef] [PubMed]
19. Trivedi, H.; Khanna, R.; Lo, W.K.; Prowant, B.F.; Nolph, K.D. Reproducibility of the peritoneal equilibration test in CAPD patients. *ASAIO J.* **1994**, *40*, M892-5. [CrossRef]
20. Krediet, R.T.; Boeschoten, E.W.; Struijk, D.G.; Arisz, L. Differences in the peritoneal transport of water, solutes and proteins between dialysis with two- and with three-litre exchanges. *Nephrol. Dial. Transplant.* **1988**, *3*, 198–204.
21. Teitelbaum, I.; Burkart, J. Peritoneal dialysis. *Am. J. Kidney Dis.* **2003**, *42*, 1082–1096. [CrossRef] [PubMed]

22. Kagan, A.; Bar-Khayim, Y.; Schafer, Z.; Fainaru, M. Kinetics of peritoneal protein loss during CAPD: I. Different characteristics for low and high molecular weight proteins. *Kidney Int.* **1990**, *37*, 971–979. [CrossRef] [PubMed]
23. Kabanda, A.; Goffin, E.; Bernard, A.; Lauwerys, R.; van Ypersele de Strihou, C. Factors influencing serum levels and peritoneal clearances of low molecular weight proteins in continuous ambulatory peritoneal dialysis. *Kidney Int.* **1995**, *48*, 1946–1952. [CrossRef] [PubMed]
24. Struijk, D.G. Monitoring of the peritoneal membrane. *NDT Plus* **2008**, *1*, 29–35. [CrossRef] [PubMed]
25. Bammens, B.; Evenepoel, P.; Verbeke, K.; Vanrenterghem, Y. Removal of middle molecules and protein-bound solutes by peritoneal dialysis and relation with uremic symptoms. *Kidney Int.* **2003**, *64*, 2238–2243. [CrossRef] [PubMed]
26. Bhasin, S.; Cunningham, G.R.; Hayes, F.J.; Matsumoto, A.M.; Snyder, P.J.; Swerdloff, R.S.; Montori, V.M. Testosterone therapy in men with androgen deficiency syndromes: An Endocrine Society clinical practice guideline. *J. Clin. Endocrinol. Metab.* **2010**, *95*, 2536–2559. [CrossRef] [PubMed]
27. Frantz, A.G.; Rabkin, M.T. Human Growth Hormone. *N. Engl. J. Med.* **1964**, *271*, 1375–1381. [CrossRef]
28. Hua, Q. Insulin: A small protein with a long journey. *Protein Cell* **2010**, *1*, 537–551. [CrossRef]
29. Clerico, A.; Del Ry, S.; Giannessi, D. Measurement of cardiac natriuretic hormones (atrial natriuretic peptide, brain natriuretic peptide, and related peptides) in clinical practice: The need for a new generation of immunoassay methods. *Clin. Chem.* **2000**, *46*, 1529–1534.
30. Malandrino, N.; Smith, R.J. Synthesis, secretion, and transport of peptide hormones. In *Principles of Endocrinology and Hormone Action*; Belfiroe, A., LeRoith, D., Eds.; Springer International Publishing: New York, NY, USA, 2018; Volume 1, pp. 29–42.
31. Kronenberg, H. *Williams Textbook of Endocrinology*, 13th ed.; Elsevier: Amsterdam, The Netherlands, 2016; Chapter 1; pp. 1–11.
32. van Swelm, R.P.; Wetzels, J.F.; Verweij, V.G.; Laarakkers, C.M.; Pertijs, J.C.; van der Wijst, J.; Thevenod, F.; Masereeuw, R.; Swinkels, D.W. Renal Handling of Circulating and Renal-Synthesized Hepcidin and Its Protective Effects against Hemoglobin-Mediated Kidney Injury. *J. Am. Soc. Nephrol.* **2016**, *27*, 2720–2732. [CrossRef]
33. Nemeth, E.; Rivera, S.; Gabayan, V.; Keller, C.; Taudorf, S.; Pedersen, B.K.; Ganz, T. IL-6 mediates hypoferremia of inflammation by inducing the synthesis of the iron regulatory hormone hepcidin. *J. Clin. Investig.* **2004**, *113*, 1271–1276. [CrossRef] [PubMed]
34. Rivera, S.; Liu, L.; Nemeth, E.; Gabayan, V.; Sorensen, O.E.; Ganz, T. Hepcidin excess induces the sequestration of iron and exacerbates tumor-associated anemia. *Blood* **2005**, *105*, 1797–1802. [CrossRef] [PubMed]
35. Kemna, E.; Pickkers, P.; Nemeth, E.; van der Hoeven, H.; Swinkels, D. Time-course analysis of hepcidin, serum iron, and plasma cytokine levels in humans injected with LPS. *Blood* **2005**, *106*, 1864–1866. [CrossRef] [PubMed]
36. Rivera, S.; Nemeth, E.; Gabayan, V.; Lopez, M.A.; Farshidi, D.; Ganz, T. Synthetic hepcidin causes rapid dose-dependent hypoferremia and is concentrated in ferroportin-containing organs. *Blood* **2005**, *106*, 2196–2199. [CrossRef] [PubMed]
37. Moretti, D.; Goede, J.S.; Zeder, C.; Jiskra, M.; Chatzinakou, V.; Tjalsma, H.; Melse-Boonstra, A.; Brittenham, G.; Swinkels, D.W.; Zimmermann, M.B. Oral iron supplements increase hepcidin and decrease iron absorption from daily or twice-daily doses in iron-depleted young women. *Blood* **2015**, *126*, 1981–1989. [CrossRef] [PubMed]
38. Hunter, H.N.; Fulton, D.B.; Ganz, T.; Vogel, H.J. The solution structure of human hepcidin, a peptide hormone with antimicrobial activity that is involved in iron uptake and hereditary hemochromatosis. *J. Biol. Chem.* **2002**, *277*, 37597–37603. [CrossRef]
39. Galesloot, T.E.; Vermeulen, S.H.; Geurts-Moespot, A.J.; Klaver, S.M.; Kroot, J.J.; van Tienoven, D.; Wetzels, J.F.; Kiemeney, L.A.; Sweep, F.C.; den Heijer, M.; et al. Serum hepcidin: Reference ranges and biochemical correlates in the general population. *Blood* **2011**, *117*, 218–225. [CrossRef]
40. Kemna, E.H.; Tjalsma, H.; Podust, V.N.; Swinkels, D.W. Mass spectrometry-based hepcidin measurements in serum and urine: Analytical aspects and clinical implications. *Clin. Chem.* **2007**, *53*, 620–628. [CrossRef]
41. Ganz, T.; Olbina, G.; Girelli, D.; Nemeth, E.; Westerman, M. Immunoassay for human serum hepcidin. *Blood* **2008**, *112*, 4292–4297. [CrossRef]

42. Schaap, C.C.; Hendriks, J.C.; Kortman, G.A.; Klaver, S.M.; Kroot, J.J.; Laarakkers, C.M.; Wiegerinck, E.T.; Tjalsma, H.; Janssen, M.C.; Swinkels, D.W. Diurnal rhythm rather than dietary iron mediates daily hepcidin variations. *Clin. Chem.* **2013**, *59*, 527–535. [CrossRef]
43. Kroot, J.J.; Hendriks, J.C.; Laarakkers, C.M.; Klaver, S.M.; Kemna, E.H.; Tjalsma, H.; Swinkels, D.W. (Pre)analytical imprecision, between-subject variability, and daily variations in serum and urine hepcidin: Implications for clinical studies. *Anal. Biochem.* **2009**, *389*, 124–129. [CrossRef] [PubMed]
44. Chan, S.; Debono, M. Replication of cortisol circadian rhythm: New advances in hydrocortisone replacement therapy. *Ther. Adv. Endocrinol. Metab.* **2010**, *1*, 129–138. [CrossRef] [PubMed]
45. Santana, M.T.; Cerini, C.; Burtey, S. Emerging Roles of Aryl Hydrocarbon Receptors in the Altered Clearance of Drugs during Chronic Kidney Disease. *Toxins* **2019**, *11*, 209. [CrossRef] [PubMed]
46. Evans, P.; Cindrova-Davies, T.; Muttukrishna, S.; Burton, G.J.; Porter, J.; Jauniaux, E. Hepcidin and iron species distribution inside the first-trimester human gestational sac. *Mol. Hum. Reprod.* **2011**, *17*, 227–232. [CrossRef] [PubMed]
47. Krediet, R.T.; Struijk, D.G.; Koomen, G.C.; Hoek, F.J.; Arisz, L. The disappearance of macromolecules from the peritoneal cavity during continuous ambulatory peritoneal dialysis (CAPD) is not dependent on molecular size. *Perit. Dial. Int.* **1990**, *10*, 147–152. [PubMed]
48. Finn, T.E.; Nunez, A.C.; Sunde, M.; Easterbrook-Smith, S.B. Serum albumin prevents protein aggregation and amyloid formation and retains chaperone-like activity in the presence of physiological ligands. *J. Biol. Chem.* **2012**, *287*, 21530–21540. [CrossRef] [PubMed]
49. Kroot, J.J.; Kemna, E.H.; Bansal, S.S.; Busbridge, M.; Campostrini, N.; Girelli, D.; Hider, R.C.; Koliaraki, V.; Mamalaki, A.; Olbina, G.; et al. Results of the first international round robin for the quantification of urinary and plasma hepcidin assays: Need for standardization. *Haematologica* **2009**, *94*, 1748–1752. [CrossRef]
50. Kroot, J.J.; van Herwaarden, A.E.; Tjalsma, H.; Jansen, R.T.; Hendriks, J.C.; Swinkels, D.W. Second round robin for plasma hepcidin methods: First steps toward harmonization. *Am. J. Hematol.* **2012**, *87*, 977–983. [CrossRef]
51. Hohlbaum, A.M.; Gille, H.; Trentmann, S.; Kolodziejczyk, M.; Rattenstetter, B.; Laarakkers, C.M.; Katzmann, G.; Christian, H.J.; Andersen, N.; Allersdorfer, A.; et al. Sustained plasma hepcidin suppression and iron elevation by Anticalin-derived hepcidin antagonist in cynomolgus monkey. *Br. J. Pharmacol.* **2018**, *175*, 1054–1065. [CrossRef]
52. Boyce, M.; Warrington, S.; Cortezi, B.; Zollner, S.; Vauleon, S.; Swinkels, D.W.; Summo, L.; Schwoebel, F.; Riecke, K. Safety, pharmacokinetics and pharmacodynamics of the anti-hepcidin Spiegelmer lexaptepid pegol in healthy subjects. *Br. J. Pharmacol.* **2016**, *173*, 1580–1588. [CrossRef]
53. van Eijk, L.T.; John, A.S.E.; Schwoebel, F.; Summo, L.; Vauléon, S.; Zöllner, S.; Laarakkers, C.M.; Kox, M.; van der Hoeven, J.G.; Swinkels, D.W.; et al. Effect of the antihepcidin Spiegelmer lexaptepid on inflammation-induced decrease in serum iron in humans. *Blood* **2014**, *124*, 2643–2646. [CrossRef] [PubMed]
54. Cooke, K.S.; Hinkle, B.; Salimi-Moosavi, H.; Foltz, I.; King, C.; Rathanaswami, P.; Winters, A.; Steavenson, S.; Begley, C.G.; Molineux, G.; et al. A fully human anti-hepcidin antibody modulates iron metabolism in both mice and nonhuman primates. *Blood* **2013**, *122*, 3054–3061. [CrossRef] [PubMed]
55. Laarakkers, C.M.; Wiegerinck, E.T.; Klaver, S.; Kolodziejczyk, M.; Gille, H.; Hohlbaum, A.M.; Tjalsma, H.; Swinkels, D.W. Improved mass spectrometry assay for plasma hepcidin: Detection and characterization of a novel hepcidin isoform. *PLoS ONE* **2013**, *8*, 75518. [CrossRef] [PubMed]
56. NCCLS; Tholen, D.W.; Kroll, M.; Astles, J.R.; Caffo, A.L.; Happe, T.M.; Krouwer, J.; Lasky, F. *Evaluation of the Linearity of Quantitative Measurement Procedures: A Statistical Approach; Approved Guideline*; Clinical Laboratory Standard Institute: Wayne, PA, USA, 2003.

6

The Efficacy of Iron Chelators for Removing Iron from Specific Brain Regions and the Pituitary—Ironing out the Brain

Robert R. Crichton [1], Roberta J. Ward [2,*] and Robert C. Hider [3]

1 Faculty of Science, Universite catholique de Louvain, 1348 Louvain-la-Neuve, Belgium; robert.crichton@uclouvain.be
2 Division of Brain Sciences, Imperial College, London W12 ONN, UK
3 Institute of Pharmaceutical Science, King's College London, London SE1 9NH, UK; robert.hider@kcl.ac.uk
* Correspondence: Rward2@ic.ac.uk

Abstract: Iron chelation therapy, either subcutaneous or orally administered, has been used successfully in various clinical conditions. The removal of excess iron from various tissues, e.g., the liver spleen, heart, and the pituitary, in beta thalassemia patients, has become an essential therapy to prolong life. More recently, the use of deferiprone to chelate iron from various brain regions in Parkinson's Disease and Friederich's Ataxia has yielded encouraging results, although the side effects, in <2% of Parkinson's Disease(PD) patients, have limited its long-term use. A new class of hydroxpyridinones has recently been synthesised, which showed no adverse effects in preliminary trials. A vital question remaining is whether inflammation may influence chelation efficacy, with a recent study suggesting that high levels of inflammation may diminish the ability of the chelator to bind the excess iron.

Keywords: iron; chelation; neurodegenerative diseases; pituitary; brain

---

1. Introduction

Iron is one of the essential elements in the body, the concentration of which is tightly regulated to prevent toxicity. Iron overload, particularly in the liver and spleen, is known to occur in several conditions, such as hereditary hemochromatosis, African iron overload, sickle cell disease, beta thalassemia, sideroblastic anaemia, enzyme deficiency (pyruvate kinase, glucose-6-phosphate dehydrogenase), and rare disorders of proteins involved in iron transport (atransferrinaemia, aceruloplasminemia). In certain conditions, e.g., sickle cell anaemia, beta thalassemia, and myelodysplasia, regular blood transfusions are an essential part of the therapy, thereby contributing to the increased iron stores, as the body is unable to excrete iron to any great extent. However, little focus has been directed at the brain iron concentrations in these conditions. Furthermore, it is also apparent that aging and neurodegenerative diseases, such as Parkinson's and Alzheimer's Disease, as well as Friederich's Ataxia, are associated with an increasing brain iron accumulation [1]. With the advent of several magnetic resonance imaging (MRI) techniques over the past 10 years it is now possible to measure pituitary and brain iron in specific brain regions and to monitor changes in its concentration after iron chelation therapy. Iron deposits are not assayed directly, but their effects on water protons as they diffuse in the magnetically inhomogeneous environment induced by iron deposition are assessed. The scanner transmits energy into the body as microwaves, followed by a waiting period, after which the energy is recalled, to be received by an antennae or coil. This process is known as relaxation and is characterised by relaxation rates R2 and R2* (measured in Hz), which are mathematically inverse of the characteristic relaxation times T2 and T2* (measured in ms).

2. Iron chelation

The chelation of excessive amounts of iron from the liver and spleen and, more recently, from the pituitary gland and the brain, has been utilised as a therapeutic approach. In what follows, we will outline the development of the most important therapeutic application of iron chelation therapy to date, namely in the treatment of thalassemia [2–5] and neurodegenerative diseases [1].

Iron Chelators in Current Clinical Use

The hexadentate chelator, deferrioxamine (DFO) (Figure 1), a bacterial hydroxamate siderophore, was introduced in the early 1970s, and initially gave poor results because it was not active by oral administration, and had a short half-life (20–30 min). However, the development of continuous subcutaneous infusion of DFO by a portable pump [6] and the establishment of sensible schedules for the optimal use of the pump [7] meant that by the 1990s markedly prolonged cardiac disease-free survival in patents, who faithfully followed the Propper and Pippard regime, could be demonstrated in three independent studies [8–10]. However, sadly, half of the patients, who could not or would not comply, developed cardiac failure or arrhythmia much more rapidly [11]. What was urgently required was a chelator which could be used more easily, thereby improving compliance, and which was both effective and orally active.

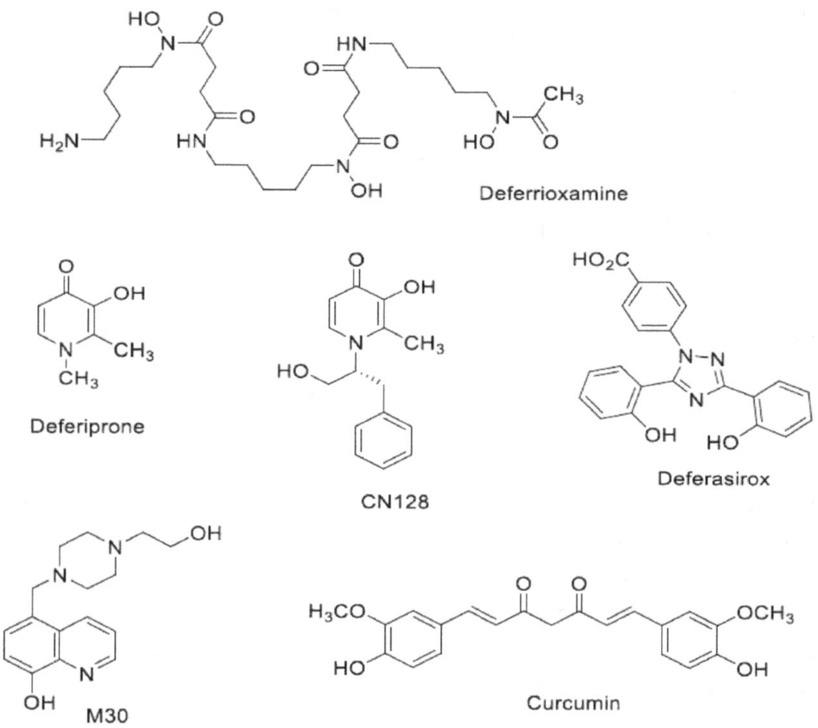

Figure 1. Chemical structures of iron chelators.

Deferiprone (DFP) a small, lipophilic bidentate chelator of the 3-hydroxypyridin-4-one family (Figure 1), was introduced into clinical practice in the 1980s [12]. Although it is orally active, its half-life is 3–4 h, which means that it must be administered three times a day at doses of 75 mg/kg/day to maintain sufficient negative iron balance equivalent to 50 mg/kg/day of DFO [13,14]. DFP has good bioavailability, but its clearance is accelerated by rapid biotransformation: approximately 85% of the drug is metabolised to a nonchelating 3-*O*-glucuronide conjugate [15]. The most important side effects of deferiprone are agranulocytosis and milder forms of neutropenia, which require appropriate monitoring [16]. However, DFP enters cells and can access intracellular chelateable iron more readily than DFO [17]. DFP possesses cardioprotective effects [18], and a multi-centre prospective comparison showed that a combined DFP + DFO regimen was more effective in removing cardiac iron than DFO, and was superior in clearing hepatic iron than either DFO or DFP monotherapy [19].

In the years that followed the introduction of DFP, the search for other orally active chelators intensified [20]. The microbial tridentate chelator, desferrithiocin, discovered in 1980, was shown to be orally active and very effective in mobilising hepatic iron in a rat model with hepatic iron loading induced by a ferrocene derivative [21], and in iron-loaded monkeys [22,23]. However, ferrithiocin itself proved to be toxic in animals [24], and although many desferrithiocin derivatives were tested and found to be more effective than desferrithiocin, toxicity remained associated with this class of chelators [25]. The clinical development of Deferasirox (DFX) (ICL670) represents an investment, the magnitude of which has no precedent in the history of chelator research. In the search for a safe tridentate chelator, a completely new chemical class of iron chelators, the bis-hydroxyphenyltriazoles, was discovered. More than forty derivatives of the triazole series were synthesised at Novartis, and evaluated, together with more than 700 chelators from other chemical classes. The tridentate chelator 4-[(3,5-Bis-(2-hydroxyphenyl)-1,2,4) triazol-1-yl]-benzoic acid (ICL670, Figure 1) emerged as the chelator which best combined high oral potency and tolerability in animals [20]. DFX has a plasma half-life of 12–16 h, which allows it to be taken once per day, effectively eliminating non-transferrin bound iron (NTBI) from the circulation [26]. In clinical studies, DFX has proven to be as effective as DFO at doses of 20–30 mg/kg [27], and in an extensive study involving 1744 patients, it was shown that fixed starting doses of DFX, based on transfusional iron intake, with dose titration guided by serum ferritin trends and safety markers, provide clinically acceptable chelation in patients with transfusional hemosiderosis from various types of anaemia [28]. Side effects are minimal, although the use of DFX is associated with rash formation and renal toxicity [29].

3. Thalassemia, Sickle-Cell Anaemia, and Haemoglobinopathies

Thalassemia, sickle-cell disease, and other hereditary disorders of haemoglobin biosynthesis are the most prevalent monogenic diseases worldwide [5]. Thalassemia results from an inherited defect in the rate of synthesis of one of the two polypeptide chains of haemoglobin, resulting in imbalance in the α,β-globin chain ratio, ineffective erythropoiesis, chronic haemolytic anaemia, and increased intestinal iron absorption. In the 1960s and 1970s, the only effective treatment for thalassemia was blood transfusion. Since humans cannot increase their iron excretion to compensate for iron loading, the transfusional iron overload, aggravated by increased intestinal iron absorption, results in massive and progressive iron overload. Each unit of transfused blood contains approximately 200 mg of iron, and since the mean transfusional loading in thalassemia major is 0.4 mg/kg/day, it comes as no surprise that most patients faced certain death before the age of 20 years from heart failure. However, the incidence of heart failure was not directly related to the cardiac iron overload, but to the level of iron loading in the liver. The explanation for this lies in the demonstration by Chaim Hershko [30] of the presence in the serum of thalassemic patients of toxic non-transferrin-bound iron (NTBI) which was responsible for the cardiac damage. When the liver iron load attains a critical level, iron is released into the circulation, and once its concentration exceeds the binding capacity of the transferrin pool, NTBI is formed. NTBI is the main source of iron accumulation in iron loading in both thalassemia and hereditary hemochromatosis, notably in the heart, pancreas, and liver [31], as well as in the brain. The influx of NTBI seems to be mediated by the ZIP14 transporter in the liver [32,33], whereas in cardiomyocytes, two calcium channels transport Fe^{2+} with an affinity similar to that of Ca^{2+} [34,35], and their expression is insensitive to cardiac iron overload.

3.1. Thalassemia-Iron Accumulation in the Pituitary

Clinical hypogonadism is common in thalassemia patients (83%) with detectable cardiac iron and is independently associated with pituitary iron deposition and gland shrinkage [36]. The pituitary gland maintains its anatomical and functional connections with the brain, yet sits outside the blood–brain barrier. Iron deposition in the anterior pituitary continues to pose a serious problem in homozygous beta thalassemia patients, particularly in terms of gonadal function. Magnetic resonance imaging (MRI) measurements are able to estimate the amount of iron in the pituitary, which can then be correlated with gonadal function. The anterior pituitary gland is particularly sensitive to free radicals produced by oxidative stress, such that exposure to these radicals injures the gland. MRI has shown that even a modest increase in iron deposition in the anterior pituitary can lead to dysfunction, such as abnormalities in the hypothalamic–pituitary growth hormone axis and growth hormone neurosecretory dysfunction, and low insulin-like growth-factor-1 levels. Abnormalities in the hypothalamic–pituitary–gonad axis will induce lower follicle stimulating hormone (FSH) and luteinizing hormone (LH) secretion, low LH/FSH response, and low sex steroid secretion from the gonads, i.e., testosterone (reviewed [37]). The spleen plays an important role in destroying abnormal red cells, sequesters 30–40% of the circulating platelet pool, and plays a role in the regulation of plasma volume. In thalassemic patients, the spleen may become enlarged, which can result in an increased propensity to recurrent infection, such that a splenectomy is required. Following splenectomy, the pituitary iron loading increases [38]. In early studies of four thalassemia patients, (Hb-E thalassemia and thalassemia major), the pituitary iron content, as assessed by MRI, was increased in all four patients compared to controls [39]. A subsequent MRI study of 84 patients with β-thalassemia established a correlation between pituitary iron overload, (evaluated by T2*) and both hepatic and cardiac iron load. In addition, pituitary MRI values correlated with serum ferritin and patient age, but not with height of the pituitary [38]. A study of 30 children and young adult thalassemic patients (13 females and 17 male patients) confirmed iron accumulation in the liver, myocardium, and the pituitary, a linear regression between pituitary iron and age in patients > 14 y, while MRI values between the pituitary and liver, and liver and myocardia, were only moderately correlated, ($r = 0.34$ and 0.42, respectively). However, no correlation was evident between pituitary and myocardial MRI results, which were of interest, since it might be considered that NTBI would be taken up by both of these organs [40]. It is clear that a therapeutic approach based on the use of iron chelators offers a solution to many of these dilemmas, associated with systemic iron overload, and their development has resulted in innumerable lives being saved, and, just as importantly, has led to an enormous improvement in the quality of life of thalassemia patients all over the world [5]. Investigations have now been extended to monitor whether excessive amounts of iron in specific brain regions and the pituitary can be removed by iron chelators.

3.2. *Iron Chelation from the Pituitary Gland*

Iron chelators, such as deferoxamine, deferiprone, or deferasirox, could be used alone or in combination to induce negative iron balance and reverse hypogonadism and endocrine complications in severely iron-overloaded thalassemic patients. Therefore, it is of interest to ascertain whether iron chelation can reduce iron overload in the pituitary as well as the liver, heart, and spleen. Berkovitch et al. [41] investigated 33 patients >15 years old with transfusion-dependent homozygous beta thalassemia, all of whom had received DFO. Anterior pituitary function (gonadotrophin releasing hormone, GnRH, stimulating test) correlated well with the MRI results for iron deposition in the anterior pituitary, although there was no correlation between the MRI measurements, the GnRH stimulation test, and the clinical status of the patients. Interestingly, 28 out of the 33 patients achieved normal puberty. The deficit in endocrine function in thalassemic patients was confirmed in a study of 78 male thalassemic patients (4–11 years) treated with frequent transfusions and long term DFO therapy, who were compared with 30 age- and sex-matched control children. The prevalence of hypogonadotropic hypogonadism in the thalassemic patients was 76.2%, with a significant increase in serum ferritin (×7), and significantly reduced the serum level of cortisol, growth hormone, stimulating hormones and testosterone [42].

Using the new oral chelator DFX for a two-year period, Wood et al. [43] investigated the pituitary iron content and volume in 31 chronically-transfused patients (28 thalassemia major and three Blackfan Diamond). MRI measurements were taken at the baseline, one, and two years. Twenty-six patients completed the study, 10 were prepubertal, 12 had achieved normal puberty, and four were hypogonadal at base line. Interestingly, the decreased pituitary volume at baseline returned to normal values after two years of DFX therapy, while pituitary iron content as assayed by R2* showed no net change. This latter result was of interest, as it was expected that with increasing age, pituitary iron would increase in parallel (predicted to be a 0.4 increase) [36].

Such studies indicate that iron chelators are able to reduce pituitary iron content as well as improve its function. It is clearly of interest to know whether brain regions are vulnerable to increased iron deposition in β-thalassemic patients. There have been three main studies which investigated other regions of the brain by quantitative MRI. In the studies of Duprez et al. [44] and Hasiloglu et al. [45], various MRI methodologies were utilised to identify an increase in iron in the choroid plexus of β-thalassemic patients. Qiu et al. [46] investigated the distribution of iron in different brain regions of 31 thalassemic patients, aged 25.3 ± 5.9 years, and 33 age matched healthy volunteers. Of the 31 patients, 27 exhibited abnormal iron deposition in one of the brain regions investigated by quantitative susceptibility, showing significantly lower susceptibility values in the globus pallidus and substantia nigra and significantly higher susceptibility in the red nucleus and choroid plexus. In the control subjects, there was a positive age effect on susceptibility value in the putamen, dentate nucleus, substantia nigra, and red nucleus. However, more information is needed with respect to the liver and heart iron deposition and the extent of chelation in each of the thalassemic patients for complete interpretation of these results. Surprisingly, there have been no studies on iron distribution in specific brain regions of thalassemic patients, before or after iron chelation. Whether continuous iron chelation in these patients will preclude such iron accumulation is unknown, nor whether there is preferential iron accumulation in specific brain regions. Further studies are clearly required.

4. Parkinson's Disease—Iron Accumulation in the Substantia Nigra

Parkinson's disease is the second most common form of motor system degeneration, and is characterised by a progressive loss of dopaminergic neurons in the substantia nigra pars compacta in the ventral midbrain. There is an increased accumulation of iron in the substantia nigra (SN) [47], with a smaller accumulation of iron in other brain regions, such as the red nuclei, globus pallidus, and the cortex of Parkinson's Disease (PD) patients. As the severity of the disease increases the total iron content increases in the SN, which correlates with motor disability [48] and microgliosis [49]. Semi-quantitative histochemical studies of the SN show that iron deposits are present within the neurons and glia of the substantia nigra, putamen, and globus pallidus, with an increase in ferritin-loaded microglia cells in the substantia nigra [50]. The increase in iron in the SN of PD patients is associated with increased ferritin and neuromelanin iron loading [50,51], as well as increased expression of divalent metal transporter 1, which may contribute to PD pathogenesis via its capacity to transport ferrous iron [52]. Intense microgliosis occurs around extra neuronal neuromelanin (released by dying neurons) in the substantia nigra of patients with Parkinson's disease [53,54], which could be an important factor in inducing iron accumulation within the microglia [49].

Preliminary reports suggested that identification of neuromelanin, NM, (rather than iron) by MRI might be feasible in patients with Parkinson's disease [55,56]. Indeed, the loss of neuromelanin in the locus coeruleus and substantia nigra, together with the associated loss in the ability to sequester iron, might be a characteristic sign of Parkinson's disease [56]. Recent studies have been able to discriminate neuromelanin in PD brains. For example, three-dimensional (3D) neuromelanin-sensitive ^{31}MRI [57] showed that signal densities and contrast ratios were significantly lower in the SN of PD patients compared to controls. Another study of 13 late stage PD patients (LSPD) and 12 de novo PD patients (2–5 years duration) showed that the signal was significantly decreased in LSPD compared to de novo PD, while in the lateral SN region, a decrease in the contrast ratios was detected in all PD groups compared to controls [58]. Interestingly, in this study, the NM signal area was significantly correlated with Hoehn Yahr Stage and Movement Disorder Society Unified Parkinson's Disease Rating Scale (MDS-UPDRS) part II, while a weak correlation was found with MDS-UPDRS part III. Such results may indicate that measurement of the neuromelanin content in the brain by MRI techniques could be an important diagnostic approach.

Chelation of Iron in the Brains of Parkinson's Disease Patients

Chelation of iron from the SN of PD brains was proposed many years ago. In our initial animal studies over 15 years ago [59,60], we showed that iron chelators (DFO and DFP) already in clinical use for the treatment of iron loading systemic diseases were able to cross the blood brain barrier (BBB), reduce the iron content in various brain regions, and induce neuroprotection in an animal model of PD. In 2010, Kwiatkowski et al. [61] reported the beneficial use of DFP in one PD patient. After one year's administration of DFP, at 30 mg/kg/day, there was an improvement in the UPDRS score and a decrease in iron accumulation in the bilateral dentate nuclei, as well as the SN [61]. It is of interest that the time period to observe a beneficial action was approximately one year. Subsequent clinical trials in 2011 and 2013 confirmed that it was necessary to administer DFP for at least nine months at a comparable dose to observe a beneficial effect, reflected by changes in the UPDRS score. Both studies [62,63] identified the beneficial effects of DFP. In the study of Devos et al. [62], R2* sequences were used to assess iron content in the SN, while UPDRS scores were acquired at various intervals to assess clinical parameters, and serum ferritin was assayed as a marker of iron stores. After six to nine months, decreases in SN iron content were quantitated by MRI, and there were improvements in both motor and UPDRS motor scores. In the second study, of six months duration [63], decreases in SN iron content were assayed by MRI T2* in patients receiving 30 mg/kg/day, and there were indications of an improvement in UPDRS. Interestingly, PD patients exhibiting high inflammatory markers in the blood, e.g., IL-6, did not respond well to iron chelation, leading to the suggestion that chelatable iron was not freely available for chelation. There was no evidence that the chelation therapy had an adverse effect on haematological parameters. Interestingly, in the study of Bastida et al. [63], the chelation of iron from other brain regions was also assessed. After three months, the caudate nucleus showed decreased iron content, while the dentate nucleus showed an iron decrease at six months. At this time there was also evidence for a decrease in substantia nigra iron content, which took up to nine months in the Davos study. Clearly, this indicates that there is a selective removal of iron from different brain regions. The major disadvantage of the use of DFP was the incidence of neutropenia and agranulocytosis, which occurred in 8% of the patients. This side effect resolved rapidly with cessation of the oral therapy. Such a side effect required that all PD patients entering the clinical trial undertook a weekly white cell count. These positive results from the clinical trials have confirmed that iron chelation therapy has potential as a therapeutic option for the treatment of PD; if the side effect could be eradicated, it would become a much more universal treatment. In addition, it remains unclear whether the long-term use of such chelators might alter oligodendrocyte function, since they have a large requirement for iron. It is therefore suggested that clinical studies that use iron chelation therapy for diseases associated with iron deposition should monitor white matter (WM) changes. A number of these diseases already report apparent hypomyelination, and further decline of WM integrity will impact the functional outcomes, since myelin integrity impacts movement and cognition. Currently, a multi-centre phase 2 clinical trial involving 300 patients from all over Europe is in place, centered at the University of Lille, France.

Over the past decade, work has been directed towards the design of hydroxypyridinones, which lack an effect on white blood count in rodents and primates. A lead compound, CN128 (Figure 1), has been identified, which possesses all of the therapeutic properties of DFP, including penetration of the blood–brain barrier, but lacks the side effects of induction of neutropenia and agranulocytosis in primates after prolonged exposure (nine months) [64]. CN128 is currently undergoing tests in a range of Parkinson's disease models.

5. Alzheimer's Disease

Alzheimer's disease (AD) is a fatal age-related neurodegenerative disease which results in cognitive decline, memory loss, and psychosis. Clinically, AD is characterised by progressive dementia. Initial symptoms are short-term memory loss, which is followed by extensive neuronal loss in the hippocampus and selected cortical and subcortical area. There is abnormal protein processing, with accumulation of the β-amyloid peptide, which is deposited extracellularly and manifests itself as neuritic amyloid plaques, and of the hyperphosphorylated tau protein, in the form of neurofibrillary tangles. Both of these abnormal protein aggregates are definitive markers of the disease in post mortem material.

There is considerable evidence that there is defective homeostasis of iron in the AD brain. Increases in the iron content of AD have been reported for over 50 years. In a recent paper, which made a comprehensive systematic meta-analysis and review of over 2556 publications, 43 eligible studies were identified where the iron content in AD serum, cerebrospinal fluid (CSF), or brain tissue had been studied. In nineteen studies, the iron content in 12 selected brain regions was analyzed by separated meta-analysis, and it was concluded that eight specific brain regions (the temporal, parietal, and frontal lobes) had higher iron concentrations, which correlated with the clinical diagnosis of AD [65]. A recent laser ablation inductively coupled mass spectroscopy study also identified increases in iron in the frontal cortex [66].

Alzheimer's Disease—Iron Chelation from the Cortex and Hippocampus

Current therapies for Alzheimer disease (AD), such as the acetylcholinesterase inhibitors and the NMDA receptor inhibitors, may provide moderate symptomatic delay at various stages of the disease, but do not arrest the disease progression or induce meaningful remission. The confirmation of altered iron homeostasis in the brain of AD patients has opened the possibility of using iron chelators as a new therapeutic approach. Various animal models of AD have been utilised to investigate the therapeutic action of iron chelators. For example, the iron chelator (-) epigallocatechin-3-gallate and M-30 (Figure 1) reduced amyloid precursor protein (APP) expression in cultured cells [67,68]. Although it is known that there is an increase in iron in various brain regions in AD patients, there has been no clinical evidence which supports the use of chelating agents as an adjunctive treatment for AD. Tea polyphenols and curcumin (Figure 1) have been advocated as metal chelators for the treatment of AD, although the efficacy of such natural products awaits further investigation.

In 1991, McLachlan showed that DFO significantly reduced the behavioral and cognitive decline of AD patients [69]. However, since this ground-breaking study it is only now that further studies are being undertaken to investigate the therapeutic efficacy of iron chelators in AD. Currently, a phase 2, randomised, placebo-controlled, multi-centre study to investigate the safety and efficacy of DFP has started recruiting. Approximately 171 participants with Prodromal Alzheimer's disease and mild Alzheimer's disease will be recruited for the study. Controlled release DFP will be used in an attempt to prevent the unwanted side effects of neutropenia and agranulocytosis. The aim of this study is to ascertain whether DFP (15 mg/kg BID orally) slows cognitive decline in Alzheimer's patients. MRI will ascertain the iron content of brain regions during the period of the study (Neuroscience Trials Australia—Clinical Trial Deferiprone to Delay orallyDementia).

Other compounds are in development for the treatment of AD, which have multitargeting properties. They include a series of (3-hydroxy-4-pyridinone)-benzofuran hybrids [70] which mimic donepezil, an inhibitor of acetylcholinesterase, and possess additional properties, such as metal chelation, radical scavenging, and the inhibition of amyloid peptide aggregation. In addition, a series of thiosemicarbazones, (pyridoxal 4-N-(1-benzylpiperidin-4-yl) thiosemicarbazone compounds exhibit very low anti-proliferative activity, substantial iron chelation efficacy, inhibition of copper-mediated amyloid-β aggregation, inhibition of oxidative stress, moderate acetylcholinesterase inhibitory activity, and autophagic induction [71]. Although such compounds show neuroprotective effects in vitro, it remains to be investigated whether they have a beneficial effect in either animal models of AD or AD patients.

6. Friederich's Ataxia

Friedreich's ataxia (FRDA) is one of a number of neurological disorders caused by the anomalous expansion of unstable nucleotide repeats in which, unlike Huntington's disease, the nucleotide expansion occurs in the non-coding part of the gene (the introns). FRDA is characterised by a progressive degeneration of large sensory neurons and cardiomyopathies [72]. Although rare, FRDA is the most frequent inherited ataxia, with an estimated prevalence of two to four people in 100,000 individuals. Most patients carry homozygous GAA expansions in the first intron of the frataxin gene on chromosome 9. Whereas the critical pathologic triplet repeat threshold is 66 repeats, the expansion can be as many as 890 GAA repeats. This results in the partial silencing of frataxin, a small mitochondrial protein which plays an essential role in iron–sulfur cluster (ISC) biogenesis, an essential metabolic pathway found in all organisms [73,74]. Frataxin interacts directly with the two central components of the ISC biogenesis machine, the NFS1/IscU complex [75]. Correct ISC synthesis in mitochondria is closely linked to cellular iron homeostasis [76], and a lack of frataxin therefore causes dysregulation of iron metabolism. As a consequence, failure to assemble mitochondrial Fe–S proteins results in increased cellular iron acquisition, mitochondrial iron overload [77], and mitochondrial iron deposits in some FRDA patients [78].

Iron Chelation from the Dentate Nucleus in Friederich's Ataxia Patients

In one clinical trial, deferiprone (10–15 mg/kg) was administered twice daily to FRDA patients in a small clinical trial over a six-month period to nine adolescent patients with no overt cardiomyopathy. Brain iron was reduced significantly in dentate nuclei. The chelator treatment caused no apparent hematologic or neurologic side effects, while reducing neuropathy and ataxic gait in the youngest patients [79]. In a second clinical trial, DFP (10 mg/kg) was administered in combination with idebenone (20 mg/kg) to 20 FRDA patients. No significant differences were observed in the total international cooperative ataxia rating score (ICARS) scores when comparing baseline status and the end of the study in the whole group of patients. Echocardiography data showed a significant reduction of the interventricular septum thickness and in the left ventricular mass index. After 11 months of treatment, iron was reduced in the dentate nuclei. However, there was a worsening of posture and gait compared to baseline [80].

7. Conclusions

The current longevity of the population will result in increasing iron loading in various brain regions, although this is not normally associated with toxicity. Exactly why and how the iron which accumulates in specific brain regions in neurodegenerative diseases is highly toxic is unclear. However, new studies of activated microglia indicate that these cells may, in part, be the source of the iron loading. Over the past 50 years chelation therapy has progressed from subcutaneous administration to oral administration, and it is hoped that toxicity that has been associated with the oral chelators will be eliminated with new formulation of the hydroxypyridinones.

Author Contributions: R.J.W. wrote the original text, which was reviewed and edited by R.R.C. and R.C.H.

Abbreviations

AD	Alzheimer's Disease
Ca^{++}	Calcium
CSF	Cerebrospinal fluid
DFO	Desferioxamine
DFP	Deferiprone
DFX	Deferasirox
$Fe2^{++}$	Ferrous
FDRA	Friederich's Ataxia
FSH	Follicle stimulating hormone
GAA	Trinucleotide repeat
GnRH	Gonadotropin-releasing hormone
GnRH stimulation	Gonadotropin-releasing hormone test.
ICARS	International Co-operative Ataxia Rating Scale
IL-6	Interleukin-6
ISC	Iron sulphur protein
LH	Luteinizing hormone
LSPD	Late stage Parkinson's Disease
MDS-UPDRS	Movement Disorder Society Unified Parkinson's Disease Rating Scale
MRI	Magnetic resonance imaging
NMDA	N-methyl-D-aspartate
NTBI	Non transferrin bound iron
PD	Parkinson's Disease
SN	Substania nigra
WM	White matter
ZIP14	Zinc transporter

References

1. Ward, R.J.; Dexter, D.T.; Crichton, R.R. Neurodegenerative diseases and therapeutic strategies using iron chelators. *J. Trace Elem. Med. Biol.* **2015**, *31*, 267–273. [CrossRef]
2. Nathan, D.G. Thalassemia: The continued challenge. *Ann. N. Y. Acad. Sci.* **2005**, *1054*, 1–10. [CrossRef]
3. Nathan, D.G. Thalassemia: A look to the future. *Ann. N. Y. Acad. Sci.* **2016**, *1368*, 11–15. [CrossRef] [PubMed]
4. Hider, R.C.; Hoffbrand, A.V. The role of deferiprone in iron chelation. *N. Engl. J. Med.* **2018**, *379*, 2140–2150. [CrossRef] [PubMed]
5. Taher, A.T.; Weatherall, D.J.; Cappellini, M.D. Thalassemia. *Lancet* **2018**, *391*, 155–167. [CrossRef]
6. Propper, R.D.; Cooper, B.; Rufo, R.R.; Nienhuis, A.W.; Anderson, W.F.; Bunn, H.F.; Rosenthal, A.; Nathan, D.G. Continuous subcutaneous administration of deferoxamine in patients with iron overload. *N. Engl. J. Med.* **1977**, *297*, 418–423. [CrossRef] [PubMed]
7. Pippard, M.J.; Callender, S.T.; Weatherall, D.J. Chelation regimens with desferrioxamine. *Lancet* **1977**, *1*, 1101. [CrossRef]
8. Brittenham, G.M.; Griffith, P.M.; Nienhuis, A.W.; McLaren, C.E.; Young, N.S.; Tucker, E.E.; Allen, C.J.; Farrell, D.E.; Harris, J.W. Efficacy of deferoxamine in preventing complications of iron overload in patients with thalassemia major. *N. Engl. J. Med.* **1994**, *331*, 567–573. [CrossRef]
9. Borgna-Pignatti, C.; Rugolotto, S.; De Stefano, P.; Zhao, H.; Cappellini, M.D.; Del Vecchio, G.C.; Romeo, M.A.; Forni, G.L.; Gamberini, M.R.; Ghilardi, R.; et al. Survival and complications in patients with thalassemia major treated with transfusion and deferoxamine. *Haematologica* **2004**, *89*, 1187–1193. [PubMed]
10. Olivieri, N.F.; Nathan, D.G.; MacMillan, J.H.; Wayne, A.S.; Liu, P.P.; McGee, A.; Martin, M.; Koren, G.; Cohen, A.R. Survival in medically treated patients with homozygous beta thalassemia. *N. Engl. J. Med.* **1994**, *331*, 574–578. [CrossRef] [PubMed]
11. Modell, B.; Khan, M.; Darlison, M. Survival in beta-thalassaemia major in the UK: Data from the UK Thalassaemia Register. *Lancet* **2000**, *355*, 2051–2052. [CrossRef]

12. Kontoghiorghes, G.J.; Aldouri, M.A.; Hoffbrand, A.V.; Barr, J.; Wonke, B.; Kourouclaris, T.; Sheppard, L. Effective chelation of iron in beta thalassaemia with the oral chelator 1,2-dimethyl-3-hydroxypyrid-4-one. *Br. Med. J. (Clin. Res. Ed.)* **1987**, *295*, 1509–1512. [CrossRef] [PubMed]
13. Olivieri, N.F.; Koren, G.; Hermann, C.; Bentur, Y.; Chung, D.; Klein, J.; St Louis, P.; Freedman, M.H.; McClelland, R.A.; Templeton, D.M. Comparison of oral iron chelator L1 and desferrioxamine in iron-loaded patients. *Lancet* **1990**, *336*, 1275–1279. [CrossRef]
14. Hoyes, K.P.; Porter, J.B. Subcellular distribution of desferrioxamine and hydroxypyridin-4-one chelators in K562 cells affects chelation of intracellular iron pools. *Br. J. Haematol.* **1993**, *85*, 393–400. [CrossRef] [PubMed]
15. Huang, X.P.; Spino, M.; Thiessen, J.J. Transport kinetics of iron chelators and their chelates in Caco-2 cells. *Pharm. Res.* **2006**, *23*, 280–290. [CrossRef] [PubMed]
16. Botzenhardt, S.; Li, N.; Chan, E.W.; Sing, C.W.; Wong, I.C.; Neubert, A. Safety profiles of iron chelators in young patients with haemoglobinopathies. *Eur. J. Haematol.* **2017**, *98*, 198–217. [CrossRef]
17. Hershko, C.; Link, G.; Pinson, A.; Peter, H.H.; Dobbin, P.; Hider, R.C. Ironmobilization from myocardial cells by 3-hydroxypyridin-4-one chelators: Studies in rat heart cells in culture. *Blood* **1991**, *77*, 2049–2053. [PubMed]
18. Anderson, L.J.; Wonke, B.; Prescott, E.; Holden, S.; Walker, J.M.; Pennell, D.J. Comparison of effects of oral deferiprone and subcutaneous desferrioxamine on myocardial iron concentrations and ventricular function in beta-thalassaemia. *Lancet* **2002**, *9332*, 516–520. [CrossRef]
19. Pepe, A.; Meloni, A.; Rossi, G.; Cuccia, L.; D'Ascola, G.D.; Santodirocco, M.; Cianciulli, P.; Caruso, V.; Romeo, M.A.; Filosa, A.; et al. Cardiac and hepatic iron and ejection fraction in thalassemia major: Multicentre prospective comparison of combined deferiprone and deferoxamine therapy against deferiprone or deferoxamine monotherapy. *J. Cardiovasc. Magn. Reson.* **2013**, *15*. [CrossRef]
20. Nick, H.; Acklin, P.; Lattmann, R.; Buehlmayer, P.; Hauffe, S.; Schupp, J.; Alberti, D. Development of tridentate iron chelators: From desferrithiocin to ICL670. *Curr. Med. Chem.* **2003**, *10*, 1065–1076. [CrossRef]
21. Longueville, A.; Crichton, R.R. An animal model of iron overload and its application to study hepatic ferritin iron mobilization by chelators. *Biochem. Pharmacol.* **1986**, *35*, 3669–3678. [CrossRef]
22. Wolfe, L.C.; Nicolosi, R.J.; Renaud, M.M.; Finger, J.; Hegsted, M.; Peter, H.; Nathan, D.G. A non-human primate model for the study of oral iron chelators. *Br. J. Haematol.* **1989**, *72*, 456–461. [CrossRef] [PubMed]
23. Bergeron, R.J.; Streiff, R.R.; Wiegand, J.; Vinson, J.R.; Luchetta, G.; Wiegand, J.; Moerker, T.; Peter, H.H. A comparative evaluation of iron clearance models. *Ann. N. Y. Acad. Sci.* **1990**, *612*, 378–393. [CrossRef] [PubMed]
24. Baker, E.; Wong, A.; Peter, H.; Jacobs, A. Desferrithiocin is an effective iron chelator in vivo and in vitro but ferrithiocin is toxic. *Br. J. Haematol.* **1992**, *81*, 424–431. [CrossRef] [PubMed]
25. Bergeron, R.J.; Wiegand, J.; McManis, J.S.; Bharti, N. Desferrithiocin: A search for clinically effective iron chelators. *J. Med. Chem.* **2014**, *57*, 9259–9291. [CrossRef] [PubMed]
26. Daar, S.; Pathare, A.; Nick, H.; Kriemler-Krahn, U.; Hmissi, A.; Habr, D.; Taher, A. Reduction in labile plasma iron during treatment with deferasirox, a once-daily oral iron chelator, in heavily loaded patients with beta-thalassaemia. *Eur. J. Haematol.* **2009**, *82*, 454–457. [CrossRef] [PubMed]
27. Cappellini, M.D.; Cohen, A.; Piga, A.; Bejaoui, M.; Perrotta, S.; Agaoglu, L.; Aydinok, Y.; Kattamis, A.; Kilinc, Y.; Porter, J.; et al. A phase 3 study of deferasirox (ICL670), a once-daily oral iron cheater in patients with best-thalassemia. *Blood* **2006**, *207*, 3455–3462. [CrossRef] [PubMed]
28. Cappellini, M.D.; Porter, J.D.; El-Beshlawy, A.; Li, C.K.; Seymour, J.F.; Elalfy, M.; Gattermann, N.; Giraudier, S.; Lee, J.W.; Chan, L.L.; et al. Tailoring iron chelation by iron intake and serum ferritin; the perspective EPIC study of deferasirox in 1744 patients with transfusion-dependent anemias. *Haematologica* **2010**, *95*, 557–566. [CrossRef] [PubMed]
29. Neufeld, E.J. Oral chelators deferasirox and deferiprone for transfusional iron overload in thalassemia major: New data, new questions. *Blood* **2006**, *107*, 3436–3441. [CrossRef] [PubMed]
30. Hershko, C.; Graham, G.; Bates, G.W.; Rachmilewitz, E.A. Non-specific serum iron in thalassaemia: An abnormal serum iron fraction of potential toxicity. *Br. J. Haematol.* **1978**, *40*, 255–263. [CrossRef] [PubMed]
31. Brissot, P.; Ropert, M.; Le Lan, C.; Loréal, O. Non-transferrin bound iron: A key role in iron overload and iron toxicity. *Biochim. Biophys. Acta* **2012**, *1820*, 403–410. [CrossRef] [PubMed]

32. Pinilla-Tenas, J.J.; Sparkman, B.K.; Shawki, A.; Illing, A.C.; Mitchell, C.J.; Zhao, N.; Liuzzi, J.P.; Cousins, R.J.; Knutson, M.D.; Mackenzie, B. Zip14 is a complex broad-scope metal-ion transporter whose functional properties support roles in the cellular uptake of zinc and nontransferrin-bound iron. *Am. J. Physiol. Cell Physiol.* **2011**, *301*, C862–C871. [CrossRef] [PubMed]
33. Jenkitkasemwong, S.; Wang, C.Y.; Coffey, R.; Zhang, W.; Chan, A.; Biel, T.; Kim, J.S.; Hojyo, S.; Fukada, T.; Knutson, M.D. SLC39A14 Is Required for the Development of Hepatocellular Iron Overload in Murine Models of Hereditary Hemochromatosis. *Cell Metab.* **2015**, *22*, 138–150. [CrossRef] [PubMed]
34. Oudit, G.Y.; Sun, H.; Trivieri, M.G.; Koch, S.E.; Dawood, F.; Ackerley, C.; Yazdanpanah, M.; Wilson, G.J.; Schwartz, A.; Liu, P.P.; et al. L-type Ca^{2+} channels provide a major pathway for iron entry into cardiomyocytes in iron-overload cardiomyopathy. *Nat. Med.* **2003**, *9*, 1187–1194. [CrossRef] [PubMed]
35. Kumfu, S.; Chattipakorn, S.; Srichairatanakool, S.; Settakorn, J.; Fucharoen, S.; Chattipakorn, N. T-type calcium channel as a portal of iron uptake into cardiomyocytes of beta-thalassemic mice. *Eur. J. Haematol.* **2011**, *86*, 156–166. [CrossRef] [PubMed]
36. Noetzli, L.J.; Panigrahy, A.; Mittelman, S.D.; Hyderi, A.; Dongelyan, A.; Coates, T.D.; Wood, J.C. Pituitary iron and volume predict hypogonadism in transfusional iron overload. *Am. J. Hematol.* **2012**, *87*, 167–171. [CrossRef] [PubMed]
37. De Sanctis, V.; Soliman, A.T.; Elsedfy, H.; Soliman, N.A.; Elalaily, R. Late onset male hypogonadism and fertility potential in thalassaemia major: Two emerging patters. *Mediterr. J. Haematol.* **2015**, *7*, e2015047.
38. Çetinçakmak, M.; Hattapoğlu, S.; Menzilcioğlu, S.; Bircan, A.; Uluca, U.; Uçar, A.; S Mura, S.; Söker, M.; Bilic, A.J. MRI-based evaluation of the factors leading to pituitary iron overload in patients with thalassemia. *J. Neuroradiol.* **2016**, *43*, 297–302. [CrossRef] [PubMed]
39. Wang, Z.; Fischer, R.; Butensky, E.; Neumayr, L.; Singer, S.T.; Lee, P.; Chu, Z.; Hunte, J.V.; Firebaugh, J.; Vichinsky, E.; et al. MRI Assessment of Pituitary Iron and Volume in Thalassemia, and Relation to Hypothalamic-Pituitary-Gonadal Axis Function (HPG): A Feasibility Study. *Blood* **2006**, *108*, 1778.
40. Christoforidis, A.; Haritandi, A.; Tsitouridis, I.; Tsatra, I.; Tsantali, H.; Karyda, S.; Dimitriadis, A.S.; Athanassiou-Metaxa, M. Correlative study of iron accumulation in liver, myocardium, and pituitary assessed with MRI in young thalassemic patients. *J. Pediatr. Hematol. Oncol.* **2006**, *28*, 311–315. [CrossRef] [PubMed]
41. Berkovitch, M.; Bistritzer, T.; Milone, S.D.; Perlman, K.; Kucharczyk, W.; Olivieri, N.F. Iron deposition in the anterior pituitary in homozygous beta thalassemia: MRI evaluation and correlation with gonadal function. *J. Pediatr. Endocrinol. Metab.* **2000**, *13*, 179–184. [CrossRef] [PubMed]
42. Abdulzahra, M.S.; Al-Hakeim, H.K.; Ridha, M.M. Study of the effect of iron overload on the function of endocrine glands in male thalassemia patients. *Asian J. Transfus. Sci.* **2011**, *5*, 127–131. [PubMed]
43. Wood, J.C.; Kang, B.P.; Thompson, A.; Giardina, P.; Harmatz, P.; Glynos, T.; Paley, C.; Coates, T.D. The effect of deferasirox on cardiac iron in thalassemia major: Impact of total body iron stores. *Blood* **2010**, *116*, 537–543. [CrossRef] [PubMed]
44. Duprez, T.; Maite, D.; Cosnard, G. Transfusional haemochromatosis of the choroid plexus in beta thalassemia major. *J. Comput. Assist. Tomogr.* **2001**, *25*, 487–488. [CrossRef] [PubMed]
45. Hasiloglu, Z.I.; Asik, M.; Ure, E.; Ertem, F.; Apak, H.; Albayram, S. The utility of susceptibility-weighted imaging to evaluate the extent of iron accumulation in the choroid plexus of patients with Î²-thalassaemiamajor. *Clin. Radiol.* **2017**, *72*, 903.e1–903.e7. [CrossRef] [PubMed]
46. Qiu, D.; Chan, G.C.; Chu, J.; Chan, Q.; Ha, S.Y.; Moseley, M.E.; Khong, P.L. MR quantitative susceptibility imaging for the evaluation of iron loading in the brains of patients with β-thalassemia major. *AJNR Am. J. Neuroradiol.* **2014**, *35*, 1085–1090. [CrossRef] [PubMed]
47. Dexter, D.T.; Wells, F.R.; Agid, F.; Agid, Y.; Lees, A.J.; Jenner, P.; Marsden, C.D. Increased nigral iron content in postmortem parkinsonian brain. *Lancet* **1987**, *21*, 1219–1220. [CrossRef]
48. Fernandez, B.; Ferrer, I.; Fernando, G.; Hilfiker, S. Biomonitorization of iron accumulation in the substantia nigra from Lewy body disease patients. *Toxicol. Rep.* **2017**, *4*, 188–193. [CrossRef]
49. Martin-Bastida, A.; Tilley, B.; Alireza, T.; Bansal, S.; Dexter, D.T.; Ward, R.J. Parkinson's, Iron and Inflammation. *Neurobiol. Dis.* **2019**, in press.
50. Jellinger, K.; Paulus, W.; Grundke-Iqbal, I.; Riederer, P.; Youdim, M.B. Brain iron and ferritin in Parkinson's and Alzheimer's diseases. *J. Neural Transm. Park. Dis. Dement. Sect.* **1990**, *2*, 327–340. [CrossRef]
51. Ben-Shachar, D.; Riederer, P.; Youdim, M.B. Iron-melanin interaction and lipid peroxidation: Implications for Parkinson's disease. *J. Neurochem.* **1991**, *57*, 1609–1614. [CrossRef] [PubMed]

52. Hadzhieva, M.; Kirches, E.; Mawrin, C. Review: Iron metabolism and the role of iron in neurodegenerative disorders. *Neuropathol. Appl. Neurobiol.* **2014**, *40*, 240–257. [CrossRef] [PubMed]
53. Zecca, L.; Wilms, H.; Geick, S.; Claasen, J.H.; Brandenburg, L.O.; Holzknecht, C.; Panizza, M.L.; Zucca, F.A.; Deuschl, G.; Sievers, J.; et al. Human neuromelanin induces neuroinflammation and neurodegeneration in the rat substantia nigra: Implications for Parkinson's disease. *Acta Neuropathol.* **2008**, *116*, 47–55. [CrossRef] [PubMed]
54. Zhang, W.; Phillips, K.; Wielgus, A.R.; Liu, J.; Albertini, A.; Zucca, F.A.; Faust, R.; Qian, S.Y.; Miller, D.S.; Chignell, C.F.; et al. Neuromelanin activates microglia and induces degeneration of dopaminergic neurons: Implications for progression of Parkinson's disease. *Neurotox. Res.* **2011**, *19*, 63–72. [CrossRef] [PubMed]
55. Nakane, T.; Nihashi, T.; Kawai, H.; Naganawa, S. Visualization of neuromelanin in the Substantia nigra and locus ceruleus at 1.5T using a 3D-gradient echo sequence with magnetization transfer contrast. *Magn. Reson. Med. Sci.* **2008**, *7*, 205–210. [CrossRef] [PubMed]
56. Sasaki, M.; Shibata, E.; Kudo, K.; Tohyama, K. Neuromelanin-Sensitive MRI. *Clin. Neuroradiol.* **2008**, *18*, 147–153. [CrossRef]
57. Prasad, S.; Stezin, A.; Lenka, A.; George, L.; Saini, J.; Yadav, R.; Pal, P.K. Three-dimensional neuromelanin-sensitive magnetic resonance imaging of the substantia nigra in Parkinson's disease. *Eur. J. Neurol.* **2018**, *25*, 680–686. [CrossRef]
58. Fabbri, M.; Reimão, S.; Carvalho, M.; Nunes, R.G.; Abreu, D.; Guedes, L.C.; Bouça, R.; Lobo, P.P.; Godinho, C.; Coelho, M.; et al. Substantia nigra neuromelanin as an imaging biomarker of disease progression in Parkinson's Disease. *J. Park. Dis.* **2017**, *7*, 491–501. [CrossRef]
59. Ward, R.J.; Dexter, D.; Florence, A.; Aouad, F.; Hider, R.; Jenner, P.; Crichton, R.R. Brain iron in the ferrocene-loaded rat: Its chelation and influence on dopamine metabolism. *Biochem. Pharmacol.* **1995**, *49*, 1821–1826. [CrossRef]
60. Dexter, D.T.; Ward, R.J.; Florence, A.; Jenner, P.; Crichton, R.R. Effects of desferrithiocin and its derivatives on peripheral iron and striatal dopamine and 5-hydroxytryptamine metabolism in the ferrocene-loaded rat. *Biochem. Pharmacol.* **1999**, *58*, 151–155. [CrossRef]
61. Kwiatkowski, J.L. Current recommendations for chelation for transfusion-dependent thalassemia. *Ann. N. Y. Acad. Sci.* **2016**, *1368*, 107–114. [CrossRef] [PubMed]
62. Devos, D.; Moreau, C.; Devedjian, J.C.; Kluza, J.; Petrault, M.; Laloux, C.; Jonneaux, A.; Ryckewaert, G.; Garçon, G.; Rouaix, N.; et al. Targeting chelatable iron as a therapeutic modality in Parkinson's disease. *Antioxid. Redox Signal* **2014**, *21*, 195–210. [CrossRef] [PubMed]
63. Martin-Bastida, A.; Ward, R.J.; Newbould, R.; Piccini, P.; Sharp, D.; Kabba, C.; Patel, M.C.; Spino, M.; Connelly, J.; Tricta, F.; et al. Brain iron chelation by deferiprone in a phase 2 randomised double-blinded placebo controlled clinical trial in Parkinson's disease. *Sci. Rep.* **2017**, *7*, 1398. [CrossRef] [PubMed]
64. Hider, R.; Liu, Z.; Liu, Y.; Li, Z. Chiral 3-Hydroxypyrid-4-one Derivative and Synthesis and Use Thereof. European Patent 2,692,724A1, 5 February 2014.
65. Tao, Y.; Wang, Y.; Rogers, J.T.; Wang, F. Perturbed iron distribution in Alzheimer's disease serum, cerebrospinal fluid, and selected brain regions: A systematic review and meta-analysis. *J. Alzheimer's Dis.* **2014**, *42*, 679–690. [CrossRef] [PubMed]
66. Hare, D.J.; Raven, E.P.; Roberts, B.R.; Bogeski, M.; Portbury, S.D.; McLean, C.A.; Masters, C.L.; Connor, J.R.; Bush, A.I.; Crouch, P.J.; et al. Laser ablation-inductively coupled plasma-mass spectrometry imaging of white and gray matter iron distribution in Alzheimer's disease frontal cortex. *NeuroImage* **2016**, *137*, 124–131. [CrossRef] [PubMed]
67. Reznichenko, L.; Amit, T.; Zheng, H.; Avarmovitch-Tirosh, Y.; Youdim, M.B.; Weinreb, O.; Mandel, S. Reduction of iron-regulated amyloid precursor protein and beta-amyloid peptide by (-)-epigallocatechin-3-gallate in cell cultures: Implications for iron chelation in Alzheimer's disease. *J. Neurochem.* **2006**, *97*, 527–536. [CrossRef] [PubMed]
68. Avramovich-Tirosh, Y.; Reznichenko, L.; Mit, T.; Zheng, H.; Fridkin, M.; Weinreb, O.; Mandel, S.; Youdim, M.B. Neurorescue activity, APP regulation and amyloid-beta peptide reduction by novel multi-functional brain permeable iron-chelating-antioxidants, M-30 and green tea polyphenol, EGCG. *Curr. Alzheimer Res.* **2007**, *4*, 403–411. [CrossRef] [PubMed]

69. McLachlan, D.R.; Smith, W.L.; Kruck, T.P. Desferrioxamine and Alzheimer's disease: Video home behavior assessment of clinical course and measures of brain aluminium. *Ther. Drug Monit.* **1993**, *15*, 602–607. [CrossRef] [PubMed]
70. Hiremathad, A.; Chand, K.; Tolayan, L.; Rajeshwari Keri, R.S.; Esteves, A.R.; Cardoso, S.M.; Chaves, S.; Santos, M.A. Hydroxypyridinone-benzofuran hybrids with potential protective roles for Alzheimer's diseasetherapy. *J. Inorg. Biochem.* **2018**, *179*, 82–96. [CrossRef]
71. Palanimuthu, D.; Poon, R.; Sahni, S.; Anjum, R.; Hibbs, D.; Lin, H.Y.; Bernhardt, P.V.; Kalinowski, D.S.; Richardson, D.R. A novel class of thiosemicarbazones show multi-functional activity for the treatment of Alzheimer's disease. *Eur. J. Med. Chem.* **2017**, *139*, 612–632. [CrossRef] [PubMed]
72. Lupoli, F.; Vannocci, T.; Longo, G.; Niccolai, N.; Pastore, A. The role of oxidative stress in Friedreich's ataxia. *FEBS Lett.* **2018**, *592*, 718–727. [CrossRef] [PubMed]
73. Adinolfi, S.; Iannuzzi, C.; Prischi, F.; Pastore, C.; Iametti, S.; Martin, S.R.; Bonomi, F.; Pastore, A. Bacterial frataxin CyaY is the gatekeeper of iron-sulfur cluster formation catalyzed by IscS. *Nat. Struct. Mol. Biol.* **2009**, *16*, 390–396. [CrossRef] [PubMed]
74. Prischi, F.; Konarev, P.V.; Iannuzzi, C.; Pastore, C.; Adinolfi, S.; Martin, S.R.; Svergun, D.I.; Pastore, A. Structural bases for the interaction of frataxin with the central components of iron-sulphur cluster assembly. *Nat. Commun.* **2010**, *1*. [CrossRef] [PubMed]
75. Prischi, F.; Pastore, A. Hybrid Methods in Iron-Sulfur Cluster Biogenesis. *Front. Mol. Biosci.* **2017**, *4*. [CrossRef] [PubMed]
76. Huang, M.L.; Lane, D.J.; Richardson, D.R. Mitochondrial mayhem: The mitochondrion as a modulator of iron metabolism and its role in disease. *Antioxid. Redox Signal* **2011**, *15*, 3003–3019. [CrossRef] [PubMed]
77. Lill, R.; Hoffmann, B.; Molik, S.; Pierik, A.J.; Rietzschel, N.; Stehling, O.; Uzarska, M.A.; Webert, H.; Wilbrecht, C.; Mühlenhoff, U. The role of mitochondria in cellular iron-sulfur protein biogenesis and iron metabolism. *Biochim. Biophys. Acta* **2012**, *1823*, 1491–1508. [CrossRef] [PubMed]
78. Ramirez, R.L.; Qian, J.; Santambrogio, P.; Levi, S.; Koeppen, A.H. Relation of cytosolic iron excess to cardiomyopathy of Friedreich's ataxia. *Am. J. Cardiol.* **2012**, *110*, 1820–1827. [CrossRef] [PubMed]
79. Boddaert, N.; Le Quan Sang, K.H.; Rötig, A.; Leroy-Willig, A.; Gallet, S.; Brunelle, F.; Sidi, D.; Thalabard, J.C.; Munnich, A.; Cabantchik, Z.I. Selective iron chelation in Friedreich ataxia: Biologic and clinical implications. *Blood* **2007**, *110*, 401–408. [CrossRef]
80. Velasco-Sánchez, D.; Aracil, A.; Montero, R.; Mas, A.; Jiménez, L.; O'Callaghan, M.; Tondo, M.; Capdevila, A.; Blanch, J.; Artuch, R.; et al. Combined therapy with idebenone and deferiprone in patients with Friedreich's ataxia. *Cerebellum* **2011**, *10*, 1–8. [CrossRef]

7

Iron Release from Soybean Seed Ferritin Induced by Cinnamic Acid Derivatives

Xuejiao Sha, Hai Chen, Jingsheng Zhang and Guanghua Zhao *

Beijing Advanced Innovation Center for Food Nutrition and Human Health, College of Food Science and Nutritional Engineering, Beijing Key Laboratory of Functional Food from Plant Resources, China Agricultural University, Beijing 100083, China; cau3060509@163.com (X.S.); chenhai2509@163.com (H.C.); zhangjingsheng@cau.edu.cn (J.Z.)

* Correspondence: gzhao@cau.edu.cn

Abstract: Plant ferritin represents a novel class of iron supplement, which widely co-exists with phenolic acids in a plant diet. However, there are few reports on the effect of these phenolic acids on function of ferritin. In this study, we demonstrated that cinnamic acid derivatives, as widely occurring phenolic acids, can induce iron release from holo soybean seed ferritin (SSF) in a structure-dependent manner. The ability of the iron release from SSF by five cinnamic acids follows the sequence of Cinnamic acid > Chlorogenic acid > Ferulic acid > *p*-Coumaric acid > *Trans*-Cinnamic acid. Fluorescence titration in conjunction with dialysis results showed that all of these five compounds have a similar, weak ability to bind with protein, suggesting that their protein-binding ability is not related to their iron release activity. In contrast, both Fe^{2+}-chelating activity and reducibility of these cinnamic acid derivatives are in good agreement with their ability to induce iron release from ferritin. These studies indicate that cinnamic acid and its derivatives could have a negative effect on iron stability of holo soybean seed ferritin in diet, and the Fe^{2+}-chelating activity and reducibility of cinnamic acid and its derivatives have strong relations to the iron release of soybean seed ferritin.

Keywords: cinnamic acid derivatives; soybean seed ferritin; iron release; binding ability; Fe^{2+}-chelating activity; reducibility

1. Introduction

Iron plays an essential role in living organisms, such as oxygen transfer, DNA synthesis, electron transport, and tricarboxylic acid and nitrogen fixation. Actually, iron deficiency is one of the most serious global nutritional problems, which affects about two billion people in the world [1]. Although the prevalence of iron deficiency anemia (IDA) is higher in developing countries, iron deficiency is still common among women and young children in industrial countries. More importantly, IDA can cause a series of consequences, such as reduced cognitive, motor development in infants and poor pregnancy outcomes. Ferritin is a natural and ubiquitous iron storage protein occurring widely in plants, animals, bacteria and fungi [2]. It consists of 24 subunits that assemble in a highly symmetric manner to a hollow protein shell with the outside diameter of about 12–13 nm and inner diameter of about 7–8 nm [3]. One ferritin molecule contains six four-fold, eight three-fold, and twelve two-fold channels (Figure 1a), which connect the inner cavity to bulk solution and serve as multiple pathways for iron entry and exit. Ferritin can store up to 4500 Fe^{3+} in its cavity, and therefore, natural ferritin, especially plant ferritin from legume seeds, has been considered as a novel alternative dietary iron supplement against IDA [1]. As compared to other iron supplements with a small size, ferritin has three major advantages: the protection of protein shell from interaction with other dietary factors, the safer form of iron stored as ferric cores rather than ferrous iron, and the possible intact absorption by receptor-mediated endocytosis [1].

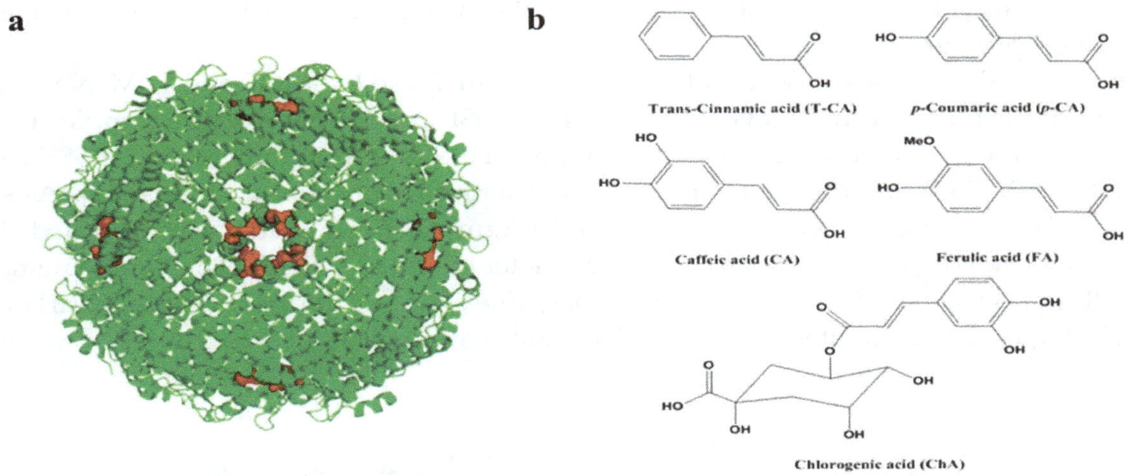

Figure 1. (**a**) Crystal structure of plant ferritin with views down the four-fold axes (channels) of the protein shell. The tryptophan residue of each subunit is highlighted in red; (**b**) Chemical structure of cinnamic acid derivatives: *Trans*-cinnamic acid (T-CA); *p*-Coumaric acid (*p*-CA); Caffiec acid (CA); Ferulic acid (FA); Chlorogenic acid (ChA).

So far, Fe^{2+} oxidation and mineral deposition in ferritin have been studied intensively and extensively [1,4]. Although some reductants such as ascorbate, 6-hydroxydopamine, 5-aminolevulinic acid, superoxide anion radical, 1,2,4-benzenetriol, benzene metabolites, NADH and anthocyanins have been shown to induce iron release from ferritin [5,6], and several iron chelators including 2, 2′-bipyridine, salicylate, citrate, nitrilotriacetate, and desferroxamine B can also induce iron release from ferritin at a slower rate [7–9]. However, there has been less attention paid to the iron release of ferritin induced by nutrients and the stability of ferritin iron core in food systems.

Phenolic acids are secondary metabolites, which are widely distributed in various plant foodstuffs. Among these phenolic acids, cinnamic acid derivatives (Figure 1b), such as caffeic, chlorogenic, *p*-coumaric and ferulic acids, are reported to possess functional activities like cancer prevention, antituberculosis, antileukaemic, hepatoprotective, antidiabetic, antioxidative, and hypocholesterolemic activities [10–12]. However, to date, whether these phenolic acids have an effect on the function of protein through intermolecular interaction has received much less attention. Based on the fact that phenolic acids such as cinnamic acid derivatives and ferritin co-exist in plant foodstuffs, and that cinnamic acid derivatives have a strong reducing activity, while ferric iron within phytoferritin exhibits a relatively strong oxidative activity, it is of special interest to know if the two kinds of molecules could interact with each other, and if so, what is the consequence of such interaction, which is the focus of this work.

2. Results and Discussion

2.1. Isolation and Characterization of SSF and rH-2

Ferritin can stay in two forms, holo and apo ferritin. Naturally occurring ferritin is a holo form which contains hydrous ferric oxide nanoparticles as iron cores within its cavity. Holo plant ferritin usually consists of two H type subunits of 26.5 (H-1) and 28.0 kDa (H-2), while their ratios vary among species. In this study, natural holo soybean seed ferritin (SSF) was used for iron release experiments because it is most extensively studied among all known plant ferritins [1,13]. However, our recent studies have showed that SSF is unstable during storage, because the extension peptide (EP) of the H-1 subunit exhibits significant serine protease-like activity, which is located at the N-terminal extremity. Consequently, recombinant soybean seed H-1 ferritin (rH-1) is prone to degradation, whereas its analogue, recombinant soybean seed H-1 ferritin (rH-2), becomes very stable under identical conditions [14]. Therefore, apo rH-2 was used to study the interaction between cinnamic acid derivatives and protein.

After purification, these two kinds of ferritins were analyzed by PAGE and TEM. Nondenaturing gel electrophoresis (native PAGE) revealed the purified SSF and rH-2 as a single complex (Figure 2a), suggesting that they have been purified to homogeneity. SDS-PAGE indicated that SSF consists of nearly 28.0 and 26.5 kD subunits, a result consistent with previous observations [15]. As expected, rH-2 was composed of only one 28.0 kD subunit (Figure 2b). TEM analyses revealed that rH-2 molecules were well dispersed with an outside diameter of ~12 nm (Figure 2c) after being negatively stained with uranyl acitate. In contrast, without negative staining, iron cores can be clearly observed in holo SSF (Figure 2d) as isolates contains ~1800 g atom of iron [1].

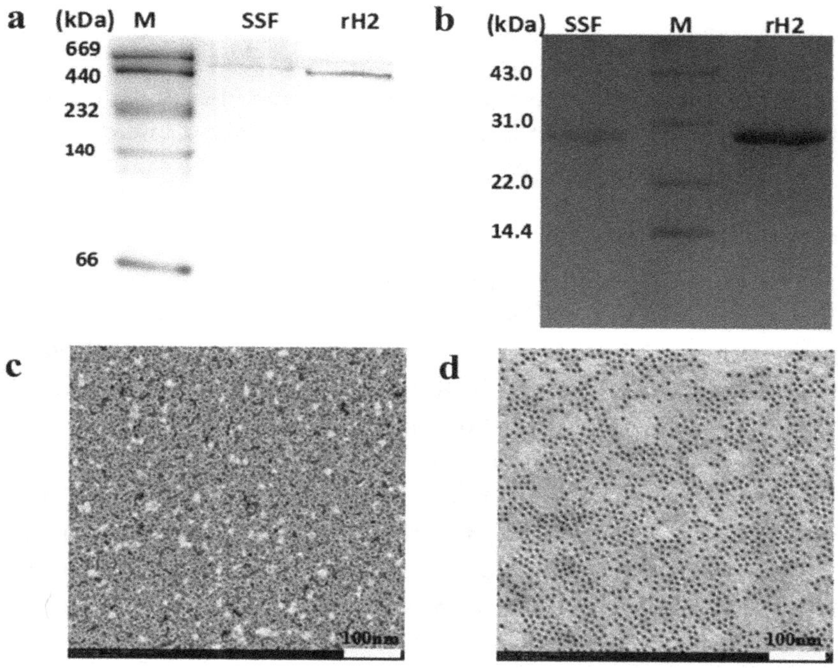

Figure 2. (**a**) Native PAGE analyses and (**b**) SDS-PAGE of soybean seed ferritin (SSF) and recombinant H2 ferritin (rH-2); (**c**) TEM picture of purified rH-2 after beingnegatively stained by 2% uranyl acetate; (**d**) TEM picture of holo soybean seed ferritin (SSF) without negative staining of uranyl acetate.

2.2. *Iron Release from SSF Induced by Cinnamic Acid Derivatives*

Subsequently, we analyzed the possibility of all cinnamic acid derivatives to induce iron release from SSF at a concentration of 25 μM [5], and results are displayed in Figure 3. It was found that all of them not only were able to cause iron release from protein shell, but also such iron release showed a structure-dependent manner. For example, CA induces iron release from SSF at the initial rate of 0.104 ± 0.006 mM/min, which is fastest among all tested compounds. The rate of iron release follows the sequence CA > ChA > FA > *p*-CA > T-CA in Mops buffer (pH 7.0) at 25 °C. CA has the higher ability to induce iron release from ferritin as compared to its analogue, ChA (0.092 ± 0.021) mM/min. This might be derived from the fact that ChA contains a sinapic acid group in its structure, thereby its large size prevents it from diffusion into the protein shell to some extent. These results suggest that the rate of iron release is inversely proportional to the size of phenolic acids, which is in agreement with a previous report [16]. Thus, it seems that the molecular size of phenolic acids plays an important role during the iron release from SSF induced by reductants.

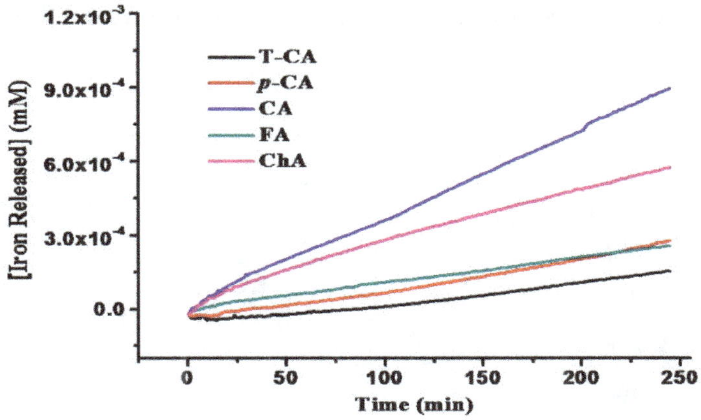

Figure 3. Kinetics of iron release from holo SSF induced by cinnamic acid derivatives. Iron release from SSF in the presence of reductants was followed by measuring the increase in absorbance at 562 nm about 250 min due to the chelation of Fe^{2+} by ferrozine. Conditions: 0.15 μM SSF, 25 μM cinnamic acids, 50 mM Mops, pH 7.0, 0.15 M NaCl, 500 μM ferrozine, 25 °C.

Besides, it was observed that the number of HO groups of cinnamic acid derivatives has a marked effect on the rate of iron release from ferritin. For example, with an increase in the number of HO from 0, 1, to 2, the rate of the iron release from ferritin increased from 0.002 ± 0.001 mM/min for T-CA, 0.014 ± 0.004 mM/min for *p*-CA, to 0.104 ± 0.006 mM/min for CA, respectively, suggesting that the number of HO group in cinnamic acid derivatives is closely associated with their ability to induce iron release from ferritin. Consistent with this idea, the rate of iron release from ferritin induced by CA was greatly decreased by ~50% after one HO group was replaced by OMe in FA (0.046 ± 0.011 mM/min) as shown in Figure 3.

2.3. *Fluorescence Quenching Analyses*

The above results demonstrated that all of these cinnamic acid derivatives are able to facilitate iron release from ferritin to different extents. To shed light on the mechanism by which iron release from ferritin was induced by these phenolic acids, we investigated the binding activity of these small molecules to ferritin through their interaction with protein. Protein intrinsic fluorescence mainly from Trp residues has been widely used to study their interaction with small molecules because of its sensitivity to microenviroment surrounding the fluorophore residue. As shown in Figure 1a, there are 24 Trp residues in one soybean seed ferritin molecule [17]. By taking advantage of this, we used intrinsic emission spectroscopy to study the interaction between these small molecules and apo rH-2, and results were shown in Figure 4. It was observed that all of cinnamic acid and its derivatives were able to quench the protein fluorescence, showing similar fluorescence quenching curves, indicative of similar interaction between cinnamic acid derivatives and apo rH-2. Thus, it seems that their interaction with apoferritin is independent of chemical structure, inconsistent with the above iron release results.

To determine whether these cinnamic acid derivatives can interact with proteins through binding, dialysis experiments were carried out wherein apo rH-2 (0.55 μM) was firstly incubated with these phenolic acids (22 μM), followed by dialysis against buffer for four times to remove free small molecules, respectively, and results are given in Figure 5. It was found that after dialysis for 5 h, the fluorescence of apo rH-2 could return to an original state upon treatment with these phenolic compounds, respectively (Figure 5). These results indicated that the fluorescence quenching of apo rH-2 caused by these compounds is dynamic, resulting from collisional encounters between the fluorophore and quencher. Instead, it is difficult to form a complex between ferritin and each of these cinnamic acid derivatives under the present experimental conditions; at most, the binding of the small compounds to apo rH-2 is very weak, and therefore, dialysis can remove them from their mixture with apo rH-2.

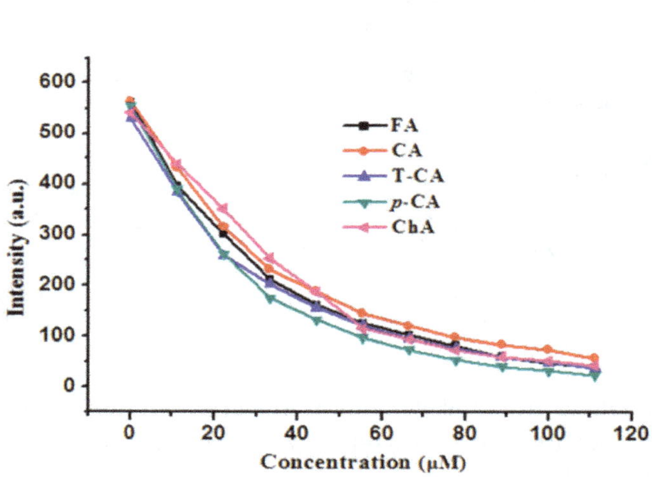

Figure 4. Comparison of cinnamic acids on the fluorescence quenching of apo rH-2. Conditions: 0.55 μM rH-2 in 50 mM Tris-HCl, [phenolic acids] = 0–110 μM, pH 7.0, 25 °C. λEx = 280 nm, slits for excitation and emission are 5 nm and 10 nm.

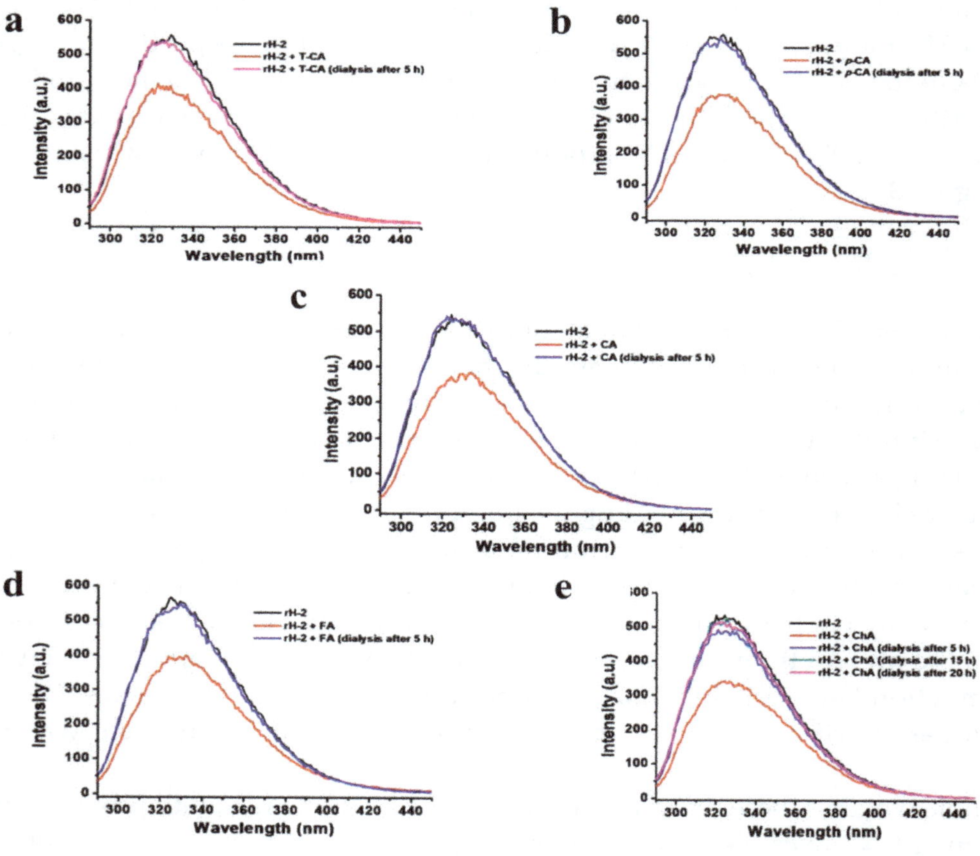

Figure 5. Dialysis study of rH-2 with cinnamic acids at pH 7.0. (**a**) *Trans*-Cinnamic acid; (**b**) *p*-Coumaric acid; (**c**) Caffeic acid; (**d**) Ferulic acid; (**e**) chlorogenic acid. Conditions: 0.55 μM rH-2 in 50 mM Tris-HCl, [cinnamic acids] = 22 μM, 25 °C. λ_{Ex} = 280 nm, slits for excitation and emission are 5 nm and 10 nm.

The weak binding activity of the cinnamic acid derivatives to ferritin might be derived from the fact that they contain less than three hydroxyl groups in the structure. Consistent with this view, our recent study showed that gallic acid, methyl gallate and propyl gallate having three HO groups can bind to rH-2 tightly, while their analogues with two HO groups cannot [18]. Thus, the number of the hydroxyl groups is closely associated with the interaction mode between phenolic acids and protein, and more hydroxyl groups in the structure favors the binding of phenolic acids to protein. Further support for this idea comes from a recent study showing that tannic acid with many hydroxyl groups can facilitate ferritn association through strong hydrogen bonds [19].

2.4. Effect of the Fe^{2+} Chelating Activity of Cinnamic Acid Derivatives on the Iron Release from Ferritin

It was previously reported that the chelating activity of reductants on iron ion was an important factor which is related to iron release from the ferritin shell [20]. Therefore, in this study, the iron chelating activity of cinnamic acid derivatives was determined, respectively, to gain insight into the mechanism of iron release from ferritin. As shown in Figure 6a, the chelating activity of cinnamic acid derivatives on ferrous ions follows the sequence of CA > ChA > FA > T-CA ≈ *p*-CA. The chelating activity of CA and ChA with catechol moiety was ~63% and 58%, respectively, which was almost six-fold stronger than their analogue, FA (~11%) where one hydroxyl group was replaced with OMe. The large difference in the chelating activity between CA/ChA and FA suggested that two hydroxyl groups in the benzene ring of CA and ChA were required for Fe^{2+} chelating, while one hydroxyl group in the benzene ring of FA is not enough to chelate iron. Agreeing with this idea, both T-CA (~7.0%) and *p*-CA (~6.5%) with zero or one hydroxyl group exhibited even much weaker chelating activity than CA or ChA. Additionally, it was found that CA and ChA exhibited nearly the same chelating activity, suggesting that the carboxyl group might not be involved in iron chelating, and at most it contributed much less to iron chelating as compared to the hydroxyl group.

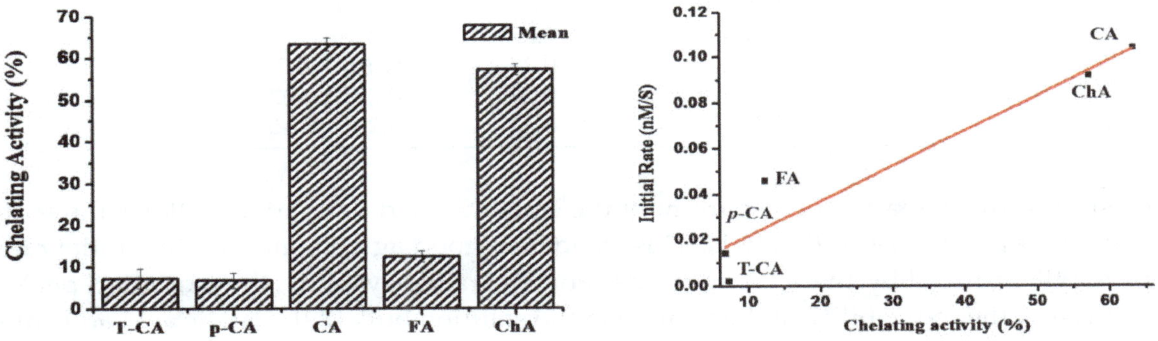

Figure 6. Chelating activity of cinnamic acid derivatives on ferrous ion. Vertical bars represent the standard error from means of three separate tests.

More importantly, it was observed that the chelating activity of these phenolic acids was in good agreement with the above iron release results (Figure 3); namely, the stronger the chelating activity, the faster rate of the iron release from ferritin. Consistent with this conclusion, there is a linear relationship between the rate of iron release from ferritin induced by these phenolic acids and their chelating activity as shown in Figure 6b. Based on these findings, it is reasonable to believe that the chelating activity of cinnamic acid derivatives has an important effect on the rate of iron release from ferritin induced by these compounds. This might be because these cinnamic acid derivatives can act as iron chelators to help iron to move out of SSF.

2.5. Effect of Reducibility of Cinnamic Acid Derivatives on the Iron Release from Ferritin

To better understand the mechanism of iron release from ferritin, we also studied the voltammetric oxidation of these phenolic acids in pH 7.0 phosphate buffer by cyclic voltammetry, and results are shown in Figure 7a. Cyclic voltammograms of CA, FA, *p*-CA and ChA at a sweep rate of 100 mM s^{-1} exhibited one anodic peak and one cathodic peak, suggesting that the oxidation process for these four investigated compounds was reversible. However, cyclic voltammograms of T-CA showed no peak, indicating that T-CA has no reducibility [21]. As shown Table 1, ChA (0.31 V) has the largest anodic peak potential among all of the five compounds.

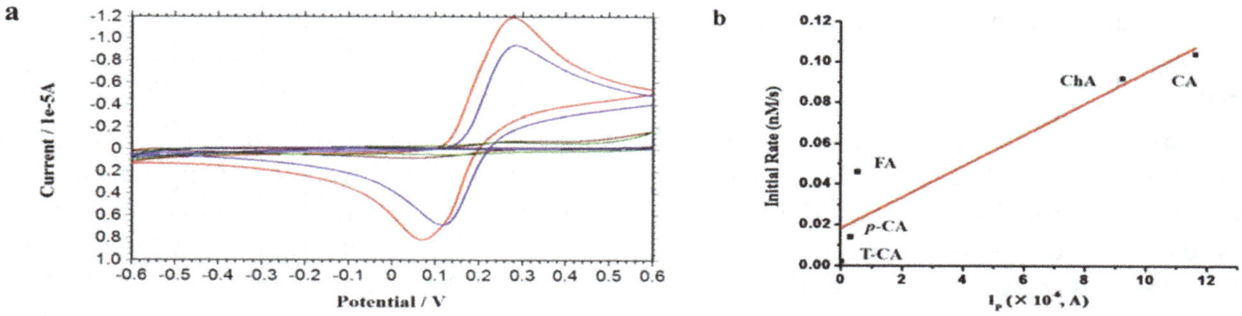

Figure 7. Cyclic voltammograms taken with a 3-mm glassy carbon electrode at 100 mVs^{-1} of: 0.5 mM cinnamic acid (mazarine line), *p*-coumaric acid (green line), caffeic acid (red line), ferulic acid (carmine red), and chlorogenic acid (blue red) in 50 mM phosphate buffer of pH 7.0.

Table 1. Evaluation of the anodic peak potentials of the studied cinnamic acid derivatives (E_P—anodic peak potential (V)) at pH 7.0, as well as the anodic peak currents at pH 7.0 (I_P—anodic peak current (A)) during the cyclic voltammetry experiment.

Phenolic Compound	E_P	I_P ($\times 10^{-6}$)
T-CA	0	0
p-CA	0.27	0.31 ± 0.12
CA	0.28	11.61 ± 0.35
FA	0.24	0.53 ± 0.07
ChA	0.31	9.23 ± 0.46

Interestingly, the oxidation peak current of the cinnamic acid derivatives follows the sequence of CA > ChA > FA > *p*-CA > T-CA (Table 1). This trend is in good agreement with the initial rate of iron release from SSF induced by these compounds. For reversible systems, the oxidation peak current, I_P could represent the reducibility of the analyte in the solution bulk [22]. Caffeic acid and chlorogenic acid with two hydroxyl groups in their benzene ring structure show the stronger oxidation peak current as compared with chlorogenic acid. In contrast, FA and *p*-CA with only one hydroxyl group have weaker oxidation peak current, while T-CA with no HO group has no reducibility. These results indicated that the reducibility of cinnamic acids can greatly influence the rate of iron release from SSF. Indeed, there is also a linear relationship between the oxidation peak current of the cinnamic acid derivatives and their ability to induce iron release from ferritin as shown in Figure 7b. Therefore, the reducibility of phenolic acids also is another important factor affecting their ability to induce iron release from the ferritin shell.

3. Materials and Methods

3.1. Chemicals

Five cinnamic acid derivatives used in this study were purchased from J&K Chemical (Beijing, China). Ferrous ion chelator 3-(2-pyridyl)-5,6-bis(4-phenylsulfonic acid)-1,2,4-triazine (ferrozine) was obtained from Sigma-Aldrich Chemical Co. (Beijing, China). Sephacryl S-300, DEAE Sepharose Fast Flow, native electrophoresis marker, and SDS electrophoresis marker were purchased from GE Healthcare Bio-Sciences AB (Beijing, China). Sodium citrate, terephthalic acid (TA) and magnesium chloride hexahydrate were obtained from Beijing Chemical Reagents Co. (Beijing, China). All other reagents used were of analytical grade or purer.

3.2. *Preparation of Soybean Seed Ferritin (SSF) and Recombinant Soybean Seed H-2 Ferritin (rH-2)*

SSF and apo rH-2 were purified as previously described with some modification [23,24]. Typically, approximately 1 kg of soybean seeds was soaked in distilled water for 8 h and mixed with three volumes of extraction buffer (50 mM KH_2PO_4, pH 7.5, 1% polyvinylpolypyrrolidone). After filtration, the filtrate was incubated for 15 min at 60 °C and then was centrifuged at 5000× *g* for 5 min to separate the insoluble material. The supernatant was adjusted to 0.5 M $MgCl_2$ and the mixture stood for 30 min at 4 °C followed by addition of sodium citrate (final concentration of 0.7 M) to complex the magnesium. After 10 h, the resultant supernatant was centrifuged at 12,000× *g* for 20 min at 4 °C. The brown precipitate thus obtained was dissolved in 50 mM KH_2PO_4•Na_2HPO_4 buffer (pH 7.5) and was dialyzed against the same buffer three times.

Escherichis coli strain BL21 (DE3) which contained rH-2 expression plasmids was grown at 37 °C. Protein expression was induced with 1 mM IPTG (isopropyl β-D-1-thiogalactopyranoside) for 7 h. The system was centrifuged and re-suspended in buffer solution (50 mM Tris-HCl, pH 8.0), followed by disruption by sonication. The supernatant of the crude extract was collected by centrifugation and further purified by ammonium sulfate fractionation (40% saturated fraction). After washed by distilled water to remove other proteins, the sediment was dissolved by solution buffer. Next the solution was dialyzed against the same buffer three times to remove the ammonium sulfate. SSF and rH-2 protein were further purified by Sephacryl S-300 gel filtration chromatography (GFC) and DEAE-Sepharose Fast Flow column, respectively. Finally, protein purity was analyzed by SDS-PAGE and Native-PAGE analysis. Protein concentrations were determined according to the Lowry method as previous reported [25].

3.3. *Kinetic Measurement of Iron Release from Holo Soybean Seed Ferritin*

The assay system (1 mL of total volume) contained 0.21 μM ferritin, 500 μM ferrozine, 0.15 M NaCl, and 25 μM cinnamic acid derivatives in 50 mM Mops buffer, pH 7.0 as previously described [5]. The same solution but just using buffer instead of cinnamic acid derivatives was used as control. Experiments were conducted at 25 °C. The iron release was measured with the development of $[Fe(ferrozine)_3]^{2+}$ at 562 nm using a Varian Cary 50 spectrophotometer, and $\varepsilon_{562} = 27.9\ mM^{-1}cm^{-1}$. The absorbance at 562 nm from the control was deducted from that of all sample mixtures. The initial rate (v_0) of iron release measured as $[Fe(ferrozine)_3]^{2+}$ formation was obtained from the linear A_1 term of third-order polynomial fitted to the experimental data as reported previously: $Y = A_0 + A_1t + A_2t^2 + A_3t^3$ and $dY/dt = A_1 + 2A_2t + 3A_3t^2$ (at t = 0, $(dY/dt)_0 = v_0$). Here t is the time in minutes and Y is the concentration of $[Fe(ferrozine)_3]^{2+}$ at time t in minutes [16].

3.4. *Fluorescence Titration Analysis*

Fluorescence titration measurements were recorded on a Cary Eclipse fluorescence spectrophotometer (Varian, Polo Alto, CA, USA), using quartz cuvettes of 1 cm path length at room temperature. In this measurement, apo rH-2 (0.55 μM, 150 mM NaCl and 50 mM Tris-HCl, pH 7.0) was titrated with 1 μL cinnamic acid derivatives (5 mM, 50 mM Tris-HCl, pH 7.0), respectively. The excitation wavelength was 280 nm, and the emission wavelength was 325 nm. Furthermore, dialysis measurements were conducted to analyze the binding affinity of cinnamic acids to apo rH-2. Typically, a mixture of apo rH-2 (0.55 μM) plus cinnamic acid derivatives (22 μM) was dialyzed (100 kDa cutoff) for 5 h against the solution buffer (50 mM Tris-HCl and 150 mM NaCl, at pH 7.0) to detect this kind of interaction [18].

3.5. *Chelating Activity of Cinnamic Acid Derivatives on Ferrous Ion*

The chelating activity of cinnamic acid derivatives on ferrous ion was measured as described previously with some modifications [5]. The reaction system (1 mL) contained 20 μM $FeSO_4$, 60 μM ferrozine, and 60 μM cinnamic acid derivatives in 50 mM Mops buffer (pH 7.0). After reaction for

5 min at 25 °C, the absorbance of system was detected at 562 nm spectrophotometrically. The ability of cinnamic acids to chelate Fe^{2+} was calculated as follows: chelating activity (%) = $\frac{A0-A}{A0} \times 100$, where A and A_0 are the absorbance in the presence or absence of the cinnamic acid derivatives, respectively.

3.6. Cyclic Voltammetry

Cyclic voltammetry experiments were performed using a potentiostat (microAutolab Type III with an Autolab Faraday Cage) and voltammograms were obtained with a scan rate of 100 mV s^{-1} with an increment potential of 2.4 mV, between −0.6 V and 0.6 V. The working electrode was a 3 mm glassy carbon disk in combination with a Metrohm tipholder, cleaned by polishing with 3 μm alumina powder during 30 s followed by fixing the potential in ultrasonication during 5 s, between acquisitions. A saturated calomel electrode was used as a reference electrode in conjunction with a platinum counter electrode. Each acquisition required 40 mL of sample. Oxygen was removed with a N_2 current flow during 5 min prior to analysis. Cyclic voltammetry experiments were controlled by the CHI600E Electrochemical Workstation. Cyclic voltammograms were taken in the absence and in the presence of cinnamic acid derivatives.

3.7. Statistical Analysis

All data analyses were performed using Origin 8.0 software and the structural formula was processed by ChemDraw 7.0. All experiments were carried out in triplicate.

4. Conclusions

The present study demonstrates that cinnamic acid derivatives, a class of naturally occurring phenolic acids, can induce iron release from holo soybean seed ferritin (SSF) in a structure-dependent manner for the first time. The ability of iron release from SSF by five cinnamic acids follows the sequence of CA > ChA > FA > *p*-CA > T-CA. Although the five phenolic acids exhibit a weak ability to bind with ferritin, they are able to induce iron release from holo ferritin through their Fe^{2+}-chelating activity and reducibility. These studies indicate that cinnamic acid and its derivatives could have a negative effect on iron absorption in humans, because they can result in loss of a certain amount of iron from holo ferritin through interactions. Therefore, the interactions between cinnamic acid derivatives and holo SSF should be avoided as much as possible during food processing.

Author Contributions: G.Z. and X.S. conceived and designed the experiments; X.S. performed the experiments; X.S., H.C. and Z.J analyzed the data; X.S. and H.C. wrote the paper.

Acknowledgments: This project was supported by the National Natural Science Foundation of China (31671805).

References

1. Zhao, G. Phytoferritin and its implications for human health and nutrition. *BBA-Gen. Subj.* **2010**, *1800*, 815–823. [CrossRef] [PubMed]
2. Theil, E.C. Iron, ferritin, and nutrition. *Annu. Rev. Nutr.* **2004**, *24*, 327–343. [CrossRef] [PubMed]
3. Harrison, P.M.; Arosio, P. The ferritins: Molecular properties, iron storage function and cellular regulation. *BBA-Bioenerg.* **1996**, *1275*, 161–203. [CrossRef]
4. Zhao, G.; Bou-Abdallah, F.; Arosio, P.; Levi, S.; Janus-Chandler, C.; Chasteen, N.D. Multiple pathways for mineral core formation in mammalian apoferritin. The role of hydrogen peroxide. *Biochemistry* **2003**, *42*, 3142–3150. [CrossRef] [PubMed]
5. Deng, J.; Cheng, J.; Liao, X.; Zhang, T.; Leng, X.; Zhao, G. Comparative study on iron release from Soybean (*Glycine max*) seed ferritin induced by anthocyanins and ascorbate. *J. Agric. Food Chem.* **2010**, *58*, 635–641. [CrossRef] [PubMed]

6. Lv, C.; Bai, Y.; Yang, S.; Zhao, G.; Chen, B. NADH induces iron release from pea seed ferritin: A model for interaction between coenzyme and protein components in foodstuffs. *Food Chem.* **2013**, *14*, 3851–3858. [CrossRef] [PubMed]
7. Castruita, M.; Elmegreen, L.A.; Shaked, Y.; Stiefel, E.I.; Morel, F.M.M. Comparison of the kinetics of iron release from a marine (*Trichodesmium erythraeum*) Dps protein and mammalian ferritin in the presence and absence of ligands. *J. Inorg. Biochem.* **2007**, *101*, 1686–1691. [CrossRef] [PubMed]
8. Crichton, R.R.; Roman, F.; Roland, F. Iron mobilization from ferritin by chelating agents. *J. Inorg. Biochem.* **1980**, *13*, 305–316. [CrossRef]
9. Laulhere, J.P.; Briat, J.F. Iron release and uptake by plant ferritin: Effects of pH, reduction and chelation. *Biochem. J.* **1993**, *290*, 693–699. [CrossRef] [PubMed]
10. De, P.; Baltas, M.; Bedos-Belval, F. Cinnamic acid derivatives as anticancer agents—A review. *Curr. Med. Chem.* **2011**, *18*, 1672–1703. [CrossRef] [PubMed]
11. Giles, F.; Fischer, T.; Cortes, J.; Garcia-Manero, G.; Beck, J.; Ravandi, F.; Masson, E.; Rae, P.; Sova, M. Antioxidant and antimicrobial activities of cinnamic acid derivatives. *Mini-Rev. Med. Chem.* **2012**, *12*, 749–767.
12. Sharma, P. Cinnamic acid derivatives: A new chapter of various pharmacological activities. *J. Chem. Pharm. Res.* **2011**, *3*, 403–423.
13. Lv, C.; Zhao, G.; Lönnerdal, B. Bioavailability of iron from plant and animal ferritins. *J. Nutr. Biochem.* **2015**, *26*, 532–540. [CrossRef] [PubMed]
14. Fu, X.; Deng, J.; Yang, H.; Masuda, T.; Goto, F.; Yoshiara, T.; Zhao, G. A novel EP-involved pathway for iron release from soya bean seed ferritin. *Biochem. J.* **2010**, *427*, 313–321. [CrossRef] [PubMed]
15. Masuda, T.; Goto, F.; Yoshihara, T. A novel plant ferritin subunit from soybean that is related to a mechanism in iron release. *J. Biol. Chem.* **2001**, *276*, 19575–19579. [CrossRef] [PubMed]
16. Hynes, M.J.; Coinceanainn, M.Ó. Investigation of the release of iron from ferritin by naturally occuring antioxidants. *J. Inorg. Biochem.* **2002**, *90*, 18–21. [CrossRef]
17. Masuda, T.; Goto, F.; Yoshihara, T.; Mikami, B. Crystal structure of plant ferritin reveals a novel metal binding site that functions as a transit site for metal transfer in ferritin. *J. Biol. Chem.* **2010**, *285*, 4049–4059. [CrossRef] [PubMed]
18. Wang, Q.; Zhou, K.; Ning, Y.; Zhao, G. Effect of the structure of gallic acid and its derivatives on their interaction with plant ferritin. *Food Chem.* **2016**, *213*, 260–267. [CrossRef] [PubMed]
19. Li, M.; Jia, X.; Yang, J.; Deng, J.; Zhao, G. Effect of tannic acid on properties of soybean (*Glycine max*) seed ferritin: A model for interaction between naturallyoccurring components in foodstuffs. *Food Chem.* **2012**, *133*, 410–415. [CrossRef] [PubMed]
20. Boyer, R.F.; McCleary, C.J. Superoxide ion as a primary reductant in ascorbate mediated ferritin iron release. *Free Radic. Biol. Med.* **1987**, *3*, 389–395. [CrossRef]
21. Madrakian, T.; Soleimani, M.; Afkhami, A. Simultaneous determination of mycophenolate mofetil and its active metabolite, mycophenolic acid, by differential pulse voltammetry using multi-walled carbon nanotubes modified glassy carbon electrode. *Mat. Sci. Eng. C* **2014**, *42*, 38–45. [CrossRef] [PubMed]
22. Hoyos-Arbeláez, J.; Vázquez, M.; Contreras-Calderón, J. Electrochemical methods as a tool for determining the antioxidant capacity of food and beverages: A review. *Food Chem.* **2017**, *221*, 1371–1381. [CrossRef] [PubMed]
23. Laulhere, J.P.; Lescure, A.M.; Briat, J.F. Purification and characterization of ferritins from maize, pea, and soyabean seeds. *J. Biol. Chem.* **1988**, *263*, 10289–10294. [PubMed]
24. Masuda, T.; Goto, F.; Yoshihara, T.; Ezure, T.; Suzuki, T.; Kobayashi, S.; Shikata, M.; Utsumi, S. Construction of homo- and heteropolymers of plant ferritin subunits using an in vitro protein expression system. *Protein Expr. Purif.* **2007**, *56*, 237–246. [CrossRef] [PubMed]
25. Lowry, O.H.; Rosebrough, N.J.; Farr, A.L.; Randall, R.J. Protein measurement with the Folin phenol reagents. *J. Biol. Chem.* **1951**, *193*, 265–275. [PubMed]

8

Iron as a Therapeutic Target in *HFE*-Related Hemochromatosis: Usual and Novel Aspects

Olivier Loréal *, Thibault Cavey, François Robin, Moussa Kenawi, Pascal Guggenbuhl and Pierre Brissot

INSERM, Univ Rennes, INRA, CHU Rennes, Institut NUMECAN (Nutrition Metabolisms and Cancer), F-35033 Rennes, France; thibault.cavey@chu-rennes.fr (T.C.); francois.robin@chu-rennes.fr (F.R.); moussa.kenawi@univ-rennes1.fr (M.K.); pascal.guggenbuhl@univ-rennes1.fr (P.G.); pierre.brissot@univ-rennes1.fr (P.B.)

* Correspondence: olivier.loreal@univ-rennes1.fr;

Abstract: Genetic hemochromatosis is an iron overload disease that is mainly related to the *C282Y* mutation in the *HFE* gene. This gene controls the expression of hepcidin, a peptide secreted in plasma by the liver and regulates systemic iron distribution. Homozygous *C282Y* mutation induces hepcidin deficiency, leading to increased circulating transferrin saturation, and ultimately, iron accumulation in organs such as the liver, pancreas, heart, and bone. Iron in excess may induce or favor the development of complications such as cirrhosis, liver cancer, diabetes, heart failure, hypogonadism, but also complaints such as asthenia and disabling arthritis. Iron depletive treatment mainly consists of venesections that permit the removal of iron contained in red blood cells and the subsequent mobilization of stored iron in order to synthesize hemoglobin for new erythrocytes. It is highly efficient in removing excess iron and preventing most of the complications associated with excess iron in the body. However, this treatment does not target the biological mechanisms involved in the iron metabolism disturbance. New treatments based on the increase of hepcidin levels, by using hepcidin mimetics or inducers, or inhibitors of the iron export activity of ferroportin protein that is the target of hepcidin, if devoid of significant secondary effects, should be useful to better control iron parameters and symptoms, such as arthritis.

Keywords: iron; genetic hemochromatosis; non transferrin bound iron; hepcidin; ferroportin; venesections

---

Iron metabolism must be tightly controlled in order to avoid deleterious situations, including iron overload diseases, especially *HFE*-related hemochromatosis. In such conditions an iron depletive treatment is engaged in order to avoid the development of complications. However, iron depletive therapy targets only iron excess and alternative, possibly complementary, novel approaches are needed.

1. Normal Iron Metabolism

1.1. The Ferroportin/Hepcidin Duo Controls Systemic Iron Metabolism

Systemic iron metabolism is characterized by a continuous distribution of iron from plasma toward cells which require its presence for participating in biological functions, including oxygen transport and enzymatic processes [1]. Plasma iron must be continuously renewed. Plasma iron originates predominantly from macrophages that recycle iron from senescent erythrocytes during the erythrophagocytosis process. The erythropoietic cells contains 70% of total body iron. The macrophages provide schematically 19 mg out of the 20 mg of iron required from the plasma by cells every day. The second source of iron is digestive absorption. Iron is absorbed in two steps from the nutrients. The first step takes place at the apical pole of the enterocytes, non-heme and heme iron being transferred from nutrients to the enterocyte cytoplasm. The transfer of non-heme iron implicates DMT1 (divalent metal transporter 1) that takes up ferrous iron [2] after reduction by the ferrireductase dCytb [3]. Heme iron is taken up through a receptor that could be HCP1 (heme carrier protein1) (controversial) [4–6]. The second step of iron absorption is the transfer of iron from the cytoplasm toward the plasma through the basal membrane of the enterocyte. This process limits the iron entry into the body, and only 1–2 mg are transferred each day toward the plasma, whereas the remaining iron is transiently stored within the cytoplasm and will be lost during enterocyte desquamation. This selective process is the classical mucosal block [7]. Ferroportin is the iron export protein that allows iron egress from enterocytes (concerning both the non-heme and heme iron absorbed at the apical side) and macrophages toward the plasma [8–10]. Once transferred into the plasma, and after its oxidation by ferroxidase enzymes—ceruloplasmin [11] and/or hephaestin [12]—ferric iron is associated to transferrin, the protein that can link up to two iron atoms and delivers iron to cells. Cellular uptake of transferrin iron is mediated by the transferrin receptor 1 (TFR1) [13]. Thereafter, endocytosis of the complex permits the transport of iron into endocytic vesicles and subsequently, its transfer to the cytosol by DMT1, that is also expressed in endocytic vesicles, after oxidation of iron by STEAP3 (*Six-Transmembrane Epithelial Antigen of the Prostate* 3) [14]. Another transferrin receptor, transferrin receptor 2 (TFR2) is expressed by cells, especially hepatocytes, but its affinity coefficient for transferrin is very low [15] so that its function is related to iron sensing rather than iron transport [16].

Hepcidin is a small cysteine rich peptide [17–19], mainly expressed by hepatocytes and secreted in the plasma, that interacts with ferroportin [20], the only known protein involved in cellular iron export. An increase of plasma hepcidin level leads to a decrease of both digestive iron absorption and iron leakage by macrophages [21]. Hepcidin decreases plasma iron concentration and the saturation of transferrin by iron. Conversely, a decrease of hepcidin expression favors cell membrane expression of ferroportin, and, in turn, the iron release from cells into the plasma, thus, increasing the transferrin saturation by iron. The regulation of hepcidin expression plays a major role in the maintenance of iron homeostasis.

1.2. Regulation of Hepcidin Expression

Hepcidin expression is regulated by many factors, including iron status [19] and inflammation [19,22] that induce an upregulation of hepcidin expression, and hypoxia/erythropoiesis activity [23–25] that decrease hepcidin expression. Mechanisms related to the induction of hepcidin expression by iron status are mainly transcriptional.

The first iron-related mechanism that regulates hepcidin expression is reported to be linked to transferrin saturation level in plasma [26,27]. This pathway involves the *HFE* gene, located on the chromosome 6, that encodes a HLA like class I protein that is expressed on cell membrane in association with the ß2-microglobulin [28]. It has been reported that HFE protein may interact either with TFR1 [29,30] or TFR2. The mechanism potentially involved in such regulation is a decrease of the physical interaction between TFR1 and HFE proteins when transferrin saturation increases [31]. This could lead to the stimulation of a MAP (mitogen-activated protein kinase) signaling pathway that promotes the hepcidin transcription level [27]. However, while the HFE/TFR2 interaction has been documented in in vitro experiments, the in vivo relevance of these findings is questionable [32]. The increase of hepcidin expression promotes ferroportin degradation, and thus, reduces plasma iron concentration and transferrin saturation by iron (Figure 1).

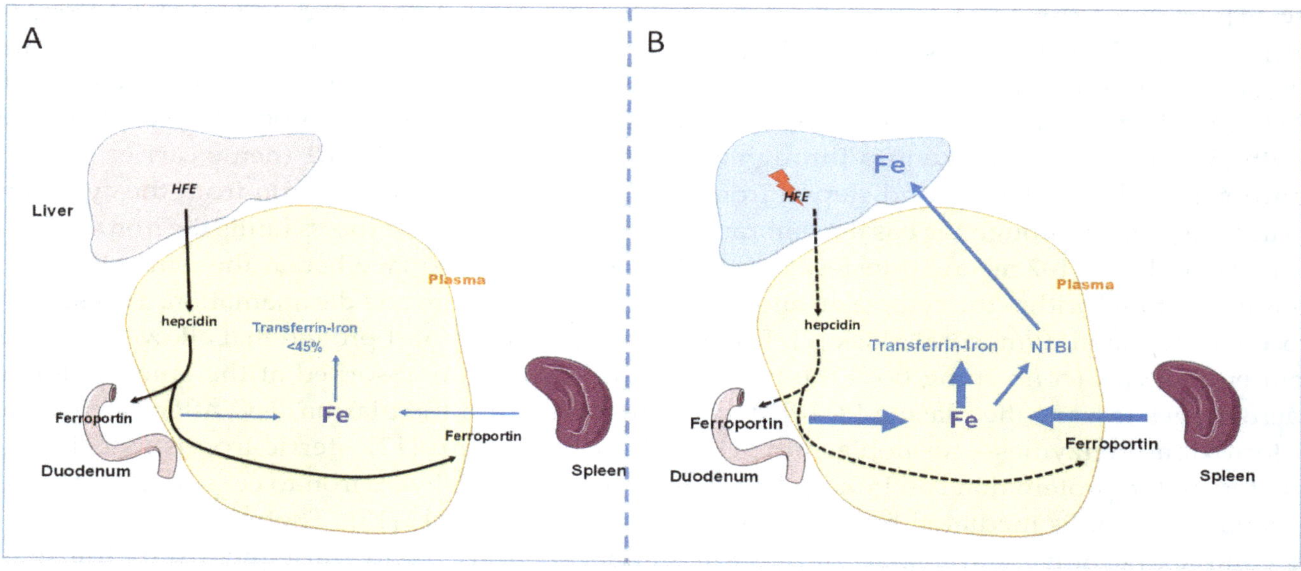

Figure 1. Schematic representation of the pathophysiological mechanisms leading to the development of iron overload during *HFE*-related hemochromatosis. (**A**): Normal situation with adequate *HFE* signaling allowing control of transferrin saturation level (<45%). (**B**): Genetic hemochromatosis with low activity of *HFE*-related signaling that limits hepcidin expression and in turn favors iron release in plasma, despite the presence of a sufficient amount of iron. Thus, the transferrin saturation increases and non-transferrin bound iron appears and targets organs such as liver, leading to abnormal iron accumulation.

The second regulatory mechanism implicates the bone morphogenetic protein/hemojuvelin/son of mothers against decapentaplegic homolog (BMP/HJV/SMAD) pathway [33–36]. When cell iron concentration increases, BMP6 and BMP2 proteins are produced and secreted by hepatocytes and more likely sinusoidal cells [37–39]. BMPs interact with BMP receptor proteins that are associated to HJV, acting as BMPs co-receptor. The interaction induces a phosphorylation of SMADs (Son of Mothers Against Decapentaplegic) 1, 5, 8 that are translocated toward the nucleus after association with SMAD4 in the nucleus [40,41]. Then, they interact with BMP-responsive element sequence within the hepcidin gene promoter and promote hepcidin transcription [35,36,42].

It is noteworthy that the hemochromatosis proteins HFE and HJV form a membrane-associated protein complex for hepcidin regulation. This suggests that the two pathways are not fully independent [43,44], and further work should help to better specify the respective roles of the different actors.

2. Pathophysiology of *HFE* Hemochromatosis

2.1. HFE Hemochromatosis

HFE hemochromatosis is a disease mainly related to homozygosity of the *C282Y* (*p.Cys282Tyr*) mutation in the *HFE* gene [45]. The *p.Cys282Tyr* mutation alters the structure of the *HFE* protein due to the substitution of a cysteine that is engaged in intra-molecular disulfide bounds, that play a role in the protein shape, by a threonine. Thus, the expression of HFE protein on cell membrane, as well as its interaction with the Beta2 microglobulin are altered [29]. Some exceptional private mutations in the *HFE* gene can also lead to hemochromatosis, when present either at the homozygous state or in association with the *C282Y* mutation [46]. Homozygosity for *H63D* (*p.His63Asp*) that is present at homozygous state in approximately 2% of the Caucasian population cannot by itself generate clinically significant iron excess, so that, when associated to iron overload, one must search for associated genetic or acquired associated factors that promote iron excess [47]. It must be pointed out that the penetrance of *HFE*-related hemochromatosis is very incomplete. In terms of clinical penetrance, some studies have estimated a prevalence of 25–60%, while a single study reported a prevalence of 28% in males and 1% in females [48]. However, in the same study the biochemical penetrance, assessed by increased ferritinemia, was much higher (82% and 55%, respectively) [48].

2.2. *Pathophysiology of Iron Overload during HFE Hemochromatosis*

In hemochromatosis, iron overload is a two-hit phenomenon.

The first hit (Figure 1), which is related to the structural change of the protein is a deficiency in hepcidin expression and secretion—meaning hepcidin deficiency—compared to the iron stores [22,26]. In other words, hepcidin expression is lower than expected when considering plasma transferrin saturation and body iron stores [49]. This hepcidin deficiency results from the mutation in the *HFE* gene that alters the efficacy of the transduction pathway regulating hepcidin expression. Consecutively, despite iron excess, ferroportin expression on cell membranes of enterocytes and macrophages remains elevated and favors an increase of both plasma iron concentration and transferrin iron saturation [20]. As previously mentioned, transferrin iron ingress into cells is modulated by the expression level of its receptor TFR1. In physiological situation, TFR1 expression on cell membranes is downregulated when cellular iron is in excess [50], in order to avoid cellular iron accumulation with subsequent toxicity, especially through the production of reactive oxygen species (ROS) [51,52]. The iron responsive element/iron regulatory protein system (IRE/IRP) regulates TFR1 and ferritin expression, adapting iron entry into the cell (TFR1) and the capacity of iron storage in cells (ferritin), to the variations of cellular iron content [50,53].

The second hit (Figure 1) involved in the development of iron overload in hemochromatosis results from the appearance of the non-transferrin-bound form of iron (NTBI) [54]. Indeed, transferrin saturation increase favors the presence of NTBI in plasma [55]. The NTBI is constituted of low molecular forms of iron linked to citrate or acetate [56]. The NTBI, in contrast to transferrin iron, constantly enters the cells, especially through the Zip14 transporter [57], even when they are already overloaded [58,59], whereas transferrin iron ingress is physiologically reduced due to the decrease of TFR1 on cell membrane [60,61]. The transporters involved in the uptake of NTBI are mainly expressed in the liver, the pancreas [57,62], and the heart, explaining that these organs are the primary targets of iron excess.

It is important to note that rare or very rare non-*HFE* mutations may also favor hepcidin deficiency. Homozygous and compound heterozygous mutations in the *HAMP* [63] or *HJV* [64] genes induce an early and severe iron overload disease (juvenile hemochromatosis) that is related to severe hepcidin deficiency with major complications that quickly impact well-being and life expectancy. In addition, mutations in the *TFR2* gene induce an hepcidin deficiency that provokes a clinical iron overload phenotype which is in between juvenile hemochromatosis and the classical *HFE*-related hemochromatosis form [65].

2.3. *Pathophysiology of Organ Damage in Hemochromatosis*

Complications of *HFE*-related genetic hemochromatosis, and more globally of hemochromatosis related to hepcidin deficiency, include hepatic damage with the development of liver fibrosis, with the risks of cirrhosis and hepatocellular carcinoma, diabetes, and at a lesser degree, heart dysfunction, which are sources of morbidity and mortality [66,67]. The risk of hepatic fibrosis increases with the severity of iron overload [68], and it is recommended to perform a liver biopsy in patients exhibiting very high levels of ferritinemia [69]. This risk is associated with the presence of sideronecrotic lesions of hepatocytes [70], that likely corresponds to the recently identified ferroptotic cell death process [71,72], a new cell death pathway in cells containing high iron content. Whereas hepatocyte iron loading is the pathophysiological basic feature of iron overload in hemochromatosis, it is noteworthy that Kupffer cell iron load finally occurs in advanced iron hemochromatosis and also represents a risk for the development of hepatic damage [70]. The role of an iron-related induction of TGF (transforming growth factor)-beta in the development of fibrosis has been reported [73,74]. It should be underlined that hepatocellular carcinoma, that mostly develops in patients with a cirrhotic liver, can also be rarely found in non-cirrhotic patients which suggests the role of iron itself [75] and/or additional cofactors in the development of hepatocellular carcinoma (HCC) (see below). Finally, patients exhibiting cirrhosis before iron depletive treatment still present a risk for developing HCC even despite completion of iron depletive treatment [67].

Other complications may include hypogonadism—mostly in juvenile hemochromatosis—and much more frequently osteoporosis and arthritis that have a strong impact on the quality of life. Arthritis is characterized by absence of systemic inflammation and sometimes presence of calcium pyrophosphate crystals in the synovial fluids and visible on X-rays (review in [76]).

The ability of excessive iron to generate oxygen reactive species (ROS) (Figure 2) through the Haber–Weiss and Fenton reactions is strongly involved in the development of tissue lesions [77]. Indeed, ROS induces peroxidation that alters lipids, proteins, and DNA, generating dysfunctions of organelles, including mitochondria and cells, thus leading to tissue and organ damage [78–80]. One of the abnormal forms of NTBI, called Labile Plasma iron-LPI (or reactive plasma iron), is found in plasma when transferrin saturation reaches 80% [81]. This iron species is highly reactive and participates strongly in oxidative stress. Labile plasma iron is considered as a major determinant in the development of organ damage during hemochromatosis [82].

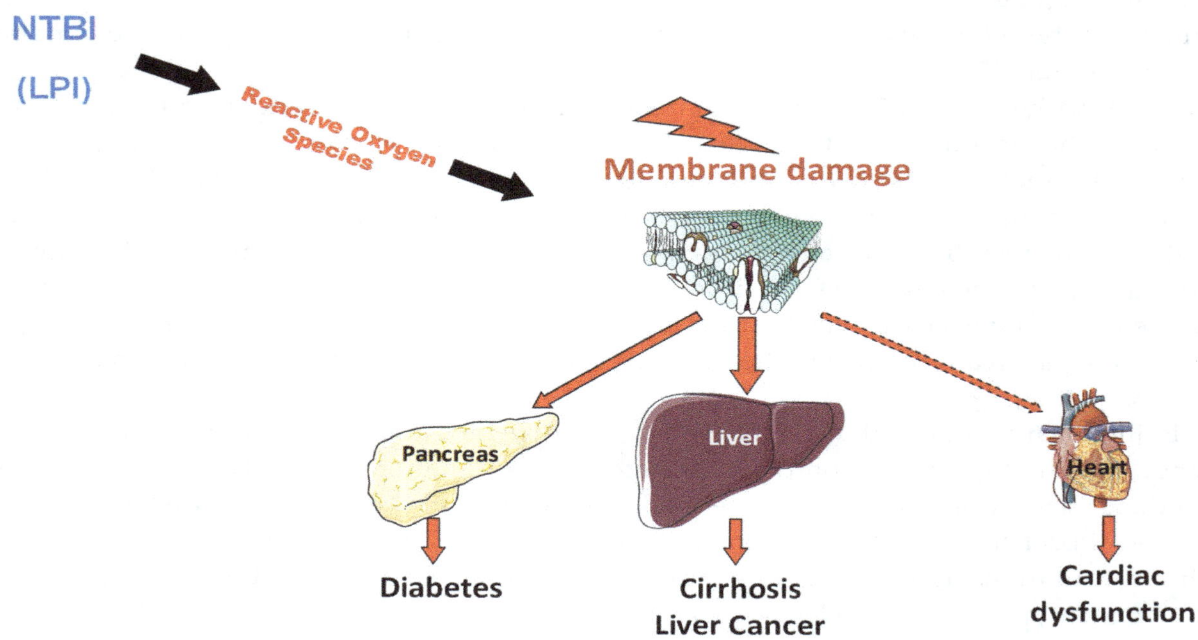

Figure 2. The appearance of non-transferrin bound forms of iron in plasma favors organ iron deposition but also the occurrence of oxidative stress that alters organelles in cells especially in iron overloaded organs.

In addition to the typical disease causing mutations associated with hemochromatosis, additional genetic modifiers have recently been described to elucidate in part, the large disparity in disease manifestations in patients. In this context, the importance of gene polymorphisms, e.g., GNPAT (glyceronephosphate O-acyltransferase) remains controversial and awaits additional confirmatory studies [83–88]. Alcohol consumption [68,89], non-alcoholic fatty liver disease [90], and viral hepatitis [91,92] may also be involved in disease penetrance, as well as a polymorphism in the *PCSK7* [93] or *PNPLA3* [94] genes.

3. Iron Is Presently the Main Therapeutic Target in *HFE*-Related Hemochromatosis

It is well known that iron depletion is a treatment of choice for hemochromatosis patients [95]. Indeed, when performed in patients prior to severe complications, the iron depletive treatment restores normal life expectancy, meaning that hepatic, pancreatic, and cardiac dysfunctions can be fully prevented [67]. In addition, partial regression of liver fibrosis after completion of iron removal has been reported [96].

3.1. Venesections Are the Mainstay Treatment for Iron Removal

The principle of repeated venesections [47,95] (Figure 3) is to remove red blood cells that are known to be very rich in iron, as part of hemoglobin. Erythropoiesis is stimulated to compensate hematocrit loss, and iron is taken up from the plasma by erythroblasts to produce new erythrocytes. In order to maintain enough plasma iron for the stimulated erythropoiesis, iron is released from macrophages and enterocytes but also from iron storage cells, including parenchymal cells such as hepatocytes. Removing iron at a faster rate than that excessively reaccumulated by intestinal absorption is critical to negative iron balance, but determining this rate prior to starting depletive treatment is difficult due to individual differences between hemochromatosis patients. It should also be recalled that hepcidin synthesis can be further suppressed by increasing erythropoiesis as a consequence of erythroferrone production. In practice, the depletive treatment includes two successive phases. The first one, called induction phase, aims at totally removing the iron excess present at the time of diagnosis. It usually consists of weekly venesections (≤7.5 mL/kg body weight per venesection). Once excess iron has been removed, the second phase, called maintenance therapy, aims to avoid recurrent iron overload using lifelong venesections, performed every 1–4 months.

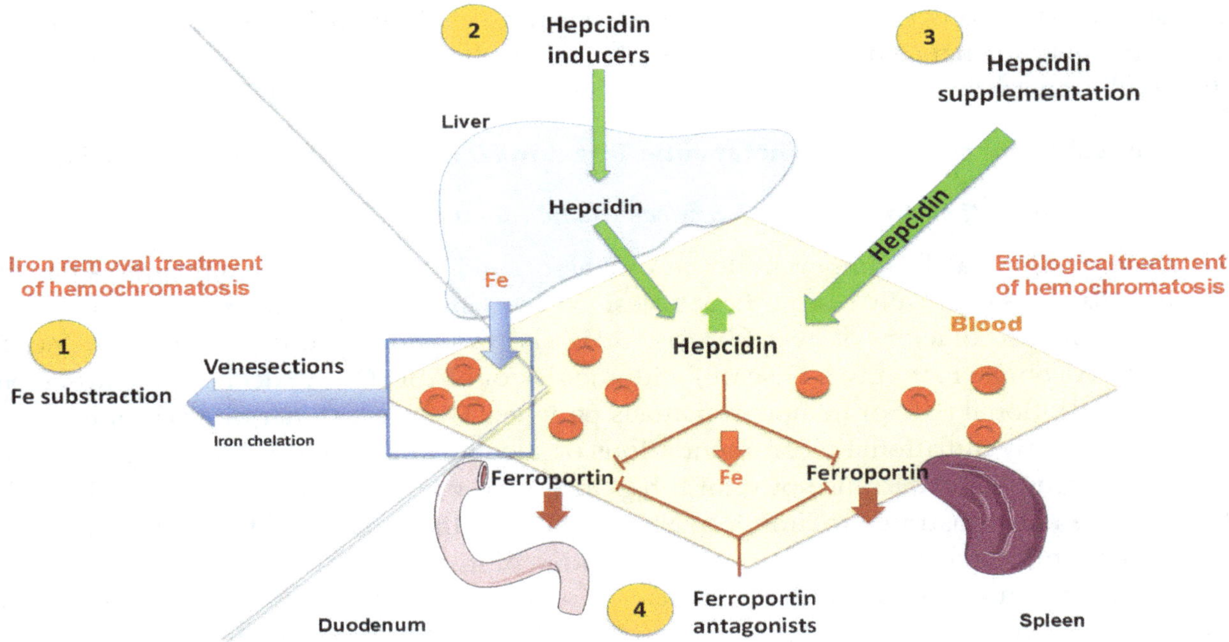

Figure 3. Schematic representation of currently used iron removal treatments during hemochromatosis and potential pathophysiological actions. (1) Iron depletive treatment is classically operated through repeated venesections that remove red blood cells. In some rare cases, iron chelators can be also used as complementary or suppletive treatment. (2) Hepcidin supplementation by endogenous or exogenous hepcidin. (3) Alternatively (4) the use of ferroportin antagonists could be also a way of treatment.

3.2. Use of Chelation Therapy

Another way to remove iron is the use of iron chelators that promote iron mobilization and excretion. However, in contrast to venesections, these drugs, including mainly today new oral iron-chelators, may have potential side effects [97]. Therefore during genetic hemochromatosis, oral chelation is only used, and as an off-label drug, in rare situations including cardiac failure, recent cerebral ischemic stroke, venous access problems limiting the possibility of venesections, or psychological intolerance to venesections.

3.3. Biochemical Follow-Up of Venesection Therapy

Three main parameters are classically followed: plasma ferritin and transferrin saturation levels that reflect the efficacy of iron depletive treatment, whereas hemoglobin levels reflect the tolerance of venesections. During the induction phase ferritinemia—that reliably reflects the amount of iron excess in hemochromatosis (provided other frequent acquired causes of hyperferritinemia have been excluded, such as inflammation, alcoholism, cytolysis or metabolic syndrome; genetic hyperferritinemia, as seen in the ferritin-cataract syndrome, is much rarer)—is the first parameter that decreases. This decrease is only slowly progressive, especially in patients exhibiting a severe iron load phenotype. Conversely, the decrease of transferrin saturation levels, that reflect plasma iron bioavailability, is a very late event. Normalization of transferrin saturation occurs only when the induction treatment is in its final phase. It is noteworthy that during hemochromatosis, despite the impressive frequency of venesections, hemoglobin levels remain stable due to the high capacity of cellular iron release by ferroportin hyperactivity, related to hepcidin deficiency. However, transient hypoxia and relative iron deficiency occurring after venesection, together with increased erythropoiesis, tend to decrease hepcidin plasma levels, thus contributing to further enhance iron entry into the plasma [98,99]. When considering NTBI during the induction therapy, its plasma concentration decreases parallel to transferrin saturation levels [55]. Altogether, these data suggest that induction therapy must be fully completed to remove iron excess, but also to prevent the appearance of toxic forms of iron, including plasma NTBI.

During the maintenance phase, it is essential to pursue the patient follow-up in order to ideally maintain both transferrin saturation and ferritin levels in the normal range [47,95].

4. Iron Removal Is not the Unique Therapeutic Target in *HFE*-Related Hemochromatosis

4.1. Other Preventive Actions to Avoid Iron Overload Complications

Besides iron removal, it is important to prevent associated causes of organ damage, as mentioned previously. This holds especially true for hepatic lesions knowing the impact of excessive alcohol intake and viral hepatitis as cofactors of liver fibrosis, cirrhosis, and hepatocellular carcinoma. Moreover, NAFLD (Non Alcoholic Fatty Liver Disease) with the risk of NASH (Non-Alcoholic Steato-Hepatitis) represents an additional risk for hemochromatosis patients. The practitioner must complete the iron removal approach by nutritional recommendations on alcohol and glucido-lipidic regimens [47,95]. Moreover, avoiding the occurrence of viral B hepatitis through vaccination is critical. In addition, tea [100] has been demonstrated to limit iron absorption, and therefore, could be used as adjuvant to avoid recurrence of excessive iron stores after completion of iron removal. In the same way, the use of therapeutic oral calcium channel blockers has also been proposed due to its positive impact on urinary iron excretion related to DMT1 activity increase in the kidney [101]. The use of proton-pump inhibitors could also represent an interesting adjunct [102].

4.2. The Development of a Pathophysiological Treatment Is a Major Goal

Iron removal is a treatment that only cures iron excess, but clearly does not correct the hepcidin deficiency that generates iron metabolism disturbances, and some clinical observations do suggest that the removal of iron excess is not sufficient to treat hemochromatosis. Considering arthropathy, it is noteworthy that, despite a well-conducted iron depletive treatment, the symptomatology may persist and even become more severe [76]. This suggests that: (i) synovial iron deposition [103] may represent an inaccessible compartment for iron depletion by venesections because synovial fluid is not contiguous with serum; (ii) synovitis, that has been documented in hemochromatosis [104,105] is irreversible despite effective iron depletion; and/or (iii) hepcidin deficiency leading to iron excess could be involved directly in symptomatic arthropathy and/or (iv) the mutations of the *HFE* gene, that encodes an HLA-like class I protein, could be involved directly in disease expression [106].

Considering the biochemical follow-up of patients, it is noteworthy that transferrin saturation levels may be found to be frequently increased during the maintenance therapeutic period, despite the absence of increased body iron stores. This could contribute to the appearance of clinical manifestations such as fatigue and arthropathy. It should be emphasized that, during the maintenance period, serum hepcidin levels are even lower than in iron overloaded patients [98,107]. Such hypohepcidinemia is expected to favor transferrin saturation increase and the appearance of NTBI that could participate in the arthritis of hemochromatosis patients.

Targeted treatment in the setting of hepcidin deficiency itself could represent an efficient way, as suggested by clinical observations obtained in hemochromatosis patients that have been transplanted for hepatocellular carcinoma [108]. The development of substitutive hepcidin treatment and/or of drugs stimulating hepcidin expression is under development and could be useful to complete the therapeutic arsenal, as suggested by results obtained with mini-hepcidins [109] and BMP known to induce hepcidin expression [110]. Clinical trials with hepcidin supplementation are ongoing (Clinical.trial.gov). Using antisense oligonucleotides for increasing hepcidin synthesis [111] or ferroportin antagonists [112] represents also further interesting innovative approaches. These different treatments could be especially indicated as an adjunct to venesections during the induction phase, and possibly as replacing venesections during maintenance therapy. Considering the overall safety and efficacy of the venesections, every putative treatment of hemochromatosis targeting iron metabolism must be without side-effects and easy to follow, suggesting especially that oral treatments providing exogenous hepcidin or inducing endogenous hepcidin synthesis might be preferable.

5. Conclusions

Iron remains the major therapeutic target during *HFE*-related hemochromatosis. However, targeting directly the iron stores by iron depletive treatment does not correct the pathophysiological defect of the disease. The development of treatments aimed at restoring iron homeostasis, especially by correcting hepcidin deficiency, could be useful to optimize the treatment, especially during the maintenance phase by controlling transferrin saturation with hopefully a favorable impact on the arthritis of hemochromatosis patients.

Acknowledgments: The authors thank the Associations Fer-Métaux Essentiels-Recherche-Santé (AFeMERS), Fédération Française des Associations de Malades de l'Hémochromatose (FFAMH) and Association Hémochromatose Ouest for their supports.

References

1. Andrews, N.C. Disorders of iron metabolism. *N. Engl. J. Med.* **1999**, *341*, 1986–1995. [CrossRef] [PubMed]
2. Gunshin, H.; Mackenzie, B.; Berger, U.V.; Gunshin, Y.; Romero, M.F.; Boron, W.F.; Nussberger, S.; Gollan, J.L.; Hediger, M.A. Cloning and characterization of a mammalian proton-coupled metal-ion transporter. *Nature* **1997**, *388*, 482–488. [CrossRef] [PubMed]
3. McKie, A.T.; Barrow, D.; Latunde-Dada, G.O.; Rolfs, A.; Sager, G.; Mudaly, E.; Mudaly, M.; Richardson, C.; Barlow, D.; Bomford, A.; et al. An Iron-Regulated Ferric Reductase Associated with the Absorption of Dietary Iron. *Science* **2001**, *291*, 1755–1759. [CrossRef] [PubMed]
4. Shayeghi, M.; Latunde-Dada, G.O.; Oakhill, J.S.; Laftah, A.H.; Takeuchi, K.; Halliday, N.; Khan, Y.; Warley, A.; McCann, F.E.; Hider, R.C.; et al. Identification of an intestinal heme transporter. *Cell* **2005**, *122*, 789–801. [CrossRef] [PubMed]
5. Qiu, A.; Jansen, M.; Sakaris, A.; Min, S.H.; Chattopadhyay, S.; Tsai, E.; Sandoval, C.; Zhao, R.; Akabas, M.H.; Goldman, I.D. Identification of an intestinal folate transporter and the molecular basis for hereditary folate malabsorption. *Cell* **2006**, *127*, 917–928. [CrossRef] [PubMed]

6. Bergamaschi, G.; Di Sabatino, A.; Pasini, A.; Ubezio, C.; Costanzo, F.; Grataroli, D.; Masotti, M.; Alvisi, C.; Corazza, G.R. Intestinal expression of genes implicated in iron absorption and their regulation by hepcidin. *Clin. Nutr. Edinb. Scotl.* **2017**, *36*, 1427–1433. [CrossRef] [PubMed]
7. Bothwell, T.H.; Pirzio-Biroli, G.; Finch, C.A. Iron absorption. I. Factors influencing absorption. *J. Lab. Clin. Med.* **1958**, *51*, 24–36. [PubMed]
8. McKie, A.T.; Marciani, P.; Rolfs, A.; Brennan, K.; Wehr, K.; Barrow, D.; Miret, S.; Bomford, A.; Peters, T.J.; Farzaneh, F.; et al. A novel duodenal iron-regulated transporter, IREG1, implicated in the basolateral transfer of iron to the circulation. *Mol. Cell* **2000**, *5*, 299–309. [CrossRef]
9. Donovan, A.; Brownlie, A.; Zhou, Y.; Shepard, J.; Pratt, S.J.; Moynihan, J.; Paw, B.H.; Drejer, A.; Barut, B.; Zapata, A.; et al. Positional cloning of zebrafish ferroportin1 identifies a conserved vertebrate iron exporter. *Nature* **2000**, *403*, 776–781. [CrossRef] [PubMed]
10. Abboud, S.; Haile, D.J. A novel mammalian iron-regulated protein involved in intracellular iron metabolism. *J. Biol. Chem.* **2000**, *275*, 19906–19912. [CrossRef] [PubMed]
11. Osaki, S.; Johnson, D.A.; Frieden, E. The possible significance of the ferrous oxidase activity of ceruloplasmin in normal human serum. *J. Biol. Chem.* **1966**, *241*, 2746–2751. [PubMed]
12. Vulpe, C.D.; Kuo, Y.M.; Murphy, T.L.; Cowley, L.; Askwith, C.; Libina, N.; Gitschier, J.; Anderson, G.J. Hephaestin, a ceruloplasmin homologue implicated in intestinal iron transport, is defective in the sla mouse. *Nat. Genet.* **1999**, *21*, 195–199. [CrossRef] [PubMed]
13. Levy, J.E.; Jin, O.; Fujiwara, Y.; Kuo, F.; Andrews, N.C. Transferrin receptor is necessary for development of erythrocytes and the nervous system. *Nat. Genet.* **1999**, *21*, 396–399. [CrossRef] [PubMed]
14. Ohgami, R.S.; Campagna, D.R.; Greer, E.L.; Antiochos, B.; McDonald, A.; Chen, J.; Sharp, J.J.; Fujiwara, Y.; Barker, J.E.; Fleming, M.D. Identification of a ferrireductase required for efficient transferrin-dependent iron uptake in erythroid cells. *Nat. Genet.* **2005**, *37*, 1264–1269. [CrossRef] [PubMed]
15. Camaschella, C.; Roetto, A.; Cali, A.; De Gobbi, M.; Garozzo, G.; Carella, M.; Majorano, N.; Totaro, A.; Gasparini, P. The gene *TFR2* is mutated in a new type of haemochromatosis mapping to 7q22. *Nat. Genet.* **2000**, *25*, 14–15. [CrossRef] [PubMed]
16. Griffiths, W.J.; Cox, T.M. Co-localization of the mammalian hemochromatosis gene product (*HFE*) and a newly identified transferrin receptor (*TFR2*) in intestinal tissue and cells. *J. Histochem. Cytochem.* **2003**, *51*, 613–624. [CrossRef] [PubMed]
17. Krause, A.; Neitz, S.; Magert, H.J.; Schulz, A.; Forssmann, W.G.; Schulz-Knappe, P.; Adermann, K. LEAP-1, a novel highly disulfide-bonded human peptide, exhibits antimicrobial activity. *FEBS Lett.* **2000**, *480*, 147–150. [CrossRef]
18. Park, C.H.; Valore, E.V.; Waring, A.J.; Ganz, T. Hepcidin, a urinary antimicrobial peptide synthesized in the liver. *J. Biol. Chem.* **2001**, *276*, 7806–7810. [CrossRef] [PubMed]
19. Pigeon, C.; Ilyin, G.; Courselaud, B.; Leroyer, P.; Turlin, B.; Brissot, P.; Loreal, O. A new mouse liver-specific gene, encoding a protein homologous to human antimicrobial peptide hepcidin, is overexpressed during iron overload. *J. Biol. Chem.* **2001**, *276*, 7811–7819. [CrossRef] [PubMed]
20. Nemeth, E.; Tuttle, M.S.; Powelson, J.; Vaughn, M.B.; Donovan, A.; Ward, D.M.; Ganz, T.; Kaplan, J. Hepcidin regulates cellular iron efflux by binding to ferroportin and inducing its internalization. *Science* **2004**, *306*, 2090–2093. [CrossRef] [PubMed]
21. Nicolas, G.; Bennoun, M.; Devaux, I.; Beaumont, C.; Grandchamp, B.; Kahn, A.; Vaulont, S. Lack of hepcidin gene expression and severe tissue iron overload in upstream stimulatory factor 2 (USF2) knockout mice. *Proc. Natl. Acad. Sci. USA* **2001**, *98*, 8780–8785. [CrossRef] [PubMed]
22. Nemeth, E.; Rivera, S.; Gabayan, V.; Keller, C.; Taudorf, S.; Pedersen, B.K.; Ganz, T. IL-6 mediates hypoferremia of inflammation by inducing the synthesis of the iron regulatory hormone hepcidin. *J. Clin. Investig.* **2004**, *113*, 1271–1276. [CrossRef] [PubMed]
23. Nicolas, G.; Viatte, L.; Bennoun, M.; Beaumont, C.; Kahn, A.; Vaulont, S. Hepcidin, A New Iron Regulatory Peptide. *Blood Cells Mol. Dis.* **2002**, *29*, 327–335. [CrossRef] [PubMed]
24. Peyssonnaux, C.; Nizet, V.; Johnson, R.S. Role of the hypoxia inducible factors HIF in iron metabolism. *Cell Cycle* **2008**, *7*, 28–32. [CrossRef] [PubMed]
25. Kautz, L.; Jung, G.; Valore, E.V.; Rivella, S.; Nemeth, E.; Ganz, T. Identification of erythroferrone as an erythroid regulator of iron metabolism. *Nat. Genet.* **2014**, *46*, 678–684. [CrossRef] [PubMed]

26. Gehrke, S.G.; Kulaksiz, H.; Herrmann, T.; Riedel, H.D.; Bents, K.; Veltkamp, C.; Stremmel, W. Expression of hepcidin in hereditary hemochromatosis: Evidence for a regulation in response to serum transferrin saturation and non-transferrin-bound iron. *Blood* **2003**, *102*, 371–376. [CrossRef] [PubMed]
27. Ramey, G.; Deschemin, J.C.; Vaulont, S. Cross-talk between the mitogen activated protein kinase and bone morphogenetic protein/hemojuvelin pathways is required for the induction of hepcidin by holotransferrin in primary mouse hepatocytes. *Haematologica* **2009**, *94*, 765–772. [CrossRef] [PubMed]
28. Feder, J.N.; Tsuchihashi, Z.; Irrinki, A.; Lee, V.K.; Mapa, F.A.; Morikang, E.; Prass, C.E.; Starnes, S.M.; Wolff, R.K.; Parkkila, S.; et al. The hemochromatosis founder mutation in HLA-H disrupts beta2-microglobulin interaction and cell surface expression. *J. Biol. Chem.* **1997**, *272*, 14025–14028. [CrossRef] [PubMed]
29. Feder, J.N.; Penny, D.M.; Irrinki, A.; Lee, V.K.; Lebron, J.A.; Watson, N.; Tsuchihashi, Z.; Sigal, E.; Bjorkman, P.J.; Schatzman, R.C. The hemochromatosis gene product complexes with the transferrin receptor and lowers its affinity for ligand binding. *Proc. Natl. Acad. Sci. USA* **1998**, *95*, 1472–1477. [CrossRef] [PubMed]
30. Schmidt, P.J.; Toran, P.T.; Giannetti, A.M.; Bjorkman, P.J.; Andrews, N.C. The transferrin receptor modulates *HFE*-dependent regulation of hepcidin expression. *Cell Metab.* **2008**, *7*, 205–214. [CrossRef] [PubMed]
31. Goswami, T.; Andrews, N.C. Hereditary hemochromatosis protein, *HFE*, interaction with transferrin receptor 2 suggests a molecular mechanism for mammalian iron sensing. *J. Biol. Chem.* **2006**, *281*, 28494–28498. [CrossRef] [PubMed]
32. Schmidt, P.J.; Fleming, M.D. Transgenic *HFE*-dependent induction of hepcidin in mice does not require transferrin receptor-2. *Am. J. Hematol.* **2012**, *87*, 588–595. [CrossRef] [PubMed]
33. Meynard, D.; Kautz, L.; Darnaud, V.; Canonne-Hergaux, F.; Coppin, H.; Roth, M.P. Lack of the bone morphogenetic protein BMP6 induces massive iron overload. *Nat. Genet.* **2009**, *41*, 478–481. [CrossRef] [PubMed]
34. Andriopoulos, B., Jr.; Corradini, E.; Xia, Y.; Faasse, S.A.; Chen, S.; Grgurevic, L.; Knutson, M.D.; Pietrangelo, A.; Vukicevic, S.; Lin, H.Y.; et al. BMP6 is a key endogenous regulator of hepcidin expression and iron metabolism. *Nat. Genet.* **2009**, *41*, 482–487. [CrossRef] [PubMed]
35. Casanovas, G.; Mleczko-Sanecka, K.; Altamura, S.; Hentze, M.W.; Muckenthaler, M.U. Bone morphogenetic protein (BMP)-responsive elements located in the proximal and distal hepcidin promoter are critical for its response to HJV/BMP/SMAD. *J. Mol. Med.* **2009**, *87*, 471–480. [CrossRef] [PubMed]
36. Island, M.L.; Jouanolle, A.M.; Mosser, A.; Deugnier, Y.; David, V.; Brissot, P.; Loreal, O. A new mutation in the hepcidin promoter impairs its BMP response and contributes to a severe phenotype in *HFE* related hemochromatosis. *Haematologica* **2009**, *94*, 720–724. [CrossRef] [PubMed]
37. Canali, S.; Zumbrennen-Bullough, K.B.; Core, A.B.; Wang, C.-Y.; Nairz, M.; Bouley, R.; Swirski, F.K.; Babitt, J.L. Endothelial cells produce bone morphogenetic protein 6 required for iron homeostasis in mice. *Blood* **2017**, *129*, 405–414. [CrossRef] [PubMed]
38. Rausa, M.; Pagani, A.; Nai, A.; Campanella, A.; Gilberti, M.E.; Apostoli, P.; Camaschella, C.; Silvestri, L. Bmp6 expression in murine liver non parenchymal cells: A mechanism to control their high iron exporter activity and protect hepatocytes from iron overload? *PLoS ONE* **2015**, *10*, e0122696. [CrossRef] [PubMed]
39. Koch, P.-S.; Olsavszky, V.; Ulbrich, F.; Sticht, C.; Demory, A.; Leibing, T.; Henzler, T.; Meyer, M.; Zierow, J.; Schneider, S.; et al. Angiocrine Bmp2 signaling in murine liver controls normal iron homeostasis. *Blood* **2017**, *129*, 415–419. [CrossRef] [PubMed]
40. Wang, R.H.; Li, C.; Xu, X.; Zheng, Y.; Xiao, C.; Zerfas, P.; Cooperman, S.; Eckhaus, M.; Rouault, T.; Mishra, L.; et al. A role of SMAD4 in iron metabolism through the positive regulation of hepcidin expression. *Cell Metab.* **2005**, *2*, 399–409. [CrossRef] [PubMed]
41. Kautz, L.; Meynard, D.; Monnier, A.; Darnaud, V.; Bouvet, R.; Wang, R.H.; Deng, C.; Vaulont, S.; Mosser, J.; Coppin, H.; et al. Iron regulates phosphorylation of Smad1/5/8 and gene expression of Bmp6, Smad7, Id1, and Atoh8 in the mouse liver. *Blood* **2008**, *112*, 1503–1509. [CrossRef] [PubMed]
42. Verga Falzacappa, M.V.; Casanovas, G.; Hentze, M.W.; Muckenthaler, M.U. A bone morphogenetic protein (BMP)-responsive element in the hepcidin promoter controls *HFE2*-mediated hepatic hepcidin expression and its response to IL-6 in cultured cells. *J. Mol. Med.* **2008**, *86*, 531–540. [CrossRef] [PubMed]

43. D'Alessio, F.; Hentze, M.W.; Muckenthaler, M.U. The hemochromatosis proteins *HFE*, *TFR2*, and *HJV* form a membrane-associated protein complex for hepcidin regulation. *J. Hepatol.* **2012**, *57*, 1052–1060. [CrossRef] [PubMed]
44. Pantopoulos, K. Iron regulation of hepcidin through *HFE* and *HJV*: Common or distinct pathways? *Hepatology* **2015**, *62*, 1922–1923. [CrossRef] [PubMed]
45. Brissot, P.; Loreal, O. Iron metabolism and related genetic diseases: A cleared land, keeping mysteries. *J. Hepatol* **2016**, *64*, 505–515. [CrossRef] [PubMed]
46. Hamdi-Roze, H.; Beaumont-Epinette, M.P.; Ben Ali, Z.; Le Lan, C.; Loustaud-Ratti, V.; Causse, X.; Loreal, O.; Deugnier, Y.; Brissot, P.; Jouanolle, A.M.; et al. Rare *HFE* variants are the most frequent cause of hemochromatosis in non-c282y homozygous patients with hemochromatosis. *Am. J. Hematol.* **2016**, *91*, 1202–1205. [CrossRef] [PubMed]
47. Brissot, P.; Pietrangelo, A.; Adams, P.C.; de Graaff, B.; McLaren, C.E.; Loréal, O. Haemochromatosis. *Nat. Rev. Dis. Primer* **2018**, *4*, 18016. [CrossRef] [PubMed]
48. Allen, K.J.; Gurrin, L.C.; Constantine, C.C.; Osborne, N.J.; Delatycki, M.B.; Nicoll, A.J.; McLaren, C.E.; Bahlo, M.; Nisselle, A.E.; Vulpe, C.D.; et al. Iron-overload-related disease in *HFE* hereditary hemochromatosis. *N. Engl. J. Med.* **2008**, *358*, 221–230. [CrossRef] [PubMed]
49. Van Dijk, B.A.C.; Laarakkers, C.M.M.; Klaver, S.M.; Jacobs, E.M.G.; van Tits, L.J.H.; Janssen, M.C.H.; Swinkels, D.W. Serum hepcidin levels are innately low in *HFE*-related haemochromatosis but differ between C282Y-homozygotes with elevated and normal ferritin levels. *Br. J. Haematol.* **2008**, *142*, 979–985. [CrossRef] [PubMed]
50. Hentze, M.W.; Kuhn, L.C. Molecular control of vertebrate iron metabolism: mRNA-based regulatory circuits operated by iron, nitric oxide, and oxidative stress. *Proc. Natl. Acad. Sci. USA* **1996**, *93*, 8175–8182. [CrossRef] [PubMed]
51. Ponka, P. Cellular iron metabolism. *Kidney Int. Suppl.* **1999**, *69*, S2–S11. [CrossRef] [PubMed]
52. Ponka, P.; Lok, C.N. The transferrin receptor: Role in health and disease. *Int. J. Biochem. Cell Biol.* **1999**, *31*, 1111–1137. [CrossRef]
53. Arosio, P.; Carmona, F.; Gozzelino, R.; Maccarinelli, F.; Poli, M. The importance of eukaryotic ferritins in iron handling and cytoprotection. *Biochem. J.* **2015**, *472*, 1–15. [CrossRef] [PubMed]
54. Hershko, C.; Peto, T.E. Non-transferrin plasma iron. *Br. J. Haematol* **1987**, *66*, 149–151. [CrossRef] [PubMed]
55. Loreal, O.; Gosriwatana, I.; Guyader, D.; Porter, J.; Brissot, P.; Hider, R.C. Determination of non-transferrin-bound iron in genetic hemochromatosis using a new HPLC-based method. *J. Hepatol.* **2000**, *32*, 727–733. [CrossRef]
56. Grootveld, M.; Bell, J.D.; Halliwell, B.; Aruoma, O.I.; Bomford, A.; Sadler, P.J. Non-transferrin-bound iron in plasma or serum from patients with idiopathic hemochromatosis. Characterization by high performance liquid chromatography and nuclear magnetic resonance spectroscopy. *J. Biol. Chem.* **1989**, *264*, 4417–4422. [PubMed]
57. Liuzzi, J.P.; Aydemir, F.; Nam, H.; Knutson, M.D.; Cousins, R.J. Zip14 (Slc39a14) mediates non-transferrin-bound iron uptake into cells. *Proc. Natl. Acad. Sci. USA* **2006**, *103*, 13612–13617. [CrossRef] [PubMed]
58. Brissot, P.; Wright, T.L.; Ma, W.L.; Weisiger, R.A. Efficient clearance of non-transferrin-bound iron by rat liver. Implications for hepatic iron loading in iron overload states. *J. Clin. Investig.* **1985**, *76*, 1463–1470. [CrossRef] [PubMed]
59. Brissot, P.; Bolder, U.; Schteingart, C.D.; Arnaud, J.; Hofmann, A.F. Intestinal absorption and enterohepatic cycling of biliary iron originating from plasma non-transferrin-bound iron in rats. *Hepatology* **1997**, *25*, 1457–1461. [CrossRef] [PubMed]
60. Hubert, N.; Lescoat, G.; Sciot, R.; Moirand, R.; Jego, P.; Leroyer, P.; Brissot, P. Regulation of ferritin and transferrin receptor expression by iron in human hepatocyte cultures. *J. Hepatol.* **1993**, *18*, 301–312. [CrossRef]
61. Sciot, R.; Verhoeven, G.; Van Eyken, P.; Cailleau, J.; Desmet, V.J. Transferrin receptor expression in rat liver: Immunohistochemical and biochemical analysis of the effect of age and iron storage. *Hepatology* **1990**, *11*, 416–427. [CrossRef] [PubMed]
62. Jenkitkasemwong, S.; Wang, C.Y.; Coffey, R.; Zhang, W.; Chan, A.; Biel, T.; Kim, J.S.; Hojyo, S.; Fukada, T.; Knutson, M.D. SLC39A14 Is Required for the Development of Hepatocellular Iron Overload in Murine Models of Hereditary Hemochromatosis. *Cell Metab.* **2015**, *22*, 138–150. [CrossRef] [PubMed]

63. Roetto, A.; Papanikolaou, G.; Politou, M.; Alberti, F.; Girelli, D.; Christakis, J.; Loukopoulos, D.; Camaschella, C. Mutant antimicrobial peptide hepcidin is associated with severe juvenile hemochromatosis. *Nat. Genet.* **2003**, *33*, 221–222. [CrossRef] [PubMed]
64. Papanikolaou, G.; Samuels, M.E.; Ludwig, E.H.; MacDonald, M.L.; Franchini, P.L.; Dube, M.P.; Andres, L.; MacFarlane, J.; Sakellaropoulos, N.; Politou, M.; et al. Mutations in *HFE2* cause iron overload in chromosome 1q-linked juvenile hemochromatosis. *Nat. Genet.* **2004**, *36*, 77–82. [CrossRef] [PubMed]
65. Bardou-Jacquet, E.; Cunat, S.; Beaumont-Epinette, M.-P.; Kannengiesser, C.; Causse, X.; Sauvion, S.; Pouliquen, B.; Deugnier, Y.; David, V.; Loréal, O.; et al. Variable age of onset and clinical severity in transferrin receptor 2 related haemochromatosis: Novel observations. *Br. J. Haematol.* **2013**, *162*, 278–281. [CrossRef] [PubMed]
66. Niederau, C.; Fischer, R.; Sonnenberg, A.; Stremmel, W.; Trampisch, H.J.; Strohmeyer, G. Survival and causes of death in cirrhotic and in noncirrhotic patients with primary hemochromatosis. *N. Engl. J. Med.* **1985**, *313*, 1256–1262. [CrossRef] [PubMed]
67. Niederau, C.; Fischer, R.; Purschel, A.; Stremmel, W.; Haussinger, D.; Strohmeyer, G. Long-term survival in patients with hereditary hemochromatosis [see comments]. *Gastroenterology* **1996**, *110*, 1107–1119. [CrossRef] [PubMed]
68. Loreal, O.; Deugnier, Y.; Moirand, R.; Lauvin, L.; Guyader, D.; Jouanolle, H.; Turlin, B.; Lescoat, G.; Brissot, P. Liver fibrosis in genetic hemochromatosis. Respective roles of iron and non-iron-related factors in 127 homozygous patients. *J. Hepatol.* **1992**, *16*, 122–127. [PubMed]
69. Guyader, D.; Jacquelinet, C.; Moirand, R.; Turlin, B.; Mendler, M.H.; Chaperon, J.; David, V.; Brissot, P.; Adams, P.; Deugnier, Y. Noninvasive prediction of fibrosis in C282Y homozygous hemochromatosis. *Gastroenterology* **1998**, *115*, 929–936. [CrossRef]
70. Deugnier, Y.M.; Loreal, O.; Turlin, B.; Guyader, D.; Jouanolle, H.; Moirand, R.; Jacquelinet, C.; Brissot, P. Liver pathology in genetic hemochromatosis: A review of 135 homozygous cases and their bioclinical correlations. *Gastroenterology* **1992**, *102*, 2050–2059. [CrossRef]
71. Dixon, S.J.; Lemberg, K.M.; Lamprecht, M.R.; Skouta, R.; Zaitsev, E.M.; Gleason, C.E.; Patel, D.N.; Bauer, A.J.; Cantley, A.M.; Yang, W.S.; et al. Ferroptosis: An iron-dependent form of nonapoptotic cell death. *Cell* **2012**, *149*, 1060–1072. [CrossRef] [PubMed]
72. Dixon, S.J.; Stockwell, B.R. The role of iron and reactive oxygen species in cell death. *Nat. Chem. Biol.* **2014**, *10*, 9–17. [CrossRef] [PubMed]
73. Houglum, K.; Bedossa, P.; Chojkier, M. TGF-beta and collagen-alpha 1 (I) gene expression are increased in hepatic acinar zone 1 of rats with iron overload. *Am. J. Physiol.* **1994**, *267*, G908–G913. [CrossRef] [PubMed]
74. Gualdi, R.; Casalgrandi, G.; Montosi, G.; Ventura, E.; Pietrangelo, A. Excess iron into hepatocytes is required for activation of collagen type I gene during experimental siderosis. *Gastroenterology* **1994**, *107*, 1118–1124. [CrossRef]
75. Deugnier, Y.M.; Guyader, D.; Crantock, L.; Lopez, J.M.; Turlin, B.; Yaouanq, J.; Jouanolle, H.; Campion, J.P.; Launois, B.; Halliday, J.W.; et al. Primary liver cancer in genetic hemochromatosis: A clinical, pathological, and pathogenetic study of 54 cases. *Gastroenterology* **1993**, *104*, 228–234. [CrossRef]
76. Guggenbuhl, P.; Brissot, P.; Loreal, O. Miscellaneous non-inflammatory musculoskeletal conditions. Haemochromatosis: The bone and the joint. *Best Pract. Res. Clin. Rheumatol* **2011**, *25*, 6649–6664. [CrossRef]
77. Wardman, P.; Candeias, L.P. Fenton chemistry: An introduction. *Radiat. Res.* **1996**, *145*, 523–531. [CrossRef] [PubMed]
78. Bacon, B.R.; Britton, R.S. Hepatic injury in chronic iron overload. Role of lipid peroxidation. *Chem. Biol. Interact.* **1989**, *70*, 183–226. [CrossRef]
79. Bacon, B.R.; Tavill, A.S.; Brittenham, G.M.; Park, C.H.; Recknagel, R.O. Hepatic lipid peroxidation in vivo in rats with chronic iron overload. *J. Clin. Investig.* **1983**, *71*, 429–439. [CrossRef] [PubMed]
80. Bacon, B.R.; O'Neill, R.; Britton, R.S. Hepatic mitochondrial energy production in rats with chronic iron overload. *Gastroenterology* **1993**, *105*, 1134–1140. [CrossRef]
81. Le Lan, C.; Loreal, O.; Cohen, T.; Ropert, M.; Glickstein, H.; Laine, F.; Pouchard, M.; Deugnier, Y.; Le Treut, A.; Breuer, W.; et al. Redox active plasma iron in C282Y/C282Y hemochromatosis. *Blood* **2005**, *105*, 4527–4531. [CrossRef] [PubMed]
82. Cabantchik, Z.I.; Breuer, W.; Zanninelli, G.; Cianciulli, P. LPI-labile plasma iron in iron overload. *Best Pr. Res. Clin. Haematol* **2005**, *18*, 277–287. [CrossRef] [PubMed]

83. Milet, J.; Dehais, V.; Bourgain, C.; Jouanolle, A.M.; Mosser, A.; Perrin, M.; Morcet, J.; Brissot, P.; David, V.; Deugnier, Y.; et al. Common variants in the *BMP2*, *BMP4*, and *HJV* genes of the hepcidin regulation pathway modulate *HFE* hemochromatosis penetrance. *Am. J. Hum. Genet.* **2007**, *81*, 799–807. [CrossRef] [PubMed]
84. De Tayrac, M.; Roth, M.-P.; Jouanolle, A.-M.; Coppin, H.; le Gac, G.; Piperno, A.; Férec, C.; Pelucchi, S.; Scotet, V.; Bardou-Jacquet, E.; et al. Genome-wide association study identifies *TF* as a significant modifier gene of iron metabolism in *HFE* hemochromatosis. *J. Hepatol.* **2015**, *62*, 664–672. [CrossRef] [PubMed]
85. McLaren, C.E.; Emond, M.J.; Subramaniam, V.N.; Phatak, P.D.; Barton, J.C.; Adams, P.C.; Goh, J.B.; McDonald, C.J.; Powell, L.W.; Gurrin, L.C.; et al. Exome sequencing in *HFE* C282Y homozygous men with extreme phenotypes identifies a GNPAT variant associated with severe iron overload. *Hepatology* **2015**, *62*, 429–439. [CrossRef] [PubMed]
86. Tchernitchko, D.; Scotet, V.; Lefebvre, T.; L'Hostis, C.; Gourlaouen, I.; Merour, M.-C.; Rebah, K.; Peoc'h, K.; Assari, S.; Ferec, C.; et al. GNPAT polymorphism rs11558492 is not associated with increased severity in a large cohort of *HFE* p.Cys282Tyr homozygous patients. *Hepatology* **2017**, *65*, 1069–1071. [CrossRef] [PubMed]
87. Levstik, A.; Stuart, A.; Adams, P.C. GNPAT variant (D519G) is not associated with an elevated serum ferritin or iron removed by phlebotomy in patients referred for C282Y-linked hemochromatosis. *Ann. Hepatol.* **2016**, *15*, 907–910. [CrossRef] [PubMed]
88. Greni, F.; Valenti, L.; Mariani, R.; Pelloni, I.; Rametta, R.; Busti, F.; Ravasi, G.; Girelli, D.; Fargion, S.; Galimberti, S.; et al. GNPAT rs11558492 is not a Major Modifier of Iron Status: Study of Italian Hemochromatosis Patients and Blood Donors. *Ann. Hepatol.* **2017**, *16*, 451–456. [CrossRef] [PubMed]
89. Fletcher, L.M.; Dixon, J.L.; Purdie, D.M.; Powell, L.W.; Crawford, D.H.G. Excess alcohol greatly increases the prevalence of cirrhosis in hereditary hemochromatosis. *Gastroenterology* **2002**, *122*, 281–289. [CrossRef] [PubMed]
90. Nelson, J.E.; Bhattacharya, R.; Lindor, K.D.; Chalasani, N.; Raaka, S.; Heathcote, E.J.; Miskovsky, E.; Shaffer, E.; Rulyak, S.J.; Kowdley, K.V. *HFE* C282Y mutations are associated with advanced hepatic fibrosis in Caucasians with nonalcoholic steatohepatitis. *Hepatology* **2007**, *46*, 723–729. [CrossRef] [PubMed]
91. Pollicino, T.; Vegetti, A.; Saitta, C.; Ferrara, F.; Corradini, E.; Raffa, G.; Pietrangelo, A.; Raimondo, G. Hepatitis B virus DNA integration in tumour tissue of a non-cirrhotic *HFE*-haemochromatosis patient with hepatocellular carcinoma. *J. Hepatol.* **2013**, *58*, 190–193. [CrossRef] [PubMed]
92. Diwakaran, H.H.; Befeler, A.S.; Britton, R.S.; Brunt, E.M.; Bacon, B.R. Accelerated hepatic fibrosis in patients with combined hereditary hemochromatosis and chronic hepatitis C infection. *J. Hepatol.* **2002**, *36*, 687–691. [CrossRef]
93. Stickel, F.; Buch, S.; Zoller, H.; Hultcrantz, R.; Gallati, S.; Österreicher, C.; Finkenstedt, A.; Stadlmayr, A.; Aigner, E.; Sahinbegovic, E.; et al. Evaluation of genome-wide loci of iron metabolism in hereditary hemochromatosis identifies PCSK7 as a host risk factor of liver cirrhosis. *Hum. Mol. Genet.* **2014**, *23*, 3883–3890. [CrossRef] [PubMed]
94. Valenti, L.; Maggioni, P.; Piperno, A.; Rametta, R.; Pelucchi, S.; Mariani, R.; Dongiovanni, P.; Fracanzani, A.L.; Fargion, S. Patatin-like phospholipase domain containing-3 gene I148M polymorphism, steatosis, and liver damage in hereditary hemochromatosis. *World J. Gastroenterol.* **2012**′ *18*, 2813–2820. [CrossRef] [PubMed]
95. Adams, P.; Altes, A.; Brissot, P.; Butzeck, B.; Cabantchik, I.; Cançado, R.; Distante, S.; Evans, P.; Evans, R.; Ganz, T.; et al. Contributors and Hemochromatosis International Taskforce Therapeutic recommendations in *HFE* hemochromatosis for p.Cys282Tyr (C282Y/C282Y) homozygous genotype. *Hepatol. Int.* **2018**, *12*, 83–86. [CrossRef] [PubMed]
96. Falize, L.; Guillygomarc'h, A.; Perrin, M.; Laine, F.; Guyader, D.; Brissot, P.; Turlin, B.; Deugnier, Y. Reversibility of hepatic fibrosis in treated genetic hemochromatosis: A study of 36 cases. *Hepatology* **2006**, *44*, 472–477. [CrossRef] [PubMed]
97. Phatak, P.; Brissot, P.; Wurster, M.; Adams, P.C.; Bonkovsky, H.L.; Gross, J.; Malfertheiner, P.; McLaren, G.D.; Niederau, C.; Piperno, A.; et al. A phase 1/2, dose-escalation trial of deferasirox for the treatment of iron overload in *HFE*-related hereditary hemochromatosis. *Hepatology* **2010**, *52*, 1671–1779. [CrossRef] [PubMed]
98. Rombout-Sestrienkova, E.; Koek, G.H.; Neslo, R.; van Kraaij, M.; Menheere, P.P.; Masclee, A.; Swinkels, D.W. Course of iron parameters in *HFE*-hemochromatosis patients during initial treatment with erythrocytapheresis compared to phlebotomy. *J. Clin. Apheresis* **2016**, *31*, 564–570. [CrossRef] [PubMed]

99. Mast, A.E.; Schlumpf, K.S.; Wright, D.J.; Johnson, B.; Glynn, S.A.; Busch, M.P.; Olbina, G.; Westerman, M.; Nemeth, E.; Ganz, T. NHLBI Retrovirus Epidemiology Donor Study-II (REDS-II) Hepcidin level predicts hemoglobin concentration in individuals undergoing repeated phlebotomy. *Haematologica* **2013**, *98*, 1324–1330. [CrossRef] [PubMed]
100. Kaltwasser, J.P.; Werner, E.; Schalk, K.; Hansen, C.; Gottschalk, R.; Seidl, C. Clinical trial on the effect of regular tea drinking on iron accumulation in genetic haemochromatosis. *Gut* **1998**, *43*, 699–704. [CrossRef] [PubMed]
101. Ludwiczek, S.; Theurl, I.; Muckenthaler, M.U.; Jakab, M.; Mair, S.M.; Theurl, M.; Kiss, J.; Paulmichl, M.; Hentze, M.W.; Ritter, M.; et al. Ca2+ channel blockers reverse iron overload by a new mechanism via divalent metal transporter-1. *Nat. Med.* **2007**, *13*, 448–454. [CrossRef] [PubMed]
102. Vanclooster, A.; van Deursen, C.; Jaspers, R.; Cassiman, D.; Koek, G. Proton Pump Inhibitors Decrease Phlebotomy Need in *HFE* Hemochromatosis: Double-Blind Randomized Placebo-Controlled Trial. *Gastroenterology* **2017**, *153*, 678–680. [CrossRef] [PubMed]
103. Schumacher, H.R. Articular cartilage in the degenerative arthropathy of hemochromatosis. *Arthritis Rheum.* **1982**, *25*, 1460–1468. [CrossRef] [PubMed]
104. Heiland, G.R.; Aigner, E.; Dallos, T.; Sahinbegovic, E.; Krenn, V.; Thaler, C.; Weiss, G.; Distler, J.H.; Datz, C.; Schett, G.; et al. Synovial immunopathology in haemochromatosis arthropathy. *Ann. Rheum. Dis.* **2010**, *69*, 1214–1219. [CrossRef] [PubMed]
105. Carroll, G.J.; Sharma, G.; Upadhyay, A.; Jazayeri, J.A. Ferritin concentrations in synovial fluid are higher in osteoarthritis patients with *HFE* gene mutations (C282Y or H63D). *Scand. J. Rheumatol.* **2010**, *39*, 413–420. [CrossRef] [PubMed]
106. Reuben, A.; Chung, J.W.; Lapointe, R.; Santos, M.M. The hemochromatosis protein *HFE* 20 years later: An emerging role in antigen presentation and in the immune system. *Immun. Inflamm. Dis.* **2017**, *5*, 218–232. [CrossRef] [PubMed]
107. Bardou-Jacquet, E.; Lainé, F.; Guggenbuhl, P.; Morcet, J.; Jézéquel, C.; Guyader, D.; Moirand, R.; Deugnier, Y. Worse Outcomes of Patients with *HFE* Hemochromatosis With Persistent Increases in Transferrin Saturation During Maintenance Therapy. *Clin. Gastroenterol. Hepatol.* **2017**, *15*, 1620–1627. [CrossRef] [PubMed]
108. Bardou-Jacquet, E.; Philip, J.; Lorho, R.; Ropert, M.; Latournerie, M.; Houssel-Debry, P.; Guyader, D.; Loreal, O.; Boudjema, K.; Brissot, P. Liver transplantation normalizes serum hepcidin level and cures iron metabolism alterations in *HFE* hemochromatosis. *Hepatology* **2014**, *59*, 839–847. [CrossRef] [PubMed]
109. Preza, G.C.; Ruchala, P.; Pinon, R.; Ramos, E.; Qiao, B.; Peralta, M.A.; Sharma, S.; Waring, A.; Ganz, T.; Nemeth, E. Minihepcidins are rationally designed small peptides that mimic hepcidin activity in mice and may be useful for the treatment of iron overload. *J. Clin. Investig.* **2011**, *121*, 4880–4888. [CrossRef] [PubMed]
110. Corradini, E.; Schmidt, P.J.; Meynard, D.; Garuti, C.; Montosi, G.; Chen, S.; Vukicevic, S.; Pietrangelo, A.; Lin, H.Y.; Babitt, J.L. BMP6 treatment compensates for the molecular defect and ameliorates hemochromatosis in *HFE* knockout mice. *Gastroenterology* **2010**, *139*, 1721–1729. [CrossRef] [PubMed]
111. Guo, S.; Casu, C.; Gardenghi, S.; Booten, S.; Aghajan, M.; Peralta, R.; Watt, A.; Freier, S.; Monia, B.P.; Rivella, S. Reducing TMPRSS6 ameliorates hemochromatosis and β-thalassemia in mice. *J. Clin. Investig.* **2013**, *123*, 1531–1541. [CrossRef] [PubMed]
112. Ross, S.L.; Biswas, K.; Rottman, J.; Allen, J.R.; Long, J.; Miranda, L.P.; Winters, A.; Arvedson, T.L. Identification of Antibody and Small Molecule Antagonists of Ferroportin-Hepcidin Interaction. *Front. Pharmacol.* **2017**, *8*, 838. [CrossRef] [PubMed]

9

Iron in Friedreich Ataxia: A Central Role in the Pathophysiology or an Epiphenomenon?

David Alsina, Rosa Purroy, Joaquim Ros and Jordi Tamarit *

Departament de Ciències Mèdiques Bàsiques, IRBLleida, Universitat de Lleida, 25198 Lleida, Spain; david.alsina@cmb.udl.cat (D.A.); rosa.purroy@irblleida.udl.cat (R.P.); joaquim.ros@cmb.udl.cat (J.R.)

* Correspondence: jordi.tamarit@cmb.udl.cat

Abstract: Friedreich ataxia is a neurodegenerative disease with an autosomal recessive inheritance. In most patients, the disease is caused by the presence of trinucleotide GAA expansions in the first intron of the frataxin gene. These expansions cause the decreased expression of this mitochondrial protein. Many evidences indicate that frataxin deficiency causes the deregulation of cellular iron homeostasis. In this review, we will discuss several hypotheses proposed for frataxin function, their caveats, and how they could provide an explanation for the deregulation of iron homeostasis found in frataxin-deficient cells. We will also focus on the potential mechanisms causing cellular dysfunction in Friedreich Ataxia and on the potential use of the iron chelator deferiprone as a therapeutic agent for this disease.

Keywords: Iron-sulfur; Friedreich Ataxia; Oxidative stress; Iron chelators

---

1. The Disease

Friedreich's Ataxia (FRDA) is a neurodegenerative disease described at the end of the 19th century by the German physician Nikolaus Friedreich from whom acquired the name. Friedreich observed in a group of patients that during the puberty a characteristic symptomatology began to manifest, specifically: ataxia, dysarthria, loss of sensitivity, muscle weakness, scoliosis, pes cavus, and heart symptoms. Later, a greater incidence of diabetes mellitus in patients than in the rest of the population was also reported [1]. It is considered a rare disease that follows a pattern of autosomal recessive inheritance. The frequency of carriers oscillates, depending on the area, between 1:50 and 1:100, while those affected by the disease are approximately 1:50,000, which makes this disease the most common form of hereditary ataxia [2].

The mutation responsible for the disease is an expansion of GAA trinucleotides in the first intron of the FXNor X25 gene (located in chromosome 9), which codes for the mitochondrial protein frataxin [3]. This expansion of triplets, which in patients can reach up to more than 1000 copies, results in a marked decrease in protein frataxin levels (below 5%–30% of normal levels) [4]. The number of GAA expansions has an inversely proportional relation to the age at which the first symptoms of the disease begin to manifest and it also determines their severity [5–7]. Besides GAA expansions, epigenetic modifications might also contribute to the variability in the onset and disease progression. Sarsero and collaborators reported differences in DNA methylation patterns between patients upstream and downstream the GAA expansion. Such differences caused variations in frataxin gene expression [8]. Finally, a small percentage of patients, around 4%, are compound heterozygous for a GAA expansion and a frataxin (FXN) point mutation or deletion [9].

2. Frataxin, an Ancestral Conserved Protein

Frataxin is a highly conserved protein throughout evolution and homologues can be found in most species. Its structure is formed by two helix alpha joined by a series of antiparallel beta sheets and is highly conserved (Figure 1). Despite the high degree of conservation in the three-dimensional structure, the stability of this protein varies significantly between species. One of the factors that are responsible for the differences in the stability of the protein is the C-terminal endpoint. While in Yfh1 (the yeast's homologue), this region is virtually nonexistent, in the human protein this fragment is found inserted between the two alpha helixes. This protects the hydrophobic nucleus of the protein and increases its stability [10].

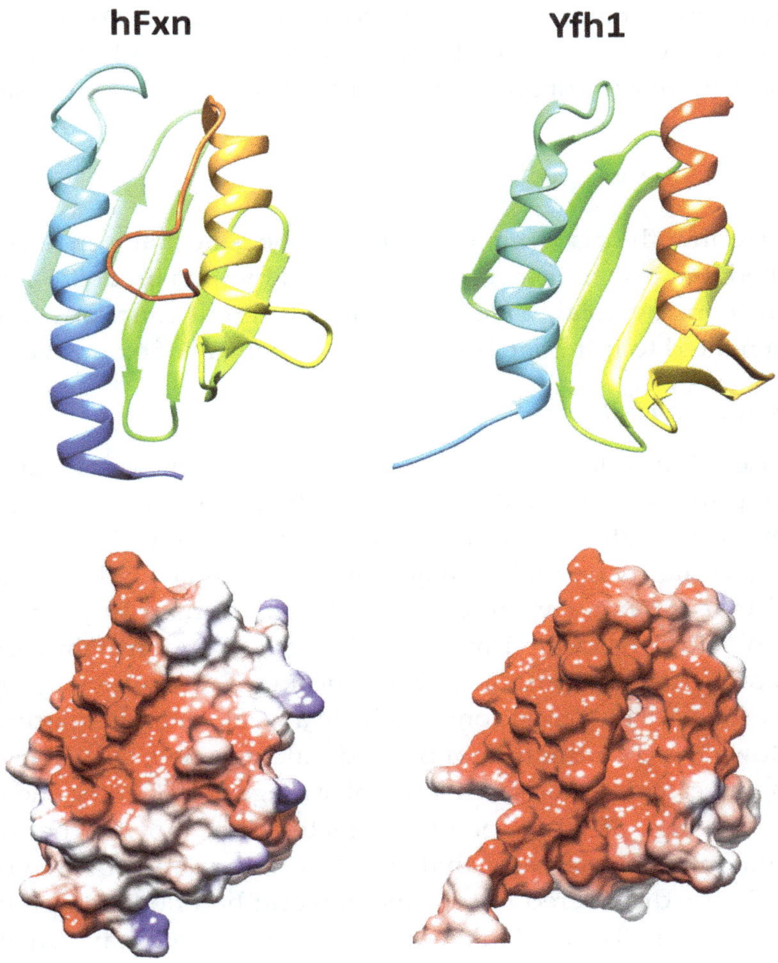

Figure 1. Structures of human frataxin (hFxn, pdb code 3s4m) and Yeast Frataxin Homologue 1 (Yfh1, pdb code 2fql). Top, ribbons representations showing the conserved alpha-beta-alpha structure. Structures are colored according to sequence, from dark blue (N-terminal) to red (C-terminal). In human frataxin the C-terminal region folds over the hydrophobic cavity formed between both alpha helices. Below, coulumbic surface coloring of the same structures. The red color indicates the presence of a marked acidic ridge, which may be involved in iron binding. Molecular graphics and analyses were performed with the UCSF Chimera package [11].

Frataxin is a mitochondrial protein, and as such, it has a signal peptide at its N-terminal end. It was soon identified, both for Yfh1 and for mouse frataxin, that Mitochondrial Processing Peptidase interacted with frataxin and was responsible for its processing [12,13]. This processing involves two sequential cleavages, which first produce an intermediate form of frataxin and subsequently the mature form. For human frataxin, the cleavage positions described are between amino acids 41–42 (intermediate form) and between amino acids 80–81 (mature form), although other less abundant forms that correspond to alternative cleavage sites (for instance, positions 55–56) have also been identified [14,15]. In these works, it was shown that the mature form of frataxin corresponds to FXN^{81-210}. This form is fully active and capable of improving the survival and phenotypes of frataxin deficient cells. Despite the demonstration that the FXN^{81-210} form is the dominant form and that it is active, there is some debate over the role that could be developed by the intermediate forms, as these forms can also be detected in certain tissues (although at low levels) [16]. It was shown that processing of the intermediate form was slower than that of the precursor form, which suggested that this could be a mechanism for controlling the levels of the different frataxin forms [17]. More recently, it has been suggested that the different forms of frataxin might play different roles. This point will be discussed in the next section. In addition to post-translational processing, alternative splicing mechanisms have also been observed that may generate different isoforms of frataxin. Work by Xia and collaborators suggested that these alternative forms could be tissue-specific and could have different functions and locations [18]. However, there are not additional evidences about the nature and relevance of these alternative forms.

3. Frataxin Function

Although very early after the discovery of frataxin as the gene that was responsible for Friedreich's Ataxia, it was established that iron homeostasis was altered by frataxin deficiency, the specific function of this protein remains controversial. Over the years, different functions have been proposed for frataxin, most of them related to iron metabolism and the control of oxidative stress in mitochondria.

3.1. Frataxin, an Iron Binding and Storage Protein

It has been proposed that frataxin could work like a metalochaperone and iron storage protein. In several studies with purified protein, it has been observed that frataxin has the ability to interact with metal ions, but the coordination environment of these metal binding sites has not been properly defined. There is also uncertainty on the number of metal ions that are bound per frataxin monomer. It has been described that frataxin can bind divalent metal ions using a group of exposed acidic residues. These amino acids are located in a specific area of the protein forming an acidic ridge, quite conserved, different from the canonical iron binding motifs where cysteine and/or histidine amino acids are usually found. This acidic zone results in a weak and non-specific electrostatic bonding of iron, which also allows the coordination of other divalent metals [19]. The estimated Kd for Fe^{2+} and Fe^{3+} of this region was calculated on the micromolar range [20]. Gentry and collaborators reported the potential presence of a high affinity iron binding site. They showed that three metal ions could be bound by each frataxin monomer, and that His86 was required for one of these binding sites. This residue is located in the disordered N-terminal tail and had not been previously reported to be involved in metal coordination. They calculated that this site would have an affinity for Fe^{2+} higher than the iron chelator ferrozine, while the remaining two sites would have lower affinities [21]. His86 is not included in most of the frataxin structures that are found in the protein data bank nor is conserved in yeast and bacterial homologues. More recently, while using NMR to investigate iron binding, it was also proposed that frataxin tightly binds a single Fe^{2+} but not Fe^{3+} [22].

Isaya and collaborators noticed that iron binding to yeast and bacterial frataxin promoted its oligomerization to complexes of high molecular weight (850–1100 kDa) [23–25]. These oligomeric forms resembled those that were formed by ferritin, the main protein responsible for iron storage in eukaryotes. Indeed, oligomeric frataxin was shown to use a ferrooxidation reaction to build a ferrihydrite mineral core inside the particles. Therefore it was proposed that frataxin could act as a mitochondrial ferritin. Although this function would be redundant in higher eukaryotes due to the presence of a mitochondrial ferritin, this hypothesis acquired some strength when subsequent studies demonstrated that the expression of mitochondrial ferritin in frataxin deficient yeast was able to partially recover some of the observed phenotypes. Specifically, the heterologous expression of mitochondrial ferritin partially prevented the accumulation of iron, the cells were more resistant to oxidizing agents and they partially recovered the activities of enzymes with iron-sulfur centers (which is a common described consequence of frataxin deficiency) [26]. Regarding human frataxin, it has been claimed that the mature form (FXN^{81-210}) does not form aggregates [27] and that only the intermediate forms FXN^{42-210} and FXN^{56-210} would be assembled into larger structures. Based on this observation, it has been suggested that different frataxin proteoforms would perform different functions. The mature form would be monomeric and involved in iron binding and delivery to biochemical pathways requiring this metal, while FXN^{56-210} and FXN^{42-210} would be able to oligomerize and store iron. A caveat to these hypotheses is that the long frataxin isoforms are not observed in most tissues by western blot. Mass spectrometry data also suggests that these long frataxin isoforms may be present at very low concentrations: data collected in the PeptideAtlas repository indicates that the theoretically likely frataxin peptides between positions 42 and 81 have never been observed, while those from the FXN^{81-210} have been observed at least 400 times. (PeptideAtlas is a publicly accessible compendium of peptides identified in mass spectrometry proteomics experiments) [28]. Recently, it has been shown that FXN^{81-210} can also undergo oligomerization under certain conditions, although the stability of these oligomers would be lower than that of bacterial frataxin [29].

Nevertheless, there are other caveats on the ferritin-like hypothesis. It has been argued that physiological conditions of calcium and magnesium stabilize the monomeric frataxin form and consequently frataxin would not oligomerize in vivo [27]. It has also been shown that mitochondrial iron in yeast strains expressing different Yfh1 concentrations, presented nearly identical chemical and biochemical characteristics [30]. Another point to take into account is which could be the contribution of frataxin to mitochondrial iron storage or trafficking from a quantitative point of view. Most iron that is present in mitochondria is found at the active sites of proteins. Despite that, non-proteinaceous labile metal iron pools have also been detected within cells. These pools are thought to be involved in cellular trafficking, regulation, signaling, and/or storage of metal ions. Due to their lability (and their presence at low concentrations), their structure and functions are not completely understood. For instance, mitochondria contain 0.7–2 mM Fe, but the proportion of labile iron is not completely known, with estimates ranging from 1 to 100 μM [31,32]. These differences in the estimates may be due to real differences between the models or experimental conditions used, but also on the methodological approaches used to analyze this elusive iron pool. Also, the nature of these nonproteinaceous metal complexes is not known. Based on the abundance of GSH within the mitochondria it has been hypothesized that could be an FeII (GSH) adduct. Citrate, which is also present in the mitochondrial matrix at high concentrations, has also been considered as a potential ligand for non-proteinaceous iron complexes (reviewed in [32]). In yeast, by using Mössbauer spectroscopy, it has been shown that the proportion and nature of these labile iron pools may vary depending on the metabolic state of the cell. Respiring mitochondria where estimated to contain ~15 μM labile non-heme high spin Fe^{2+}, while this pool in fermenting mitochondria increased to ~150 μM. The concentration of yeast frataxin in mitochondria has been estimated to be three orders of magnitude lower, around 35 nM [33].

Therefore, as monomeric frataxin has been claimed to bind three iron atoms, it cannot contribute significantly to store iron in a non-reactive easy deliverable form. However, it could play a role in iron trafficking as a temporary carrier or catalyzing its speciation between different forms. For instance, it could bind Fe^{2+} and promote its controlled oxidation to Fe^{3+}, which would be then stored in the form of Fe^{3+}-phosphate nanoparticles. Regarding oligomeric frataxin, the mineralization process would allow for this protein to bind much more iron atoms per subunit. The yeast 48 subunit oligomer can store ~50–75 iron atoms per subunit in 1–2 nm cores [34]. This raises the iron potentially bound by frataxin up to the μM range, but still this amount may not be a significant contribution to the whole mitochondrial iron pool. In comparison, around 35% of mitochondrial iron in fermenting mitochondria may be stored in the form of Fe^{3+} nanoparticles [33]. That said, the contribution of mitochondrial ferritin to iron storage in mitochondria is also intriguing, as the concentration of this protein according to the PaxDb database is much lower than that of frataxin (PaxDB is a database that contains protein abundance information across organisms and tissues) [35].

3.2. *Frataxin in the Biosynthesis of Iron Containing Proteins*

It has also been proposed that frataxin could participate in the biosynthesis of both heme groups and of iron-sulfur centers. This hypothesis has several fundamentals: (a) frataxin deficiency leads to a loss in proteins which contain iron-sulfur centers or heme groups; (b) frataxin has the ability to bind iron atoms; and, (c) several studies have shown the ability of frataxin to interact with proteins that areinvolved in heme or iron-sulfur biosynthesis.

3.2.1. Biosynthesis of Heme Groups

The incorporation of the iron atom into protoporphyrin IX is the last step in the biosynthesis of heme groups. This step is catalyzed by ferrochelatase, but it is not known how iron is provided to this enzyme. In in vitro studies, it was shown that there was a physical interaction between frataxin and ferrochelatase with a 1 to 2 stoichiometry, which seems logical, since ferrochelatase functions as a dimer. In addition, this interaction resulted in the formation of heme groups [36]. A study in which NMR spectroscopy was used to analyze the binding between both of the proteins suggested that ferrochelatase interacted with frataxin in a manner that included its iron-binding interface [37]. More recently, Söderberg and collaborators presented a model of the interaction of trimeric Yfh1 (yeast frataxin) and ferrochelatase in which one of the subunits of the Yfh1 trimer interacted with one subunit of the ferrochelatase dimer, whereas another trimer subunit was positioned for iron delivery [38]. These results support the hypothesis of frataxin acting as an iron donor in the biosynthesis of heme groups. However, heme deficiency is not always observed in frataxin-deficient cells and anemia has not been shown to be a symptom of FRDA. Indeed, no alterations where observed in heme synthesis in erythroid progenitor stem cells that were obtained from FRDA patients [39]. Moreover, experiments using either conditional frataxin-deficient T-Rex-293 cells or yeasts have shown that heme deficiency is a late consequence of frataxin deficiency [40,41]. These observations suggest that heme deficiency may be an epiphenomenon observed in certain frataxin-deficient cells which could be caused by poor iron availability or by metabolic remodeling. In this regard, we have shown in frataxin-deficient yeast that heme deficiency could be caused by the induction of Cth2, a protein induced in response to iron limitation, which promotes the degradation of mRNAs from iron-containing proteins [42].

3.2.2. Biosynthesis of Iron-Sulfur Centers

In addition to interacting with ferrochelatase, frataxin also interacts with the proteins that form the central biosynthesis machinery of iron-sulfur centers: IscU (Isu1 in yeast), Nfs1, and Isd11 [43,44]. Several authors have shown that this interaction facilitates the formation of an iron-sulfur center into IscU, the scaffold protein where these cofactors are first assembled. It was initially suggested that frataxin would act as an iron donor in the biosynthesis of these centers [45]. More recently, it has been suggested that frataxin would participate in the biosynthesis of iron-sulfur centers as an allosteric regulator and not as an iron donor. In works that were carried out in vitro with the CyaY protein (bacterial homologue of frataxin), it was shown that this protein had an inhibitory effect on the production of iron-sulfur centers. As this effect was increased in response to iron concentration, the authors suggested that frataxin could adapt the production of iron-sulfur to the number of final acceptor proteins [46]. Surprisingly, studies with human proteins demonstrated that eukaryotic frataxins would have a contrary effect. In this case, they stimulated the production of iron-sulfur centers by favoring the desulfurase activity of Nfs1 [47–49].

Today, despite the intense debate that is generated around the function or functions of frataxin, this non-essential activity in the metabolism of iron as an allosteric regulator of the biosynthesis of iron-sulfur centers has strong support from in vitro biochemical data and is the most accepted hypothesis. A detailed explanation of this complex biochemical process can be found in recent reviews [50,51]. However, this hypothesis also presents caveats when exposed to in vivo biological data. Remarkably, iron-sulfur cluster deficiency is not observed in several models of frataxin deficiency, such as flies [52], patient fibroblasts [53], or rat cardiac myocytes [54]. Moreover, detailed analysis of the cellular events that are caused by frataxin deficiency in yeast, have shown that iron-sulfur deficiency is an epiphenomenon that is caused by a metabolic remodeling program activated in response to disrupted iron homeostasis [41,55]. These observations question the role of frataxin in iron-sulfur biogenesis or at least suggest the possibility of additional functions for frataxin beyond iron-sulfur biogenesis. From these observations, it also becomes obvious that frataxin is not essential for iron-sulfur biogenesis.

3.3. Control of Oxidative Stress and the Generation of Ros

One of the phenotypes most consistently observed in frataxin-deficient cells is sensitivity to oxidizing agents [56,57]. Some authors have linked such sensitivity to oxidative stress to impaired biosynthesis of iron-sulfur centers. This hypothesis suggests that a vicious cycle would be created in which the deficient formation of iron-sulfur clusters would increase mitochondrial free iron that would increase the production of reactive oxygen species (ROS) through Fenton reaction. Then, ROS would further damage iron-sulfur clusters and promote the formation of more free iron. In fact, increased presence of labile iron has been reported in frataxin deficient yeast [58], T-Rex-293 cells [40] and in a mouse model of hepatic FXN deficiency [59]. However, no differences where observed between the mitochondrial iron pools from human lymphoblasts and fibroblasts that were obtained from either controls or FRDA patients [31]. Nevertheless, some observations suggest that oxidative stress could be the cause (and not the consequence) of iron-sulfur deficiency. For instance, in fibroblasts or lymphocytes from patients [53], or in frataxin-deficient cardiac myocytes [54], oxidative stress could be observed while the activities of iron-sulfur proteins remained unaltered. Moreover, there are evidences that iron-sulfur deficiency can be modulated by oxygen concentration or antioxidant treatment. In this regard, frataxin is not required for iron-sulfur biogenesis in yeasts grown at low oxygen tensions [60,61]. In some fly models, iron-sulfur deficiency is only observed under hyperoxic conditions [52], while in other models it can be prevented by antioxidants [62].

Which could be the origin of oxidative stress? Since frataxin has the ability to bind iron, a redox active metal, and oxidize it to Fe^{3+}, it has been proposed that frataxin could prevent oxidative stress by limiting the presence of free Fe^{2+} through its binding and the subsequent controlled oxidation to Fe^{3+}. This reaction would prevent the formation of reactive oxygen species through the reaction of Fe^{2+} with oxygen [63,64]. Therefore, the vicious cycle would have its origin in free iron than would then generate oxidative stress that would damage iron-sulfur clusters and generate more free iron. Another potential source of reactive oxygen species in frataxin-deficient cells could be the OXPHOS system. In this regard, an interaction was described between frataxin and mitochondrial electron transport chain proteins [65]. Also, decreased activity of the mitochondrial electron transport chain has been observed in several biological models of frataxin deficiency [53,66,67]. Any alteration in the OXPHOS system that was caused by frataxin deficiency could increase electron leakage and thus generate ROS [68].

Rustin and collaborators observed that frataxin-deficient cells could not properly activate the NRF2 signaling pathway in response to oxidative damage and in consequence they had a deficient response to oxidative insults and hypersensitivity to oxidative stress. They hypothesized that this impairment was related to actin remodeling [69]. This phenomenon has also been described in frataxin-deficient motor neurons [70], and in the frataxin-deficient YG8R mouse model where transcriptomic analysis showed a downregulation of NRF2-dependent antioxidant enzymes [71].

4. Evidences of Iron Accumulation and Its Relation to Pathophysiology in FRDA

Iron accumulation in a frataxin deficient cell model was first described in yeast *yfh1* mutants [72]. This early observation has been subsequently confirmed by several other researchers. Using Mössbauer spectroscopic analysis, Dancis and collaborators showed that in *Dyfh1* mitochondria iron was present as amorphous nano-particles of ferric phosphate [73]. Iron accumulation is caused by increased iron uptake due to activation of the iron sensor Aft1 [58], but the mechanisms leading to such activation are not completely understood. It has been assumed that it would be caused by iron-sulfur cluster loss, as Aft1 is known to be regulated by the presence of these cofactors. However, previous research from our group using conditional Yfh1 mutants provided two observations that challenged this hypothesis: (i) activation of Aft1 was observed earlier than iron-sulfur loss [41]; and, (ii) loss of iron-sulfur containing proteins in Yfh1 deficient yeasts was not observed in *cth2* cells. Therefore iron-sulfur loss was an epiphenomenon mainly caused by Cth2, which is an Aft1 target that binds to mRNAs from iron-containing proteins and promotes its degradation [42]. Moreover, we have also observed that nitric oxide can prevent Aft1 activation in Yfh1-deficient cells, but not in cells that are deficient in iron-sulfur biogenesis [74]. This observation also indicates that in Yfh1 deficient yeast Aft1 may be activated by a mechanism different than iron-sulfur cluster deficiency. Besides yeast, iron deposits or accumulation have also been clearly observed in frataxin deficient flies [75,76] and in cardiac muscles from frataxin deficient mice [77] and FRDA patients [78]. Iron in the heart from cardiac KO conditional mouse (the MCK mutant) was found in mitochondrial aggregates 100–400 nm in diameter, markedly different from those observed for mammalian ferritin. Energy-dispersive X-ray analysis showed that, in addition to iron, phosphorus and sulfur were present in these aggregates. Mössbauer spectra also confirmed that these aggregates where different than mammalian ferritin. The absorption profile observed was consistent with paramagnetic high-spin Fe(III) [79]. These observations are consistent with those that were obtained in frataxin-deficient yeast, and suggest that iron could be in the form of ferric-phosphate nanoparticles in both models. In other tissues or mammalian cell types, iron accumulation is not consistently observed. For instance, in fibroblasts or lymphoblasts from patients, there are no evidences of iron accumulation [31], while some authors have observed it in the nervous system [80]. Changes in the iron-responsive proteins, ferritin, divalent metal transporter 1 (DMT1), transferrin receptor 1 (TfR1), and ferroportin have been reported in the dentate nucleus of affected individuals [81]. Similar to yeast, iron deregulation in mammals might be caused by Iron-responding protein 1 (IRP1) activation [82,83], but the mechanisms causing this activation are not completely understood. It could be caused by deficiencies in iron supply to mitochondrial iron-dependent pathways that would activate the mechanisms of response to iron deficiency [59]. Frataxin has also been shown to interact with IRP1 and modulate the switch between its aconitase and RNA-binding forms. This function would be carried on by a cytosolic form of frataxin [84]. However, some authors are skeptical about the existence of an extra mitochondrial form of frataxin, and therefore question the physiological relevance of the observed interaction between IRP1 and frataxin.

As indicated above, many evidences support that frataxin deficiency causes a dysregulation in iron homeostasis, and it has also been shown in several models that the modulation of iron homeostasis ameliorates several phenotypes caused by frataxin deficiency [74,85]. However, the contribution of iron accumulation to the pathophysiology of FRDA has not been clearly determined. In this regard, several hypotheses have been formulated. It has been proposed that iron accumulation would be toxic and could be contributing to the formation of reactive oxygen species through the Fenton reaction. Iron overload could be also inducing the synthesis of sphingolipids, which, through the Pdk1/Mef2 pathway, would trigger neurodegeneration [76,80]. Iron toxicity could be also related to the formation of iron-phosphate aggregates that would compromise phosphate availability [86]. Nevertheless, it has also been suggested that iron accumulation would not be toxic per se, and that pathological consequences of frataxin deficiency would be mostly related to deficient iron supply to iron-dependent proteins. In this regard, it has been shown that IRP1 activation has a protective effect in a mouse model of hepatic FXN deficiency, as it contributes to sustain mitochondrial iron needs and mitochondrial function in these mice [59]. It has also been observed that dietary iron supplementation limits cardiac hypertrophy in MCK mutant mice [79].

These contradictory observations suggest that the pathological mechanisms could be more complex and specific for different models and tissues. For instance, in yeast, we have observed that activation of Aft1 causes the overexpression of Cth2, an mRNA binding protein that downregulates the expression of most iron-binding proteins that are required for aerobic growth. Thus, the activation of such pathway has a strong contribution to the alterations observed in yeast [42]. Beyond yeast, there are several evidences that frataxin deficiency may be causing perturbations in signaling pathways that could contribute to pathology. For instance, as mentioned before, neurodegeneration has been linked to the activation of the Pdk1/Mef2 pathway [76,80]. Cardiac hypertrophy could be related to the activation of the NFAT/calcineurin pathway, which has been observed in rat frataxin deficient cardiac myocytes [87]. Therefore, pathophysiology could be related to the pathways activated in different cells and tissues in response to the perturbations caused by frataxin deficiency.

Besides iron, some authors have reported deregulation of the homeostasis of other metals as a consequence of frataxin deficiency. In frataxin deficient yeast, we observed a decrease in manganese content and limited copper availability [58,88]. Subsequent studies using a conditional frataxin mutant indicated that manganese deficiency was caused by downregulation of Smf2, a Mn transporter that was degraded in response to iron accumulation [41]. In frataxin deficient flies it was found that the levels of zinc, copper, and manganese were increased, and that copper and zinc chelation improved the impaired motor performance of these flies [89]. In Dorsal Root Ganglia from FRDA patients, zinc and iron related proteins displayed major shifts in their cellular localization [90]. Alterations in calcium homeostasis have also been reported in several models of FRDA [87,91]. These alterations are mostly considered to be consequences of the deregulation of iron homeostasis, which may impact other metals. Nevertheless, frataxin is known to have also the capacity to chelate metals that are different than iron, such as manganese or copper [92]. The biological significance of these interactions has not been explored yet.

5. Targeting Iron as a Therapeutic Approach in FRDA

There is currently no cure for FRDA but several therapeutic approaches are being investigated. Some drugs have already entered clinical trials. Briefly, therapeutic approaches can be divided into compounds that improve mitochondrial function and reduce oxidative stress, drugs that modulate the altered metabolic pathways, and strategies to increase the expression or content of frataxin, either by promoting its expression, by supplying it through gene therapy (reviewed in [93]) or by protein replacement strategies [94].

Due to the alterations that were observed in iron homeostasis in different models and patients of FRDA, the use of iron chelators as a treatment to eliminate the excess iron accumulating in mitochondria was proposed many years ago. Deferoxamine was not considered to be a suitable iron chelator for depleting the intracellular iron deposits found in FRDA, as it does not cross the blood brain barrier and poorly penetrates biological membranes. It also has a high affinity for iron, which could compromise iron availability. The proposed alternative was deferiprone, an orally administered, lipidsoluble iron chelator that had been previously used to treat iron overload in polytransfused individuals with hemoglobinopathies. This compound can easily cross the blood–brain barrier and cellular membranes and therefore reach intracellular (or mitochondrial) iron deposits. In addition, since its affinity for iron is lower than that of transferrin, it has been shown that it can redistribute iron from intracellular iron deposits to this protein [95]. Indeed, the cellular properties that are affected by frataxin deficiency in HEK-293 cells were corrected by deferiprone treatment [96].

Several clinical trials have been performed with deferiprone in FRDA patients. In summary, these studies suggested that low doses of deferiprone would be beneficial on cardiac parameters. Higher doses of the drug worsened the condition and could result in agranulocytosis (reviewed in [97]). We can speculate that this dose dependent effect could be a consequence of different pathological mechanisms that are exerted by frataxin deficiency. Some of them would be caused by iron accumulation, while others would be caused by deficient iron availability. Therefore, low doses of the chelator would partially prevent the toxic effects that are caused by iron accumulation, while higher doses of deferiprone would compromise iron availability, and therefore worsen those pathological conditions caused by inefficient iron availability. Nevertheless, it has been proposed that deferiprone at low doses could be combined with other drugs. A pilot study with five FRDA patients suggested that combined therapy of deferiprone and idebenone (a Q10 analogue) was relatively safe and it could provide some benefits on neurological function and heart hypertrophy [98].

6. Concluding Remarks

Many evidences indicate that the lack of frataxin leads to alterations in iron cellular homeostasis. However, the precise mechanism(s) causing iron deregulation in frataxin-deficient cells are not completely understood. Several hypotheses have been formulated, but although most of them are well supported by in vitro data, all of them present caveats when exposed to biological data. In Figure 2, we have summarized two potential mechanisms which in our opinion could explain iron accumulation and oxidative stress: (1) the iron-sulfur hypothesis proposes that frataxin contributes to iron-sulfur biogenesis and its deficiency activates cellular iron sensors that would promote iron uptake; and, (2) the iron toxicity hypothesis assumes that frataxin would be involved in controlled iron ferrooxidation, and its deficiency would lead to ROS generation and the increased formation of ferric-phosphate nanoparticles. The iron-sulfur hypothesis is well supported by in vitro data, but its major caveat is the absence of iron-sulfur deficiency in many models of frataxin deficiency. On the other hand, the iron toxicity hypothesis does not provide a clear explanation for the activation of iron sensors.

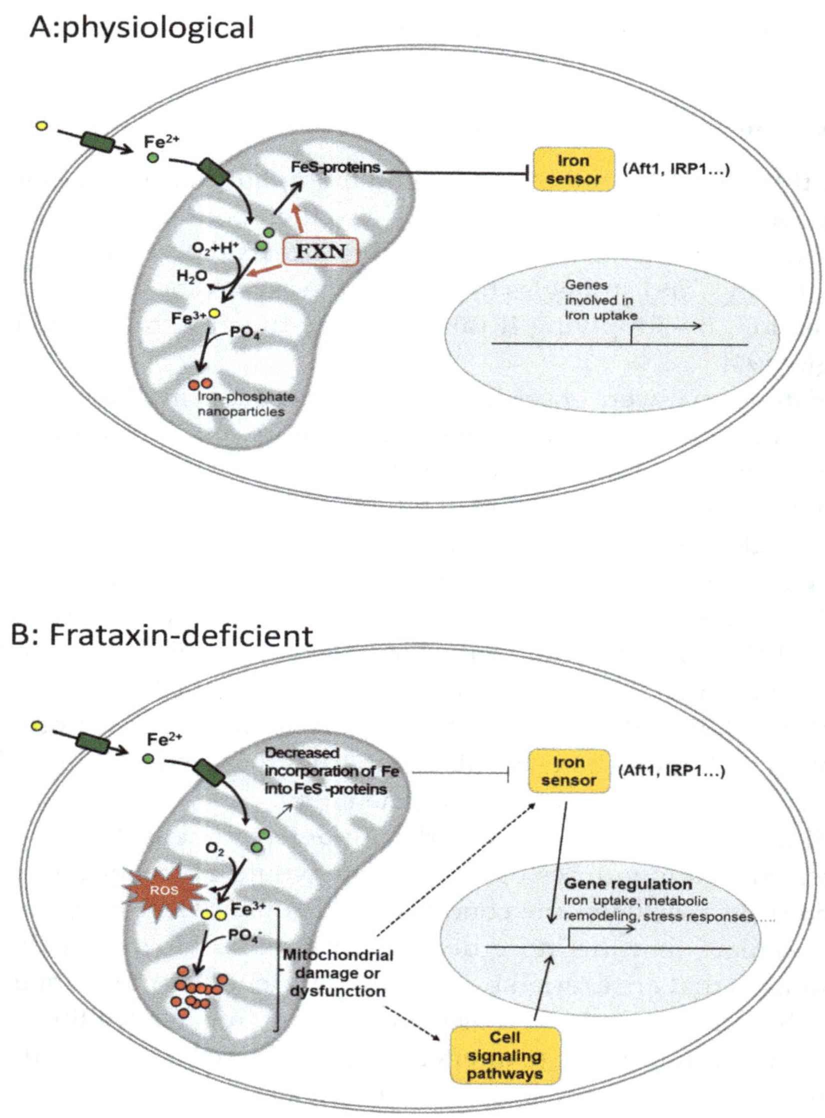

Figure 2. Potential contribution of frataxin to iron homeostasis and cellular consequences of its deficiency. (**A**), physiological: frataxin (FXN) binds Fe^{2+} and contributes to its controlled oxidation to

Fe^{3+} and/or to incorporate it into Fe-containing proteins. These Fe-containing proteins (notably FeS proteins) keep the iron sensor inactive and genes involved in iron uptake are not expressed. Oxidized iron (Fe^{3+}) is stored in the form of ferric-phosphate nanoparticles. (**B**), frataxin-deficient: loss of frataxin leads to decreased incorporation of iron into Fe-proteins and/or uncontrolled oxidation of Fe^{2+} by O_2. Such events lead to reactive oxygen species (ROS) generation, decreased phosphate availability, and mitochondrial dysfunction. Iron sensors and other cell signaling pathways are activated and regulate the expression of genes involved in iron uptake and/or other cell-specific pathways involved on metabolic remodeling, hypertrophy or neurodegeneration.

Also, it is not clear the contribution of iron to FRDA pathology, which could be related either to iron accumulation or to limited iron availability. Indeed, iron homeostasis deregulation could be an epiphenomenon that is not linked to pathology. In fact, many evidences suggest that the mechanisms causing cellular dysfunction could be tissue or model specific. They could also be related to the signaling pathways activated in response to the alterations that are caused by frataxin deficiency. This complexity may explain the limited effects of iron chelators on clinical trials, as these compounds would only prevent certain pathological mechanisms in a limited number of tissues.

Acknowledgments: Molecular graphics and analyses were performed with the UCSF Chimera package. Chimera is developed by the Resource for Biocomputing, Visualization, and Informatics at the University of California, San Francisco (supported by NIGMS P41-GM103311).

References

1. Ashby, D.W.; Tweedy, P.S. Friedreich's ataxia combined with diabetes mellitus in sisters. *Br. Med. J.* **1953**, *1*, 1418–1421. [CrossRef] [PubMed]
2. Koeppen, A.H. Friedreich's ataxia: Pathology, pathogenesis, and molecular genetics. *J. Neurol. Sci.* **2011**, *303*, 1–12. [CrossRef] [PubMed]
3. Campuzano, V.; Montermini, L.; Molto, M.D.; Pianese, L.; Cossee, M.; Cavalcanti, F.; Monros, E.; Rodius, F.; Duclos, F.; Monticelli, A.; et al. Friedreich's ataxia: Autosomal recessive disease caused by an intronic GAA triplet repeat expansion. *Science* **1996**, *271*, 1423–1427. [CrossRef] [PubMed]
4. Campuzano, V.; Montermini, L.; Lutz, Y.; Cova, L.; Hindelang, C.; Jiralerspong, S.; Trottier, Y.; Kish, S.J.; Faucheux, B.; Trouillas, P.; et al. Frataxin is Reduced in Friedreich Ataxia Patients and is Associated with Mitochondrial Membranes. *Hum. Mol. Genet.* **1997**, *6*, 1771–1780. [CrossRef] [PubMed]
5. Filla, A.; De Michele, G.; Cavalcanti, F.; Pianese, L.; Monticelli, A.; Campanella, G.; Cocozza, S. The relationship between trinucleotide (GAA) repeat length and clinical features in Friedreich ataxia. *Am. J. Hum. Genet.* **1996**, *59*, 554–560. [PubMed]
6. Isnard, R.; Kalotka, H.; Dürr, A.; Cossée, M.; Schmitt, M.; Pousset, F.; Thomas, D.; Brice, A.; Koenig, M.; Komajda, M. Correlation between left ventricular hypertrophy and GAA trinucleotide repeat length in Friedreich's ataxia. *Circulation* **1997**, *95*, 2247–2249. [CrossRef] [PubMed]
7. McDaniel, D.O.; Keats, B.; Vedanarayanan, V.; Subramony, S.H. Sequence variation in GAA repeat expansions may cause differential phenotype display in Friedreich's ataxia. *Mov. Disord.* **2001**, *16*, 1153–1158. [CrossRef] [PubMed]
8. Evans-Galea, M.V.; Carrodus, N.; Rowley, S.M.; Corben, L.A.; Tai, G.; Saffery, R.; Galati, J.C.; Wong, N.C.; Craig, J.M.; Lynch, D.R.; et al. FXN methylation predicts expression and clinical outcome in Friedreich ataxia. *Ann. Neurol.* **2012**, *71*, 487–497. [CrossRef] [PubMed]
9. Galea, C.A.; Huq, A.; Lockhart, P.J.; Tai, G.; Corben, L.A.; Yiu, E.M.; Gurrin, L.C.; Lynch, D.R.; Gelbard, S.; Durr, A.; et al. Compound heterozygous *FXN* mutations and clinical outcome in friedreich ataxia. *Ann. Neurol.* **2016**, *79*, 485–495. [CrossRef] [PubMed]
10. Adinolfi, S.; Nair, M.; Politou, A.; Bayer, E.; Martin, S.; Temussi, P.; Pastore, A. The factors governing the thermal stability of frataxin orthologues: How to increase a protein's stability. *Biochemistry* **2004**, *43*, 6511–6518. [CrossRef] [PubMed]

11. Pettersen, E.F.; Goddard, T.D.; Huang, C.C.; Couch, G.S.; Greenblatt, D.M.; Meng, E.C.; Ferrin, T.E. UCSF Chimera—A visualization system for exploratory research and analysis. *J. Comput. Chem.* **2004**, *25*, 1605–1612 [CrossRef] [PubMed]
12. Koutnikova, H.; Campuzano, V.; Koenig, M. Maturation of wild-type and mutated frataxin by the mitochondrial processing peptidase. *Hum. Mol. Genet.* **1998**, *7*, 1485–1489. [CrossRef] [PubMed]
13. Branda, S.S.; Cavadini, P.; Adamec, J.; Kalousek, F.; Taroni, F.; Isaya, G. Yeast and human frataxin are processed to mature form in two sequential steps by the mitochondrial processing peptidase. *J. Biol. Chem.* **1999**, *274*, 22763–22769. [CrossRef] [PubMed]
14. Condò, I.; Ventura, N.; Malisan, F.; Rufini, A.; Tomassini, B.; Testi, R. In vivo maturation of human frataxin. *Hum. Mol. Genet.* **2007**, *16*, 1534–1540. [CrossRef] [PubMed]
15. Schmucker, S.; Argentini, M.; Carelle-Calmels, N.; Martelli, A.; Puccio, H. The in vivo mitochondrial two-step maturation of human frataxin. *Hum. Mol. Genet.* **2008**, *17*, 3521–3531. [CrossRef] [PubMed]
16. Gakh, O.; Bedekovics, T.; Duncan, S.F.; Smith, D.Y.; Berkholz, D.S.; Isaya, G. Normal and Friedreich ataxia cells express different isoforms of frataxin with complementary roles in iron-sulfur cluster assembly. *J. Biol. Chem.* **2010**, *285*, 38486–38501. [CrossRef] [PubMed]
17. Cavadini, P.; Adamec, J.; Taroni, F.; Gakh, O.; Isaya, G. Two-step Processing of Human Frataxin by Mitochondrial Processing Peptidase. *J. Biol. Chem.* **2000**, *275*, 41469–41475. [CrossRef] [PubMed]
18. Xia, H.; Cao, Y.; Dai, X.; Marelja, Z.; Zhou, D.; Mo, R.; Al-Mahdawi, S.; Pook, M.A.; Leimkühler, S.; Rouault, T.A.; et al. Novel frataxin isoforms may contribute to the pathological mechanism of Friedreich ataxia. *PLoS ONE* **2012**, *7*, e47847. [CrossRef] [PubMed]
19. Pastore, A.; Puccio, H. Frataxin: A protein in search for a function. *J. Neurochem.* **2013**, *126*, 43–52. [CrossRef] [PubMed]
20. Yoon, T.; Cowan, J.A. Iron−Sulfur Cluster Biosynthesis. Characterization of Frataxin as an Iron Donor for Assembly of [2Fe^{-2}S] Clusters in ISU-Type Proteins. *J. Am. Chem. Soc.* **2003**, *125*, 6078–6084. [CrossRef] [PubMed]
21. Gentry, L.E.; Thacker, M.A.; Doughty, R.; Timkovich, R.; Busenlehner, L.S. His86 from the N-Terminus of Frataxin Coordinates Iron and Is Required for Fe-S Cluster Synthesis. *Biochemistry* **2013**, *52*, 6085–6096. [CrossRef] [PubMed]
22. Cai, K.; Frederick, R.O.; Tonelli, M.; Markley, J.L. Interactions of iron-bound frataxin with ISCU and ferredoxin on the cysteine desulfurase complex leading to Fe-S cluster assembly. *J. Inorg. Biochem.* **2018**, *183*, 107–116. [CrossRef] [PubMed]
23. Adamec, J.; Rusnak, F.; Owen, W.G.; Naylor, S.; Benson, L.M.; Gacy, M.; Isaya, G. Iron-dependent self-assembly of recombinant yeast frataxin: Implications for Friedreich ataxia. *Am. J. Hum. Genet.* **2000**, *67*, 549–562. [CrossRef] [PubMed]
24. Cavadini, P.; O'Neill, H.A.; Benada, O.; Isaya, G. Assembly and iron-binding properties of human frataxin, the protein deficient in Friedreich ataxia. *Hum. Mol. Genet.* **2002**, *11*, 217–227. [CrossRef] [PubMed]
25. Schagerlof, U.; Elmlund, H.; Gakh, O.; Nordlund, G.; Hebert, H.; Lindahl, M.; Isaya, G.; Al-Karadaghi, S. Structural basis of the iron storage function of frataxin from single-particle reconstruction of the iron-loaded oligomer. *Biochemistry* **2008**, *47*, 4948–4954. [CrossRef] [PubMed]
26. Campanella, A.; Isaya, G.; O'Neill, H.A.; Santambrogio, P.; Cozzi, A.; Arosio, P.; Levi, S. The expression of human mitochondrial ferritin rescues respiratory function in frataxin-deficient yeast. *Hum. Mol. Genet.* **2004**, *13*, 2279–2288. [CrossRef] [PubMed]
27. Adinolfi, S.; Trifuoggi, M.; Politou, A.S.; Martin, S.; Pastore, A. A structural approach to understanding the iron-binding properties of phylogenetically different frataxins. *Hum. Mol. Genet.* **2002**, *11*, 1865–1877. [CrossRef] [PubMed]
28. Desiere, F.; Deutsch, E.W.; King, N.L.; Nesvizhskii, A.I.; Mallick, P.; Eng, J.; Chen, S.; Eddes, J.; Loevenich, S.N.; Aebersold, R. The PeptideAtlas project. *Nucleic Acids Res.* **2006**, *34*, D655–D658. [CrossRef] [PubMed]
29. Ahlgren, E.C.; Fekry, M.; Wiemann, M.; Söderberg, C.A.; Bernfur, K.; Gakh, O.; Rasmussen, M.; Højrup, P.; Emanuelsson, C.; Isaya, G.; et al. Iron-induced oligomerization of human FXN81-210 and bacterial CyaY frataxin and the effect of iron chelators. *PLoS ONE* **2017**, *12*, e0188937. [CrossRef] [PubMed]
30. Seguin, A.; Sutak, R.; Bulteau, A.L.; Garcia-Serres, R.; Oddou, J.L.; Lefevre, S.; Santos, R.; Dancis, A.; Camadro, J.; Latour, J.; et al. Evidence that yeast frataxin is not an iron storage protein in vivo. *Biochim. Biophys. Acta-Mol. Basis Dis.* **2010**, *1802*, 531–538. [CrossRef] [PubMed]

31. Sturm, B.; Bistrich, U.; Schranzhofer, M.; Sarsero, J.P.; Rauen, U.; Scheiber-mojdehkar, B.; de Groot, H.; Ioannou, P.; Petrat, F. Friedreich's Ataxia, No Changes in Mitochondrial Labile Iron in Human Lymphoblasts and Fibroblasts A Decrease in Antioxidative Capacity? *J. Biol. Chem.* **2004**, *280*, 6701–6708. [CrossRef] [PubMed]
32. Lindahl, P.A.; Moore, M.J. Labile Low-Molecular-Mass Metal Complexes in Mitochondria: Trials and Tribulations of a Burgeoning Field. *Biochemistry* **2016**, *55*, 4140–4153. [CrossRef] [PubMed]
33. Garber-Morales, J.; Holmes-Hampton, G.P.; Miao, R.; Guo, Y.; Münck, E.; Lindahl, P.A. Biophysical characterization of iron in mitochondria isolated from respiring and fermenting yeast. *Biochemistry* **2010**, *49*, 5436–5444. [CrossRef] [PubMed]
34. Park, S.; Gakh, O.; O'Neill, H.; Mangravita, A.; Nichol, H.; Ferreira, G.C.; Isaya, G. Yeast frataxin sequentially chaperones and stores iron by coupling protein assembly with iron oxidation. *J. Biol. Chem.* **2003**, *278*, 31340–31351. [CrossRef] [PubMed]
35. Wang, M.; Herrmann, C.J.; Simonovic, M.; Szklarczyk, D.; von Mering, C. Version 4.0 of PaxDb: Protein abundance data, integrated across model organisms, tissues, and cell-lines. *Proteomics* **2015**, *15*, 3163–3168. [CrossRef] [PubMed]
36. Yoon, T.; Cowan, J.A. Frataxin-mediated iron delivery to ferrochelatase in the final step of heme biosynthesis. *J. Biol. Chem.* **2004**, *279*, 25943–25946. [CrossRef] [PubMed]
37. He, Y.; Alam, S.L.; Proteasa, S.V.; Zhang, Y.; Lesuisse, E.; Dancis, A.; Stemmler, T.L. Yeast frataxin solution structure, iron binding, and ferrochelatase interaction. *Biochemistry* **2004**, *43*, 16254–16262. [CrossRef] [PubMed]
38. Soderberg, C.G.; Gillam, M.E.; Ahlgren, E.C.; Hunter, G.A.; Gakh, O.; Isaya, G.; Ferreira, G.C.; Al-Karadaghi, S. The Structure of the Complex between Yeast Frataxin and Ferrochelatase: Characterization and pre-Steady State Reaction of Ferrous Iron Delivery and Heme Synthesis. *J. Biol. Chem.* **2016**, *291*, 11887–11898. [CrossRef] [PubMed]
39. Steinkellner, H.; Singh, H.N.; Muckenthaler, M.U.; Goldenberg, H.; Moganty, R.R.; Scheiber-Mojdehkar, B.; Sturm, B. No changes in heme synthesis in human Friedreich's ataxia erythroid progenitor cells. *Gene* **2017**, *621*, 5–11. [CrossRef] [PubMed]
40. Lu, C.; Cortopassi, G. Frataxin knockdown causes loss of cytoplasmic iron-sulfur cluster functions, redox alterations and induction of heme transcripts. *Arch. Biochem. Biophys.* **2007**, *457*, 111–122. [CrossRef] [PubMed]
41. Moreno-Cermeno, A.; Obis, E.; Belli, G.; Cabiscol, E.; Ros, J.; Tamarit, J. Frataxin Depletion in Yeast Triggers Up-regulation of Iron Transport Systems before Affecting Iron-Sulfur Enzyme Activities. *J. Biol. Chem.* **2010**, *285*, 41653–41664. [CrossRef] [PubMed]
42. Moreno-Cermeno, A.; Alsina, D.; Cabiscol, E.; Tamarit, J.; Ros, J. Metabolic remodeling in frataxin-deficient yeast is mediated by Cth2 and Adr1. *Biochim. Biophys. Acta* **2013**, *1833*, 3326–3337. [CrossRef] [PubMed]
43. Schmucker, S.; Martelli, A.; Colin, F.; Page, A.; Wattenhofer-Donze, M.; Reutenauer, L.; Puccio, H. Mammalian Frataxin: An Essential Function for Cellular Viability through an Interaction with a Preformed ISCU/NFS1/ISD11 Iron-Sulfur Assembly Complex. *PLoS ONE* **2011**, *6*, e16199. [CrossRef] [PubMed]
44. Wang, T.; Craig, E.A. Binding of yeast frataxin to the scaffold for Fe-S cluster biogenesis. *J. Biol. Chem.* **2008**, *283*, 12674–12679. [CrossRef] [PubMed]
45. Gerber, J.; Muhlenhoff, U.; Lill, R. An interaction between frataxin and Isu1/Nfs1 that is crucial for Fe/S cluster synthesis on Isu1. *EMBO Rep.* **2003**, *4*, 906–911. [CrossRef] [PubMed]
46. Adinolfi, S.; Iannuzzi, C.; Prischi, F.; Pastore, C.; Iametti, S.; Martin, S.R.; Bonomi, F.; Pastore, A. Bacterial frataxin CyaY is the gatekeeper of iron-sulfur cluster formation catalyzed by IscS. *Nat. Struct. Mol. Biol.* **2009**, *16*, 390–396. [CrossRef] [PubMed]
47. Bridwell-Rabb, J.; Fox, N.G.; Tsai, C.L.; Winn, A.M.; Barondeau, D.P. Human frataxin activates Fe-S cluster biosynthesis by facilitating sulfur transfer chemistry. *Biochemistry* **2014**, *53*, 4904–4913. [CrossRef] [PubMed]
48. Tsai, C.L.; Barondeau, D.P. Human frataxin is an allosteric switch that activates the Fe-S cluster biosynthetic complex. *Biochemistry* **2010**, *49*, 9132–9139. [CrossRef] [PubMed]
49. Parent, A.; Elduque, X.; Cornu, D.; Belot, L.; Le Caer, J.P.; Grandas, A.; Toledano, M.B.; D'Autréaux, B. Mammalian frataxin directly enhances sulfur transfer of NFS1 persulfide to both ISCU and free thiols. *Nat. Commun.* **2015**, *6*, 5686. [CrossRef] [PubMed]

50. Rouault, T.A.; Maio, N. Biogenesis and functions of mammalian iron-sulfur proteins in the regulation of iron homeostasis and pivotal metabolic pathways. *J. Biol. Chem.* **2017**, *292*, 12744–12753. [CrossRef] [PubMed]
51. Braymer, J.J.; Lill, R. Iron-sulfur cluster biogenesis and trafficking in mitochondria. *J. Biol. Chem.* **2017**, *292*, 12754–12763. [CrossRef] [PubMed]
52. Llorens, J.; Navarro, J.; Martínez-Sebastián, M.J.; Baylies, M.K.; Schneuwly, S.; Botella, J.; Moltó, M.D. Causative role of oxidative stress in a Drosophila model of Friedreich ataxia. *FASEB J.* **2007**, *21*, 333–344. [CrossRef] [PubMed]
53. Rötig, A.; de Lonlay, P.; Chretien, D.; Foury, F.; Koenig, M.; Sidi, D.; Munnich, A.; Rustin, P. Aconitase and mitochondrial iron-sulphur protein deficiency in Friedreich ataxia. *Nat. Genet.* **1997**, *17*, 215–217. [CrossRef] [PubMed]
54. Obis, È.; Irazusta, V.; Sanchís, D.; Ros, J.; Tamarit, J. Frataxin deficiency in neonatal rat ventricular myocytes targets mitochondria and lipid metabolism. *Free Radic. Biol. Med.* **2014**, *73*, 21–33. [CrossRef] [PubMed]
55. Gabrielli, N.; Ayte, J.; Hidalgo, E. Cells lacking pfh1, a fission yeast homolog of Mammalian frataxin protein, display constitutive activation of the iron starvation response. *J. Biol. Chem.* **2012**, *287*, 43042–43051. [CrossRef] [PubMed]
56. Tamarit, J.; Obis, È.; Ros, J. Oxidative stress and altered lipid metabolism in Friedreich ataxia. *Free Radic. Biol. Med.* **2016**, *100*, 138–146. [CrossRef] [PubMed]
57. Bayot, A.; Santos, R.; Camadro, J.M.; Rustin, P. Friedreich's ataxia: The vicious circle hypothesis revisited. *BMC Med.* **2011**, *9*, 112–119. [CrossRef] [PubMed]
58. Irazusta, V.; Obis, E.; Moreno-Cermeño, A.; Cabiscol, E.; Ros, J.; Tamarit, J. Yeast frataxin mutants display decreased superoxide dismutase activity crucial to promote protein oxidative damage. *Free Radic. Biol. Med.* **2010**, *48*, 411–420. [CrossRef] [PubMed]
59. Martelli, A.; Schmucker, S.; Reutenauer, L.; Mathieu, J.R.R.; Peyssonnaux, C.; Karim, Z.; Puy, H.; Galy, B.; Hentze, M.W.; Puccio, H. Iron Regulatory Protein 1 Sustains Mitochondrial Iron Loading and Function in Frataxin Deficiency. *Cell Metab.* **2015**, *21*, 311–322. [CrossRef] [PubMed]
60. Bulteau, A.L.; Dancis, A.; Gareil, M.; Montagne, J.J.; Camadro, J.M.; Lesuisse, E. Oxidative stress and protease dysfunction in the yeast model of Friedreich ataxia. *Free Radic. Biol. Med.* **2007**, *42*, 1561–1570. [CrossRef] [PubMed]
61. Gibson, T.J.; Koonin, E.; Musco, G.; Pastore, A.; Bork, P. Friedreich's ataxia protein: Phylogenetic evidence for mitochondrial dysfunction. *Trends Neurosci.* **1996**, *19*, 465–468. [CrossRef]
62. Anderson, P.R.; Kirby, K.; Orr, W.C.; Hilliker, A.J.; Phillips, J.P. Hydrogen peroxide scavenging rescues frataxin deficiency in a Drosophila model of Friedreich's ataxia. *Proc. Natl. Acad. Sci. USA* **2008**, *105*, 611–616. [CrossRef] [PubMed]
63. O'Neill, H.A.; Gakh, O.; Park, S.; Cui, J.; Mooney, S.M.; Sampson, M.; Ferreira, G.C.; Isaya, G. Assembly of human frataxin is a mechanism for detoxifying redox-active iron. *Biochemistry* **2005**, *44*, 537–545. [CrossRef] [PubMed]
64. Gakh, O.; Park, S.; Liu, G.; Macomber, L.; Imlay, J.A.; Ferreira, G.C.; Isaya, G. Mitochondrial iron detoxification is a primary function of frataxin that limits oxidative damage and preserves cell longevity. *Hum. Mol. Genet.* **2006**, *15*, 467–479. [CrossRef] [PubMed]
65. Gonzalez-Cabo, P.; Vazquez-Manrique, R.P.; Garcia-Gimeno, M.A.; Sanz, P.; Palau, F. Frataxin interacts functionally with mitochondrial electron transport chain proteins. *Hum. Mol. Genet.* **2005**, *14*, 2091–2098. [CrossRef] [PubMed]
66. Koutnikova, H.; Campuzano, V.; Foury, F.; Dolle, P.; Cazzalini, O.; Koenig, M. Studies of human, mouse and yeast homologues indicate a mitochondrial function for frataxin. *Nat. Genet.* **1997**, *16*, 345–351. [CrossRef] [PubMed]
67. Lodi, R.; Rajagopalan, B.; Blamire, A.M.; Cooper, J.M.; Davies, C.H.; Bradley, J.L.; Styles, P.; Schapira, A. Cardiac energetics are abnormal in Friedreich ataxia patients in the absence of cardiac dysfunction and hypertrophy: An in vivo 31P magnetic resonance spectroscopy study. *Cardiovasc. Res.* **2001**, *52*, 111–119. [CrossRef]
68. Armstrong, J.S.; Khdour, O.; Hecht, S.M. Does oxidative stress contribute to the pathology of Friedreich's ataxia? A radical question. *FASEB J.* **2010**, *24*, 2152–2163. [CrossRef] [PubMed]

69. Paupe, V.; Dassa, E.P.; Goncalves, S.; Auchere, F.; Lonn, M.; Holmgren, A.; Rustin, P. Impaired nuclear Nrf2 translocation undermines the oxidative stress response in Friedreich ataxia. *PLoS ONE* **2009**, *4*, e4253. [CrossRef] [PubMed]
70. D'Oria, V.; Petrini, S.; Travaglini, L.; Priori, C.; Piermarini, E.; Petrillo, S.; Carletti, B.; Bertini, E.; Piemonte, F. Frataxin deficiency leads to reduced expression and impaired translocation of NF-E2-related factor (Nrf2) in cultured motor neurons. *Int. J. Mol. Sci.* **2013**, *14*, 7853–7865. [CrossRef] [PubMed]
71. Shan, Y.; Schoenfeld, R.A.; Hayashi, G.; Napoli, E.; Akiyama, T.; Carstens, M.; Carstens, E.E.; Pook, M.A.; Cortopassi, G.A. Frataxin deficiency leads to defects in expression of antioxidants and Nrf2 expression in dorsal root ganglia of the Friedreich's ataxia YG8R mouse model. *Antioxid. Redox Signal.* **2013**, *19*, 1481–1493. [CrossRef] [PubMed]
72. Babcock, M.; de Silva, D.; Oaks, R.; Davis-Kaplan, S.; Jiralerspong, S.; Montermini, L.; Pandolfo, M.; Kaplan, J. Regulation of mitochondrial iron accumulation by Yfh1p, a putative homolog of frataxin. *Science* **1997**, *276*, 1709–1712. [CrossRef] [PubMed]
73. Lesuisse, E.; Santos, R.; Matzanke, B.F.; Knight, S.A.B.; Camadro, J.M.; Dancis, A. Iron use for haeme synthesis is under control of the yeast frataxin homologue (Yfh1). *Hum. Mol. Genet.* **2003**, *12*, 879–889. [CrossRef] [PubMed]
74. Alsina, D.; Ros, J.; Tamarit, J. Nitric oxide prevents Aft1 activation and metabolic remodeling in frataxin-deficient yeast. *Redox Biol.* **2018**, *14*, 131–141. [CrossRef] [PubMed]
75. Soriano, S.; Llorens, J.V.; Blanco-Sobero, L.; Gutiérrez, L.; Calap-Quintana, P.; Morales, M.P.; Moltó, M.D.; Martínez-Sebastián, M.J. Deferiprone and idebenone rescue frataxin depletion phenotypes in a Drosophila model of Friedreich's ataxia. *Gene* **2013**, *521*, 274–281. [CrossRef] [PubMed]
76. Chen, K.; Lin, G.; Haelterman, N.A.; Ho, T.S.Y.; Li, T.; Li, Z.; Duraine, L.; Graham, B.H.; Jaiswal, M.; Yamamoto, S.; et al. Loss of Frataxin induces iron toxicity, sphingolipid synthesis, and Pdk1/Mef2 activation, leading to neurodegeneration. *Elife* **2016**, *5*, e16043. [CrossRef] [PubMed]
77. Whitnall, M.; Rahmanto, Y.S.; Sutak, R.; Xu, X.; Becker, E.M.; Mikhael, M.R.; Ponka, P.; Richardson, D.R. The MCK mouse heart model of Friedreich's ataxia: Alterations in iron-regulated proteins and cardiac hypertrophy are limited by iron chelation. *Proc. Natl. Acad. Sci. USA* **2008**, *105*, 9757–9762. [CrossRef] [PubMed]
78. Ramirez, R.L.; Qian, J.; Santambrogio, P.; Levi, S.; Koeppen, A.H. Relation of Cytosolic Iron Excess to Cardiomyopathy of Friedreich's Ataxia. *Am. J. Cardiol.* **2012**, *110*, 1820–1827. [CrossRef] [PubMed]
79. Whitnall, M.; Rahmanto, Y.S.; Huang, M.L.H.; Saletta, F.; Lok, H.C.; Gutierrez, L.; Lázaro, F.J.; Fleming, A.J.; St. Pierre, T.G.; Mikhael, M.R.; et al. Identification of nonferritin mitochondrial iron deposits in a mouse model of Friedreich ataxia. *Proc. Natl. Acad. Sci. USA* **2012**, *109*, 20590–20595. [CrossRef] [PubMed]
80. Chen, K.; Ho, T.S.Y.; Lin, G.; Tan, K.L.; Rasband, M.N.; Bellen, H.J. Loss of Frataxin activates the iron/sphingolipid/PDK1/Mef2 pathway in mammals. *Elife* **2016**, *5*, e20732. [CrossRef] [PubMed]
81. Koeppen, A.H.; Michael, S.C.; Knutson, M.D.; Haile, D.J.; Qian, J.; Levi, S.; Santambrogio, P.; Garrick, M.D.; Lamarche, J.B. The dentate nucleus in Friedreich's ataxia: The role of iron-responsive proteins. *Acta Neuropathol.* **2007**, *114*, 163–173. [CrossRef] [PubMed]
82. Seznec, H.; Simon, D.; Monassier, L.; Criqui-Filipe, P.; Gansmuller, A.; Rustin, P.; Koenig, M.; Puccio, H. Idebenone delays the onset of cardiac functional alteration without correction of Fe-S enzymes deficit in a mouse model for Friedreich ataxia. *Hum. Mol. Genet.* **2004**, *13*, 1017–1024. [CrossRef] [PubMed]
83. Stehling, O.; Elsässer, H.P.; Brückel, B.; Mühlenhoff, U.; Lill, R. Iron-sulfur protein maturation in human cells: Evidence for a function of frataxin. *Hum. Mol. Genet.* **2004**, *13*, 3007–3015. [CrossRef] [PubMed]
84. Condò, I.; Malisan, F.; Guccini, I.; Serio, D.; Rufini, A.; Testi, R. Molecular control of the cytosolic aconitase/IRP1 switch by extramitochondrial frataxin. *Hum. Mol. Genet.* **2010**, *19*, 1221–1229. [CrossRef] [PubMed]
85. Navarro, J.A.; Botella, J.A.; Metzendorf, C.; Lind, M.I.; Schneuwly, S. Mitoferrin modulates iron toxicity in a Drosophila model of Friedreich's ataxia. *Free Radic. Biol. Med.* **2015**, *85*, 71–82. [CrossRef] [PubMed]
86. Seguin, A.; Santos, R.; Pain, D.; Dancis, A.; Camadro, J.M.; Lesuisse, E. Co-precipitation of phosphate and iron limits mitochondrial phosphate availability in Saccharomyces cerevisiae lacking the yeast frataxin homologue (YFH1). *J. Biol. Chem.* **2011**, *286*, 6071–6079. [CrossRef] [PubMed]
87. Purroy, R.; Britti, E.; Delaspre, F.; Tamarit, J.; Ros, J. Mitochondrial pore opening and loss of Ca^{2+} exchanger NCLX levels occur after frataxin depletion. *Biochim. Biophys. Acta-Mol. Basis Dis.* **2018**, *1864*, 618–631. [CrossRef] [PubMed]

88. Irazusta, V.; Cabiscol, E.; Reverter-Branchat, G.; Ros, J.; Tamarit, J. Manganese is the link between frataxin and iron-sulfur deficiency in the yeast model of Friedreich ataxia. *J. Biol. Chem.* **2006**, *281*, 12227–12232 [CrossRef] [PubMed]
89. Soriano, S.; Calap-Quintana, P.; Llorens, J.V.; Al-Ramahi, I.; Gutiérrez, L.; Martínez-Sebastián, M.J.; Botas, J.; Moltó, M.D. Metal Homeostasis Regulators Suppress FRDA Phenotypes in a Drosophila Model of the Disease. *PLoS ONE* **2016**, *11*, e0159209. [CrossRef] [PubMed]
90. Koeppen, A.H.; Kuntzsch, E.C.; Bjork, S.T.; Ramirez, R.; Mazurkiewicz, J.E.; Feustel, P.J. Friedreich ataxia: Metal dysmetabolism in dorsal root ganglia. *Acta Neuropathol. Commun.* **2013**, *1*, 26. [CrossRef] [PubMed]
91. Mincheva-Tasheva, S.; Obis, E.; Tamarit, J.; Ros, J. Apoptotic cell death and altered calcium homeostasis caused by frataxin depletion in dorsal root ganglia neurons can be prevented by BH4 domain of Bcl-xL protein. *Hum. Mol. Genet.* **2013**, *23*, 1829–1841. [CrossRef] [PubMed]
92. Han, T.H.L.; Camadro, J.M.; Santos, R.; Lesuisse, E.; Chahine, J.M.; Ha-Duong, N.T. Mechanisms of iron and copper-frataxin interactions. *Metallomics* **2017**, *9*, 1073–1085. [CrossRef] [PubMed]
93. Tai, G.; Corben, L.A.; Yiu, E.M.; Milne, S.C.; Delatycki, M.B. Progress in the treatment of Friedreich ataxia. *Neurol. Neurochir. Pol.* **2018**, *52*, 129–139. [CrossRef] [PubMed]
94. Britti, E.; Delaspre, F.; Feldman, A.; Osborne, M.; Greif, H.; Tamarit, J.; Ros Salvador, J. Frataxin-deficient neurons and mice models of Friedreich ataxia are improved by TAT-MTScs-FXN treatment. *J. Cell. Mol. Med.* **2017**, *22*, 834–848. [CrossRef] [PubMed]
95. Sohn, Y.S.; Breuer, W.; Munnich, A.; Cabantchik, Z.I. Redistribution of accumulated cell iron: A modality of chelation with therapeutic implications. *Blood* **2008**, *111*, 1690–1699. [CrossRef] [PubMed]
96. Kakhlon, O.; Manning, H.; Breuer, W.; Melamed-Book, N.; Lu, C.; Cortopassi, G.; Munnich, A.; Cabantchik, Z. Cell functions impaired by frataxin deficiency are restored by drug-mediated iron relocation. *Blood* **2008**, *112*, 5219–5227. [CrossRef] [PubMed]
97. Pandolfo, M.; Hausmann, L. Deferiprone for the treatment of Friedreich's ataxia. *J. Neurochem.* **2013**, *126*, 142–146. [CrossRef] [PubMed]
98. Elincx-Benizri, S.; Glik, A.; Merkel, D.; Arad, M.; Freimark, D.; Kozlova, E.; Cabantchik, I.; Hassin-Baer, S. Clinical Experience With Deferiprone Treatment for Friedreich Ataxia. *J. Child Neurol.* **2016**, *31*, 1036–1040. [CrossRef] [PubMed]

10

Twenty Years of Ferroportin Disease: A Review or An Update of Published Clinical, Biochemical, Molecular and Functional Features

L. Tom Vlasveld [1], Roel Janssen [2], Edouard Bardou-Jacquet [3], Hanka Venselaar [4], Houda Hamdi-Roze [5], Hal Drakesmith [6] and Dorine W. Swinkels [2,*]

1 Department of Internal Medicine, Haaglanden MC-Bronovo, 2597AX The Hague, The Netherlands
2 Department of Laboratory Medicine, Translational Metabolic Laboratory, Radboud University Medical Center, P.O. Box 9101, 6500 HB Nijmegen, The Netherlands
3 Liver Diseases Department, French Reference Centre for Rare Iron Overload Diseases of Genetic Origin, University Hospital Pontchaillou, 35033 Rennes, France
4 Centre for Molecular and Biomolecular Informatics, Radboud Institute for Molecular Life Sciences, Radboud, University Medical Center, P.O. Box 9191, 6500 HB Nijmegen, The Netherlands
5 Molecular Genetics Department, French Reference Centre for Rare Iron Overload Diseases of Genetic Origin, University Hospital Pontchaillou, 35033 Rennes, France
6 MRC Human Immunology Unit, Weatherall Institute of Molecular Medicine, University of Oxford, Oxford OX39DS, UK
* Correspondence: dorine.swinkels@radboudumc.nl

Abstract: Iron overloading disorders linked to mutations in ferroportin have diverse phenotypes in vivo, and the effects of mutations on ferroportin in vitro range from loss of function (LOF) to gain of function (GOF) with hepcidin resistance. We reviewed 359 patients with 60 ferroportin variants. Overall, macrophage iron overload and low/normal transferrin saturation (TSAT) segregated with mutations that caused LOF, while GOF mutations were linked to high TSAT and parenchymal iron accumulation. However, the pathogenicity of individual variants is difficult to establish due to the lack of sufficiently reported data, large inter-assay variability of functional studies, and the uncertainty associated with the performance of available in silico prediction models. Since the phenotypes of hepcidin-resistant GOF variants are indistinguishable from the other types of hereditary hemochromatosis (HH), these variants may be categorized as ferroportin-associated HH, while the entity ferroportin disease may be confined to patients with LOF variants. To further improve the management of ferroportin disease, we advocate for a global registry, with standardized clinical analysis and validation of the functional tests preferably performed in human-derived enterocytic and macrophagic cell lines. Moreover, studies are warranted to unravel the definite structure of ferroportin and the indispensable residues that are essential for functionality.

Keywords: SLC40A1; ferroportin; iron overload; non-HFE; ferritin; hemochromatosis

---

1. Introduction

Hereditary hemochromatosis (HH) type 4 or ferroportin disease (OMIM-code: 606069 Orphanet-code: 139491) is associated with variants in *SLC40A1* and inherited in an autosomal-dominant manner. Since 1999, ferroportin disease was classified into two entities [1–3], based on experimental in vitro models of genetic variants found in patients [4–10]. Classical ferroportin disease (Type 4A) is associated with loss-of-function (LOF) variants with diminished cell surface expression of ferroportin and lower iron export capacity, and is characterized by macrophage iron retention and iron restriction for erythropoiesis. It is clinically recognized by the presence of high serum ferritin concentrations with low to normal transferrin saturation (TSAT) and poor tolerance to phlebotomy. Non-classical (atypical, type 4B) ferroportin disease is associated with gain-of-function (GOF) variants that render ferroportin protein resistant to hepcidin, resulting in continued iron export, and leading to a phenotype that mimics classical HFE HH characterized by parenchymal (hepatocellular) iron overload with elevated serum ferritin and TSAT.

Systematic and narrative reviews on ferroportin disease revealed the great variety in iron parameters among patients with ferroportin variants and emphasize the poor correlation between iron export capacity in functional studies and clinical characteristics (phenotype) [7,9–11] and question the pathogenicity of various variants [8,12].

To better guide the management of this disorder, a better understanding of the clinical and biochemical features of ferroportin disease and its underlying pathological mechanisms is required. In this report, we evaluated and describe clinical and laboratory data of patients reported between 1999 and June 2019, in whom the identified ferroportin variant was assumed to be associated with the defined state of iron overload. The relation between patient's clinical features and the functional in vitro features of underlying variants is assessed in context of current knowledge on the function and structure of ferroportin and its regulatory mechanisms. We comment on the shortcomings of describing the phenotype based on case and family reports, and review the limited applicability of functional studies and available in silico prediction models to determine pathogenicity. We recommend the institution of a global registry with a (1) standardized diagnostic protocol, (2) validated functional tests, and (3) studies to establish the definite secondary and tertiary structure of ferroportin and residues involved in its binding with hepcidin for ubiquitination and to ferroportin for iron transport.

2. Methods

2.1. Data Collection and Selection

Identification, Demographic Characteristics, and Iron Parameters

A literature search was done using Medline and Embase (searching strategy: #1 (SLC40A1 or ferroportin or IREG or IREG-1 or FPN or FPN1 or non-HFE hemochromatosis), #2 (mutation or variant) from 1999 to June 2019. Papers with only an abstract in English were also selected. We included all the cases (including family studies) of ferroportin variants that are associated with unexplained elevated serum ferritin concentration. Since the aim of this analysis was to evaluate the relation between the clinical features and the functional in vitro characteristics in experimental cell lines of the various potentially pathogenic variants, we excluded variants for which these functional studies have not been performed, e.g., variants in promoter and untranslated regions, splicing variants as well as variants leading to synonymous amino acids such as Iso109Iso, Leu129Leu, and Val221Val [13–17]. In addition, we excluded patients with previously established neutral or (possibly) iron-modifying polymorphisms with a variant population frequency $> 1\%$, such as the African Gln248His variant and variants in residues Leu348 and Leu384 [7,18–21].

Only patients with reported numerical value of at least transferrin saturation (TSAT) or ferritin concentration were selected. Demographic features, presenting symptoms, blood test results (hemoglobin (Hb), mean corpuscular volume (MCV), serum iron, TSAT, ferritin, and alanine aminotransferase (ALT)), hepatic iron content and hepatic histology, data on tolerability of phlebotomy (including the amount of iron removed), and the presence of p.Cys282Tyr and p.His63Asp HFE variants and other potential confounders, such as alcohol consumption and signs of metabolic syndrome, were collected. Organ iron accumulation as assessed by MRI and histologic examination was evaluated. Hepatic damage was histologically scored using the Meta-analysis of Histological Data in Viral Hepatitis (METAVIR) score (0 = no fibrosis, 1 = mild fibrosis (portal fibrosis without septa), 2 = moderate fibrosis (portal fibrosis and few septa), 3 = severe fibrosis (numerous septa without cirrhosis), and 4 = cirrhosis). Differences between categorical variables were compared with the Chi-square test with Yates correction while the comparison of continuous variables was done with the Mann-Whitney U-test and Student's–t -test of independent means. A two-sided p-value < 0.05 was considered significant. The correlation between variables was determined by the Pearson correlation coefficient.

2.2. *Variant Classification Based on Functional In Vitro Studies*

Functional studies on iron export and/or ferroportin expression were performed in cell lines transfected with the ferroportin protein variant. We reviewed the reported functional studies on iron export capacity and ferroportin expression that were performed in cell lines transfected with the wild-type and the variant ferroportin protein. We assigned a variant as an LOF variant when the iron export capacity was significantly reduced, in comparison to the wild-type (WT) protein. The variant was assigned as a GOF variant when the iron transport capacity was preserved. When the addition of hepcidin significantly inhibited the iron export capacity and/or ferroportin expression, the variant was defined as hepcidin-sensitive, and the variant was hepcidin-resistant in the absence of a modulating effect of hepcidin. A variant was scored as "non-classified" when no relevant functional data were available, and as "conflicting" when data on the hepcidin effect were inconsistent or inconclusive.

2.3. *Bioinformatics Prediction Software Analysis*

To assess co-segregation in multiple affected family members, the simplified method of segregation analysis (SISA) was applied [22,23] and classified according to recent recommendations to define co-segregation to fit the guidelines of the American College of Medical Genetics and Genomics and the Association for Molecular Pathology (ACMG-AMP) [22,24]. Briefly, to determine the co-segregation we used the classification suggested by Jarvik et al. and the method to calculate the probability that the phenotype of a variant carrier is caused by chance rather than genotype, as suggested by Moller et al. [22,23]. This probability is described as $(1/2)^n$, wherein n is the number of informative meiosis and will be the number of the carriers with the affected phenotype of interest and all the carriers in between them, minus one. The genome aggregation data base (gnomAD), was applied to determine of the allele frequency of a variant. In order to further determine the potential pathogenicity of the various variants three commonly used algorithms were applied [25]. Polyphen2 predicts the impact of amino acid substitution on the structure and function of human protein using physical and comparative considerations [26]. The method "Sorts intolerant from Tolerant" (SIFT) (http://www.blocks.fhcrc.org/sift/SIFT.html) classifies non-synonymous single nucleotide polymorphisms on the basis of the evolutionary conservation of amino acids within protein families [27]. Align-GVGD predicts variants in the query sequence based on a combination of Grantham Variation (GV) which measures the evolutionary variation at a particular position in the alignment and Grantham Deviation (GD), measuring the biochemical difference between the reference and amino acid encoded by the variant [28].

3. Evaluation and Analysis

3.1. *Description of the Phenotype of Patients (Including Related Family Members) in Relation Findings in Functional Studies*

3.1.1. Patients Characteristics

Ferroportin Disease Occurs in Different Parts of the World and Has no Specific Symptoms

We retrieved 359 individuals with 60 variants (59 missense variants and one deletion) in the ferroportin protein (Table 1). The reported patients, were predominantly male and of European descent. When reported, fatigue and arthralgia were the major presenting symptoms. Overall, patients had normal Hb and MCV with a serum iron level and TSAT at the upper range of normal and moderately elevated ferritin levels.

Table 1. Patient Characteristics. MCV: mean corpuscular volume, TSAT: transferrin saturation.

Characteristics	*n*	Value (Median)	Range
Patients	359		
Probands		68	
Relatives from probands		191	
Individual patients		88	
Gender	342		
Female		131	
Male		211	
Age (years)	322	41	2–87
Continent	352		
Europe		258	
North–South America		37	
Asia		44	
Australia/Oceania		13	
Presenting clinical symptoms	71		
Fatigue		34	
Elevated liver enzymes / hepatomegaly		30	
Joint complaints/arthralgia		36	
Miscellaneous		47	
Referral because of high ferritin level	131		
Hematological Parameters			
Hemoglobin (g/dL)#			
Female	60	13.1	7.5–16.3
Male	92	15.0	6.5–18.4
MCV (fl)			
Female	38	91	77–107
Male	46	91	70–108
Serum iron (μmol/L)			
Female	34	20.9	6.7–94.0
Male	56	26.3	6.2–86.0
TSAT (%)			
Female	116	31.5	2.0–100.0
Male	180	38.0	7.0–104.0
Ferritin (μg/L)			
Female	122	1026	4–8943
Male	201	1514	12–18695

Iron Parameters are Determined by Gender and Age. #Significant difference between females and males ($p < 0.05$, also after correcting for multiple testing according to Bonferroni (<0.01).

Women had significantly lower Hb, TSAT, and serum ferritin concentration (Table 1). There was a weak correlation between age and TSAT ($r = 0.1796$) and serum ferritin ($r = 0.3461$) (Figure S1a–c). Probands were significantly older than affected family members (45.5 versus 34 years) with significantly higher (1896 versus 948 μg/L) serum ferritin levels (Table S1). Ten percent (20/191) of affected family's members (6/14 males/females, median age 42 years) had no biochemical signs of iron overload (ferritin level ≤ 200 μg/L and normal TSAT).

Modification by Additional Hereditary and Acquired Conditions

We found no effect of the presence of p.Cys282Tyr (13 heterozygotes) and p.His63Asp (35 heterozygotes, five homozygotes) HFE variants on iron parameters (Table S2). In only 84 patients, the current alcohol consumption was reported without demonstrable effect (Table S3). The reported clinical data were insufficient for the proper determination of the presence of metabolic syndrome to explore its modifying effect.

3.2. Relation between In Vitro Functional Studies of Ferroportin Variants on Clinical Features

We identified 27 different GOF variants (110 patients), 21 LOF variants (205 patients), and 12 unclassified variants (33 patients) (Table 2). A total of 355 cases involved heterozygosity for ferroportin variants. One homozygous Gly204Ser GOF variant was reported in a 52-year-old female with ferritin concentration of 5236 μg/L, TSAT of 100%, and symptoms of hepatic fibrosis revealed by radiology [15]. A patient with homozygosity for the GOF variant Arg561Gly had biochemical signs of severe iron overload reflected by a serum ferritin of 2750 μg/L and TSAT of 84% [29].

Table 2. Functional and phenotypical characteristics of 359 patients with 60 ferroportin variants. GOF: gain of function, LOF: loss of function.

Protein	Iron Export		Hepcidin Effect on				TSAT		
Variant	Expression	Capacity	Expression	Export Capacity	Fate of Hepcidin	Patients (n)	Normal	High	Reference%
Tyr64Asn	PM	=	no	no	↓↓ubiquitination/uptake	8	-	8	[11,30–36]
Cys326Ser	PM	=	no	no	↓binding/no uptake	7	-	6	[30,32,34,37,38]
Cys326Tyr	PM	=	no	no	↓/no uptake	4	-	4	[8,31,34,35,39–44]
Tyr333His	PM	=	no	no		5	-	5	[45]
Tyr501Cys	PM	=	no	no	↓binding	7	2	5	[30,33,46]
Asp504Asn	PM	=	no	no	↓binding/uptake	2	-	2	[8,30]
His507Arg	PM	=	no	no	↓↓ubiquitination	4	-	4	[30,41,47]
Sum: 7	GOF		Hepcidin Resistant			37	2	34	
ILe180Thr	PM	=	yes	–	normal uptake	3	2	1	[8,48,49]
Thr230Asn	PM	=	yes	–	normal uptake	1	1	-	[8]
Met266Thr	PM	=	yes	–	normal uptake	1	1	-	[8]
Leu345Phe	PM	=	yes	–	normal uptake	1	1	-	[8]
Ile351Val	PM	=	yes	–	↑uptake	1	1	-	[8]
Pro443Leu	PM	=	yes	–	↑uptake	1	-	-	[8]
Arg561Gly	PM	=	yes	–	normal uptake	4	1	2	[8,29,50]
Sum: 7	GOF		Hepcidin Sensitive: Neutral			12	7	3	
Ala69Thr	PM	=	–	↓!	–	4	2	2	[42,51,52]
Val72Phe	PM	=	yes	↓!	↓binding	5	2	3	[30,53]
Asn144Asp	PM	=#	conflicting	no#	↓binding/uptake	2	-	1	[30–32,35,54]
Asn144His	PM	=	conflicting	yes	↓uptake	20	13	7	[3,6,31,34,35,39,40,42,55–59]
Asn144Thr	PM	=	conflicting	yes#	↓uptake	1	-	1	[6,31,32,34,60]
Gln182His	PM	=	conflicting	yes	normal uptake	2	1	-	[55,56,61]
Gly204Arg~	PM	=	no$	no$	–	1	-	1	[51]
Gly204Ser	PM	=	conflicting	no#	↓ubiquitination	14	4	10	[9,11,15,30]
Ser209Leu	PM	=	no$	no$	–	7	7	-	[62,63]
Asp270Val	PM	=#	yes	↓!	‡ubiquitination	2	1	1	[14,30,64]
Arg296Gln~	PM	=	no$	‡	–	1	1	-	[51]
Ser338Arg	PM	=	yes	↓!	‡ubiquitination	1	-	1	[6,30,65]
Arg371Gln	IC/PM	=	no	yes	–	1	1	-	[11]

Table 2. *Cont.*

Protein	Iron Export		Hepcidin Effect on				TSAT		
Variant	Expression	Capacity	Expression	Export Capacity	Fate of Hepcidin	Patients (n)	Normal	High	Reference[%]
Sum: 13	GOF		Uncertain/Conflicting/Unknown			61	32	27	
Asp84Glu	–	↓	no	–	–	1	-	-	[43]
Val162del	IC/↓PM	↓	no	no	↓↓uptake	50	39	2	[6,8,35,43,51,55,56,66–79]
Asp181Asn	PM	↓	no	no	–	6	6	-	[51]
Asp181Val	↓PM	↓	no	no	–	10	10	-	[8,42,46,80]
Gly490Asp	IC/PM	↓	no	no	no uptake	12	9	3	[8,34,55,81]
Sum: 5	LOF		Hepcidin Resistant			79	64	5	
Arg88Gly	IC/PM	↓	yes	–	–	7	3	3	[8,11,82]
Leu129Pro	PM	↓	yes	ǂyes	–	5	3	2	[83]
Arg178Gln	PM	↓	yes	–	–	26	17	-	[75,82,84,85]
Asn185Asp	PM	↓	yes	–	–	19	4	6	[9,11,86]
Sum: 4	LOF		Hepcidin Sensitive			57	27	11	
Ala77Asp	IC/PM	↓	conflicting	not reliable@	no uptake	26	15	11	[1,2,8,11,34,35,39,41,42,56,57,66, 71,73,87–90]
Gly80Ser	↓PM	↓&	not reliable@	not reliable@	normal uptake&	24	15	3	[8,57,73,87,88,91,92]
Ile152Phe	PM	↓	↓	↓	–	2	-	-	[39,93]
Asp157Gly	IC/PM	↓	conflicting	no&	–	4	3	1	[8,34,55,56,61]
Asp157Tyr	↓PM	↓	–	–	–	2	1	1	[8,94]
Trp158Cys	IC	↓	not reliable@	not reliable@	–	4	4	-	[41,62]
Trp158Leu	IC	↓	not reliable@	not reliable@	–	2	2	-	[11]
Asn174Ile	IC/PM	↓	conflicting	not reliable@	↓uptake	3	1	2	[34,39,46,87,88]
Leu233Pro	IC/↓PM	↓	not reliable@	–	–	3	1	2	[8,55,93]
Gly323Val	IC/PM	↓	conflicting	not reliable@	↓↓uptake	1	-	-	[34,55,56,61]
Arg489Lys	IC	↓	–	–	–	6	4	-	[40]
Gly490Ser	↓PM	↓	–	–	–	3	2	1	[8,35,82]

Table 2. *Cont.*

Protein	Iron Export		Hepcidin Effect on			TSAT			
Variant	Expression	Capacity	Expression	Export Capacity	Fate of Hepcidin	Patients (n)	Normal	High	Reference%
Sum: 12	LOF		Uncertain/Conflicting/Unknown			80	48	21	
Tyr64His						1	-	1	[95]
Gly80Val						2	2	-	[80]
Arg88Thr						7	3	4	[48]
Asp157Ala						5	2	3	[96–98]
Asp157Asn						5	5	-	[45,53]
Ala232Asp						2	2	-	[99]
Lys240Glu						1	-	1	[100]
Gly267Asp						1	1	-	[80]
Cys326Phe						1	-	1	[101]
Gly468Ser						3	3	-	[102]
Arg489Ser						4	2	2	[94,103]
Val511Ile						1	-	1	[45]
Sum: 12	Non-Classified					33	20	13	
Sum: 60						359	200	114	

%reference before the comma refers to reports on functional data; reference after the comma points to reports on clinical data; PM plasma membrane; IC intracellular; = comparable; – no data available; ~ discrepancy in the classification with respect to the original report [51], ! dependent on the dose of hepcidin and time of exposure; # data not fully consistent; $ not strongly established; ^ In one study [104], this variant had diminished iron efflux; ↓↓ severe; ↓moderate/mild, ǂ borderline impaired; @ interpretation is hampered since the variant is mainly localized intracellularly in the experiments; & data of de Domenico et al. [55,87] were disregarded in view of an unexpected discrepancy with other reports.

3.2.1. Clear Distinct Phenotypical Features in Patients with GOF and LOF Variants

Patients with GOF variants had significantly lower ferritin (755 μg/L versus 1595 μg/L) concentration (Table 3) and higher serum iron (36.0 μmol/L versus 17.5 μmol/L) concentration and TSAT (62% versus 32%) than patients with LOF variants. Inter-individual variation in TSAT levels was high in both LOF and GOF patients (Figure 1). In contrast to previous reports [7,105] and the prevailing opinion [10], patients with LOF and GOF variants were found to have a comparable Hb and prevalence of anemia (according to the World Health Organization criteria). While hepatic iron content was similar in patients with LOF and GOF variants, patients with LOF variants display iron deposition predominantly in macrophages (Kupffer cells), while the iron in GOF patients is predominantly present in hepatocytes, and is associated with more hepatic damage as reflected by the significantly higher serum ALT and amount of fibrosis (scored according to the METAVIR scale).

Table 3. Phenotypic features by ferroportin functional gene variant.

Phenotypic Features	Gain-of-Function (n = 110)	Loss-of-Function (n = 216)	p
Age (years) median (range)	n = 93 46 (2–80)	n = 203 36 (6–87)	0.032[&] 0.055[&&]
Gender (n) Female Male	 35 66	 82 126	 ns
Hb (g/dL) median (range)	n = 39 14.4 (9.5–16.5)	n = 104 14.4 (10.1–18.4)	 ns
Anemia Yes No	 4 35	 14 90	 ns
MCV (fl) median (range)	n = 29 93 (70–108)	n = 50 91 (73–98)	 ns
Serum iron (μmol/L) median (range)	n = 45 36.0 (8.0–74.0)	n = 51 15.7 (6.2–94.0)	0.0002[&] 0.00017[&&]
TSAT (%) median (range)	n = 105 62 (2–104)	n = 174 32 (5–99)	< 0.0001[&] < 0.0001[&&]
Ferritin (μg/L) median (range)	n = 100 755 (4–15000)	n = 208 1595 (24–21665)	< 0.0001[&] 0.0013[&&]
Iron Removed (g) median (range)	n = 10 10.2 (2–24.4)	n = 31 8.0 (1.6–80.0)	 ns
Tolerance to Phlebotomy (n) Good Poor	 16 2	 38 13	 ns

Table 3. *Cont.*

Phenotypic Features	Gain-of-Function (n = 110)	Loss-of-Function (n = 216)	p
HIC(µg/g)	n = 19	n = 53	
median (range)	11718 (925–38665)	10052 (307–58590)	ns
Grade of fibrosis			
0–2	14	20	
3–4	10	2	0.012
Hepatic Iron distribution			
Hepatic (predominant)	18	7	< 0.00001[@]
Macrophagic (predominant)	0	28	
Mixed	10	16	< 0.00001[@@]
ALT (IU/L)	n = 31	n = 48	0.0026[&]
median (range)	52.0 (14.0–304.0)	29.5 (6.0–98.0)	0.004[&&]

HIC, hepatic iron content; ALT, alanine aminotransferase. [&]Mann–Whitney U-test, [&&]Student's t-test of independent means, p is significant < 0.0033 when corrected for multiple testing according to Bonferroni. [@]difference between hepatic and macrophagic, [@@]difference between hepatic, macrophagic, and mixed.

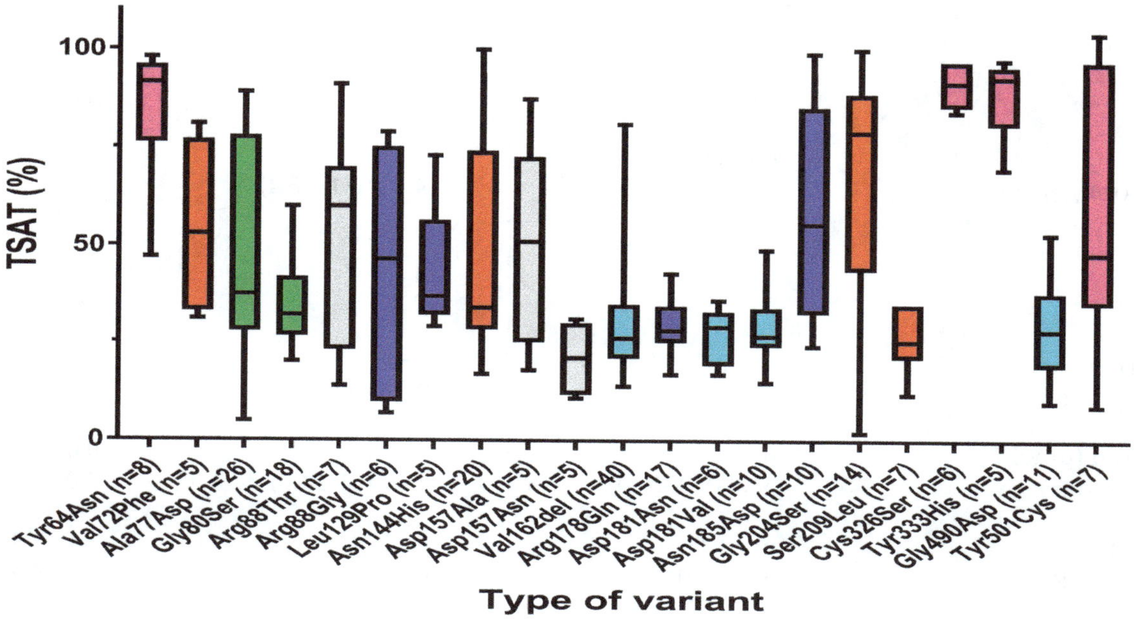

Figure 1. Box plots (Whiskers: min to max) of transferrin saturation (TSAT) in individuals with ferroportin variants. Only the variants with at least five reported TSAT levels in patients are included. Red: GOF without or conflicting data about hepcidin sensitivity; Pink: GOF hepcidin-resistant variants; Green: LOF without or conflicting data about hepcidin sensitivity; Light blue: LOF hepcidin-resistant variants; Blue: LOF hepcidin-sensitive variants; Gray: No data available.

Long-term follow-up information and data to determine a difference in clinical course between GOF and LOF variant patients are limited [12,106]. We found three documented deaths related to ferroportin disease: fatal hepatocellular carcinoma in one GOF and one LOF variant patient [48,82]. One patient with a GOF mutation died of multiorgan failure due to widespread iron deposition [50].

3.2.2. Strong Association of Hepcidin Sensitivity of Ferroportin Functional Gene Variants with Serum Iron Parameters

In vitro hepcidin sensitivity studies were performed in 45 variants. We identified seven hepcidin-resistant and seven hepcidin-sensitive GOF variants, and five hepcidin-resistant and four hepcidin-sensitive LOF variants (Table 2). Twelve LOF and 13 GOF variants were designated as uncertain/conflicting/unknown, including those variants with partial resistance or sensitivity.

Patients with hepcidin-resistant LOF variants had significantly lower TSAT (27% versus 35%) and serum iron (14.1 μmol/L versus 28.7 μmol/L) but higher ferritin (1810 μg/L versus 1066 μg/L) than patients with a hepcidin-sensitive LOF variant (Table S4, Figure 2).

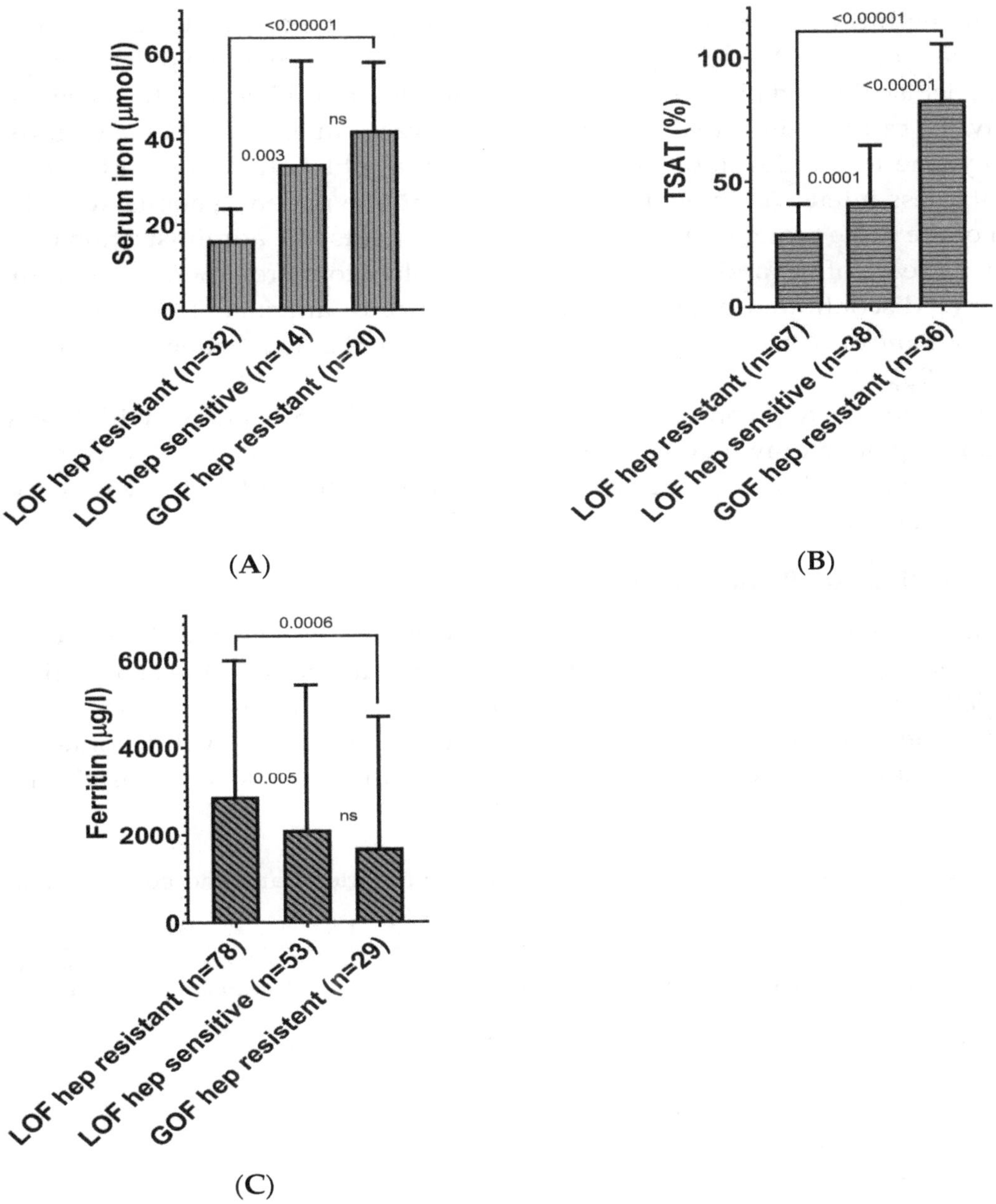

Figure 2. Iron parameters for the different ferroportin variants. Mean (+ SD) of (**A**) serum iron, (**B**) transferrin saturation, and (**C**) ferritin as measured in patient samples for the function of variant (LOF = loss-of-function, GOF = gain-of-function) and the effect of hepcidin (hep resistant = hepcidin-resistant, hep sensitive = hepcidin-sensitive) on the iron transport capacity, as assessed by in vitro functional tests. TSAT = transferrin saturation. The Student's t-test was applied to determine the difference between serum iron and TSAT, while the Mann–Whitney U-test test was applied for ferritin. Displayed p values, serum iron, and TSAT are according to the Student's t-test. Displayed p values ferritin according to the Mann–Whitney U-test.

However, patients with hepcidin-resistant GOF variants had highly significant higher serum iron (44.0 μmol/L versus 14.0 μmol/L) and TSAT (92% versus 28%) and lower ferritin (642 μg/L versus

1810 µg/L) concentration than patients with hepcidin-resistant LOF variants (Table S5, Figure 2). All seven patients with a hepatocyte predominant iron deposition carried a hepcidin-resistant GOF variant, while all nine patients with a macrophage predominant iron deposition had a hepcidin-resistant LOF variant.

3.3. Therapeutic Considerations

In patients with primary iron overload, phlebotomy is the cornerstone of treatment. In 93 of 102 patients who were reported to be phlebotomized, the tolerance of the phlebotomy was reported. A total of 73 patients tolerated phlebotomy without side effects. In 17 of 20 patients with poor tolerance to phlebotomy, the cause of the intolerance could be analyzed. In 12 of the 14 patients with intolerance to phlebotomy due to the development of early anemia, phlebotomy could be continued by the application of a less intensive phlebotomy schedule. In one patient, anemia subsided despite the continuation of the same regimen. In three additional patients, the administration of erythropoietin resulted in an increase of Hb and continuation of the phlebotomy regimen [59,107]. In two patients, phlebotomy was discontinued because of the occurrence of anemia. Treatment with deferasirox resulted in a dramatic decrease in serum ferritin concentration in two patients, but was not successful in another [52,76,96].

In contrast to the current consensus [1,2,4,6,8,40,71,83,92,105], patients with LOF variants were not less tolerant to phlebotomy than patients with GOF variants (Table 3). Nevertheless, in five of 22 (23%) patients with hepcidin-resistant LOF variants the reported phlebotomy was poorly tolerated (Table S5) due to early anemia.

4. Critical Annotations on Pathogenicity of Variants

In Table 4, we depicted the potential pathogenicity of the various variants derived from available clinical, epidemiological, and genetic data from the original reports. We scored the likelihood of the pathogenicity of a variant based on the available data from the genome aggregation data base (gnomAD), data derived from the functional tests, at the molecular level in context of the current knowledge of the function and structure of the ferroportin molecule, and based on three in silico predicting models.

Table 4. Likelihood of pathogenicity derived from the reported data, and current databases and prediction models.

Variant	Pheno-Type	Co-Segregation	VO/Controls	gnomAD	Functional	Molecular	In silico Prediction		
							Poly-phen2	SIFT	Align-GVGD
Tyr64Asn	+++	+++	0/100		++++	++	++	0	0
Tyr64His	+++&					++	++	0	0
Ala69Thr	+++&	0			++	0	++	+	0
Val72Phe	+	+			+++	0	++	0	0
Ala77Asp	+++	++,+++#	0/100		+++	0	++	+	0
Gly80Ser	++		0/734		+++	+	++	+	0
Gly80Val	++		0/100			+	++	+	0
Asp84Glu	+++&				++	+	++	+	0
Arg88Gly	+++		0/734		++	+	++	+	0
Arg88Thr	++	+++	0/60			+	++	+	0
Leu129Pro	Ø	+			++++	0	++	+	+++
Asn144Asp	+++				+++	+	++	0	0
Asn144His	Ø	+++	0/200		+++	+	+	0	0
Asn144Thr	0&		0/100		+++	+	++	0	0
Ile152Phe	+++	+			+++	+	++	0	0
Asp157Ala	++	++				+	++	+	0
Asp157Asn	++	0				+	++	0	0
Asp157Gly	+++		0/80, 0/734		+++	+	+	0	0
Asp157Tyr	+++		0/734		+	+	++	+	+
Trp158Cys	+++	**0,+**	0/50		+++	0	++	+	++
Trp158Leu	+++				+++	0	+	0	0
Val162del	++	+,+++	0/100, 0/103, 0/734		++++	0	@	@	@

Table 4. *Cont.*

Variant	Pheno-Type	Co-Segregation	VO/Controls	gnomAD	Functional	Molecular	In silico Prediction Poly-phen2	SIFT	Align-GVGD
Asn174Ile	+++				**+++**	+	++	+	+++
Arg178Gln	**+++**	**0–+++**$^{\#\#}$			++	+++	++	0	0
Ile180Thr	0	0	0/100	7.076^{-5}	++	0	++	+	+++
Asp181Asn	**++**				**++**	+	++	+	+
Asp181Val	**++**	**+,++**	0/100, 0/734		**++**	+	++	+	+++
Gln182His	+++		0/80		+++	0	++	+	+
Asn185Asp	**+++**	**+,+++**	0/50		+	0	++	+	+
Gly204Arg	+++$^{\&}$				++	0	++	+	+++
Gly204Ser	**+**	+++	2/100	7.955^{-6}	+++	0	++	0	0
Ser209Leu	**0**	++		1.485^{-4}	+++	0	0	0	+
Thr230Asn	0$^{\&}$		0/734	1.096^{-4}	++	0	+	0	0
Ala232Asp	0			4.95^{-5}		0	+	0	+
Leu233Pro	+++	0	0/734		++	0	++	+	+++
Lys240Glu	+++$^{\&}$		0/50			0	0	+	0
Met266Thr	0$^{\&}$		0/734		++	0	0	+	0
Gly267Asp	++$^{\&}$		0/100	4.382^{-5}		0	+	0	0
Asp270Val	+		4/100, 1/516	7.09^{-5}	+++	0	0	0	0
Arg296Gln	0$^{\&}$				++	0	+	0	++
Gly323Val	+++$^{\&}$		0/80		**+++**	0	++	+	+++
Cys326Phe	+++$^{\&}$	0				++	++	0	+
Cys326Ser	**+++**	+++			**++++**	+++	+	0	0
Cys326Tyr	+++		0/800		**++++**	++	+	0	0
Tyr333His	**+++**		0/40		++	+	++	+	+++
Ser338Arg	+++$^{\&}$				**+++**	0	0	0	0
Leu345Phe	0$^{\&}$		0/734		++	0	++	0	0
Ile351Val	0$^{\&}$		0/734	2.125^{-5}	++	0	0	0	0
Arg371Gln	0$^{\&}$			2.388^{-5}	+++	0	0	0	0
Pro443Leu	0$^{\&}$		0/734	5.87^{-4}	++	0	0	0	0
Gly468Ser	++	0		4.005^{-6}		0	++	0	+
Arg489Lys	**+++**	+++	0/50		+	+	++	+	+++
Arg489Ser	+		0/734			+	++	+	+++
Gly490Asp	**+++**	0	0/734		**++++**	0	++	0	0
Gly490Ser	+++		0/734		+	0	++	0	0
Tyr501Cys	**+**		0/200	3.184^{-5}	**++++**	+++	+	0	+
Asp504Asn	+++		0/734		++++	+++	++	0	0
His507Arg	+++	**+**	0/50		++++	++	++	0	0
Val511Ile	+++$^{\&}$					0	++	+	++
Arg561Gly	+		0/734	1.638^{-3}	++	0	0	0	0

Open space: no data available. **Phenotype:** bold: at least five patients; 0 = < 50%, + = 51–80%, ++ = 81–99%, +++ =100% presence of an elevated TSAT in GOF patients and elevated ferritin in LOF patients. Variants in italic are unclassified; + = elevated TSAT and/or ferritin (but not in all patients), ++ = elevated TSAT or ferritin in all patients, +++ = elevated TSAT and ferritin in all patients. & only one reported patient. # enumeration of a limited number of studies; ## range in multiple studies. **Co-segregation** from pedigrees in the original reports using the simplified method of segregation analysis (SISA) according to the following scoring system: single family: 0 = no evidence, + = ≤1/8 (supporting), ++ = ≤ 1/16 (moderate), +++ = ≤ 1/32 (strong); bold: multiple family studies: 0 = no evidence, + = ≤ 1/4 (supporting), ++ = ≤ 1/8 (moderate), +++ = ≤ 1/16 (strong); all according to the recommendations of Jarvik et al. [22] to define co-segregation as criteria to fit the ACMG-AMP guidelines [24]. **VO/Controls:** Variant Occurrence in controls reported in the original reports. **GnomAD:** allele frequency derived from GnomAD data base [25]; the variants for which no allele frequency are given are absent in the database and thus extremely rare. **Functional:** + = effect of hepcidin not performed, ++ = effect of hepcidin established only on membrane expression or iron transport, +++ = conflicting or unreliable results on the effect of hepcidin, with reported fate of hepcidin, ++++ = established effect of hepcidin on membrane expression and iron export with/without reported fate of hepcidin; Bold = ≥ 3 independent studies. **Molecular:** 0 = variant present on a site without established role in ferroportin molecule, + = variant present at a site potentially involved in the formation of the intracellular and extracellular gate, internalization and degradation of the ferroportin molecule or at a site potentially involved in iron binding or egress, ++ = variant present at a site with established function in hepcidin binding, +++ = variant present at a site leading to established conformational changes in the structure of the ferroportin molecule as predicted in the available three-dimensional (3D) models. **In silico prediction:** Polyphen 2: 0 = benign, + = possibly damaging, ++ = probably damaging; "Sorts intolerant from Intolerant" (SIFT): 0 = tolerated, + = deleterious; Align-GVGD: 0 = class 0, + = Class 15, ++ = Class 25 and 35, +++ = Class 55 and 65; @ = It is not possible to test deletions in Polyphen2, SIFT, and Align-GVGD.

4.1. Shortcomings in Description of Clinical Phenotypes

The collected data to describe the clinical phenotype were derived from extensively documented family studies to isolated patients with minimal reported clinical data as part of national surveys of patients with iron overload. So, the available clinical, biochemical, radiological, and histological data were the most heterogenous. In addition, in family studies, relatives were more than 10 years younger with a milder phenotype, including 11% with normal iron parameters. In many patients, a genetic diagnosis was made after referral, and reported iron parameters may potentially have been affected by previous phlebotomies. The demonstrated lack of effect on the presence of additional acquired iron-modulating conditions must be interpreted with caution in view of insufficient reported data. The presence of polymorphisms in ferroportin may affect the degree of iron overload in homozygotic patients for p.Cys282Tyr variants in the HFE molecule [13]. The lack of effect of presence of HFE variants on the iron parameters in our analysis is likely to be explained by the absence of patients with homozygotic p.Cys282Tyr HFE variants.

The phenotype of a number of reported variants raised doubt on the pathogenicity of these variants. An elevated TSAT is considered to be the hallmark of GOF variants. In 41 of 116 GOF patients, TSAT was normal. Since 13 of them also had a ferritin level ≤ 200 μg/L, 11% of GOF patients had normal serum iron parameters, especially patients with Asn144His (8/20 pts) and Val72Phe (2/5 pts) variants. Also, 7/9 reported patients with the seven hepcidin-sensitive GOF variants had a normal TSAT. The Gly204Ser GOF variant displayed evident pathologic iron parameters in a homozygous patient with normal iron parameters in the two heterozygous relatives, and four of 14 additional reported patients had normal TSAT. Six of 197 LOF patients had normal reported ferritin level including 3/5 Leu129Pro variant patients. In a 10-year follow-up study of a proband and his father with a Arg489Ser variant, the serum iron spontaneously decreased with a slight reduction in the MRI estimated HIC [12].

4.2. *Shortcomings in Establishment of Pathogenicity*

4.2.1. Co-Segregation with Disease in the Family

SISA was applicable for 26 variants and hampered by the small pedigrees in most reports. In 13 variants, there was no or only supporting evidence for pathogenicity; in nine variants, evidence was moderate or strong, and for four variants, the score for pathogenicity was inconclusive (Table 4).

4.2.2. Variant Occurrence and Allele Frequency

In the original reports, variant occurrence in healthy controls was determined for 37 variants in relatively small cohorts (range 40 to 734 persons) with an established occurrence of < 1/100 for 26 variants. In the genome aggregation data base (gnomAD, [25]), 213 missense variants were observed with subsequent determination of the allele frequency. Of these, only 13 variants displayed clinical symptoms to be reported and analyzed in the current review. Notably, 47/60 variants in our analysis are so rare that the allele frequency is not depicted in gnomAD.

4.2.3. Limitations of Functional In Vitro Tests

In most of the transfection studies HEK293T, a human embryonic kidney cell line, was used [6,8,11,31–33,35,39–42,46,55–57,83,87,93] and occasionally *Xenophus* oocytes, colon carcinoma CaCo-2, or hepatoma HuH7 cell lines [6,57,66]. Protocols are not standardized. Iron loading was done with 1 to 2 mg/mL of holotransferrin [8,41], 1 to 4 mg/mL of ^{55}Fe [8,33,35,39,46], 20 to 40 μg/mL of ^{59}Fe bound to transferrin [31,40,42], nitrilotriacetate [46] or ascorbate [66], or 10 to 100 μM of ferric ammonium citrate [6,32,55,57,83,93] for 24 h before to 48 h [8,31–33,39,40,42,46,55,66,83,87] after transfection. Cells were lysed 4 to 72 h after iron loading [8,31,33,46,56]. Iron export capacity was determined either by the measurement of radioactive Fe [8,31,33,35,39,40,42,46,56,66] or ferritin concentration [6,8,11,32,33,35,41,42,55,57,83,87,93] in lysed cells [6,32,33,35,40,42,57,93] or in the supernatant [8,11,31,33,35,39,46,56,83]. Results obtained in cells transfected with the variant ferroportin were compared with results in untransfected cells and in cells transfected with wild-type ferroportin. The effect of hepcidin on iron export capacity and the expression of the variant ferroportin protein were analyzed. Experimental conditions are also not standardized; specific differences include: (i) applied hepcidin concentration, which varied between 0.01 and 10 μM, and (ii) incubation times, which varied between 3 and 56 h [11,31–34,39,41,42,55,56,83,87,93]. The membrane expression of variant ferroportin proteins was determined by surface biotinylation and Western blotting [8,39], immunofluorescence [6,31–33,40,42,46,55–57,65,87] and confocal microscopy [11,34,41,83], or flow cytometry [31,35,41,42,56]. These differences may be responsible for the variable results reported on the effect of hepcidin on the membrane expression and iron export capacity of cells transfected with WT ferroportin.

In a significant number of the tested variants, the effect of hepcidin was determined by means of ferroportin expression and not by changes in iron export. Furthermore, in the vast majority of the transfected LOF variants, the membrane expression of the protein was strongly reduced or even absent, and therefore the effect of hepcidin is difficult to determine reliably. In a number of variants, the inhibitory effect of hepcidin was tested at various concentrations of hepcidin and/or exposure times, which resulted in a time and/or concentration dependent effect, ranging from hepcidin resistant to more or less hepcidin sensitive [6,30,42,65]. Therefore it is not unthinkable that the same variant is considered hepcidin resistant by one investigator and hepcidin sensitive by the other, depending on the design of the applied assay.

So, large inter-assay variation may not only lead to conflicting results in ferroportin variants tested in multiple studies, but also to reluctance to draw firm conclusions for data obtained in a single study. In addition, our definition of LOF (i.e. a significant reduced iron transport in functional tests) and hepcidin sensitivity (i.e. a significant reduction in iron transport or ferroportin expression in functional assays upon the addition of hepcidin) may lead to discrepancies in the interpretation of the functional characterization of some individual variants such as Gly204Arg and Arg296Gln, between us and the authors of the original publication [51].

4.2.4. Lack of Concordance between Various In Silico Prediction Models

As illustrated in Table 4, the concordance between the three methods is poor, with a weak albeit significant correlation between SIFT and Align-GVGD ($r = 0.5441$), polyphen2 and SIFT ($r = 0.3832$), and polyphen2 and Align-GVGD ($r = 0.3066$).

4.3. Assessment of Pathogenicity of Ferroportin Variants on Molecular Level in Context of Current Knowledge on the Function and Structure of Ferroportin

4.3.1. Ferroportin, the Protein, Its Variants, and Function: Current Knowledge

Ferroportin is a 571 amino acid cation transporter of the major facilitator superfamily (MFS) encoded by the *SLC40A1* gene [46,108–111]. It is the only known cellular iron exporter, and primarily expressed in the basolateral membrane of duodenal enterocytes, macrophages, and hepatocytes [108,110–112]. In the most widely accepted secondary structure, ferroportin comprises 12 helices located in 12 transmembrane (TM) domains bound via six extracellular (ES) and five intracellular (IS) segments with a large intracellular loop between the sixth and seventh transmembrane helix and intracellularly located N and C terminus [6,8,34,46,56,113]. Although the amount of polymerization is still a matter of debate, most investigators assume that ferroportin is expressed on the membrane as a dimer [6,34,35,55,114]. Available three-dimensional models are based on comparison with ferroportin from other species with only 10-24% sequence homology and 40% similarity [8,39,46,115]. Recent studies reveal an open-inward and an open-outward structure with an intracellular and extracellular gate between the sixth and seventh transmembrane domain. Extrapolating the experimental model to the human protein reveals that residues Asp84, Arg88, Asp157, Asn174, Gln481, Glu486, and Arg489, which are located at IS1, IS2 and IS5, are important in intracellular gate interaction, while the residues Phe44, Val48, Val 51, Leu58, Asp325, Thr329, Leu342, and Phe520, which are located at TM1, TM12, ES1 and ES4, are involved in extracellular gate interaction (Figure 3) [46,115]. It is postulated that intracellular iron is transported outside the cell, and that extracellular hepcidin is transported inside the cell through this gate via a so called "rocker-switch" mechanism [46,115,116].

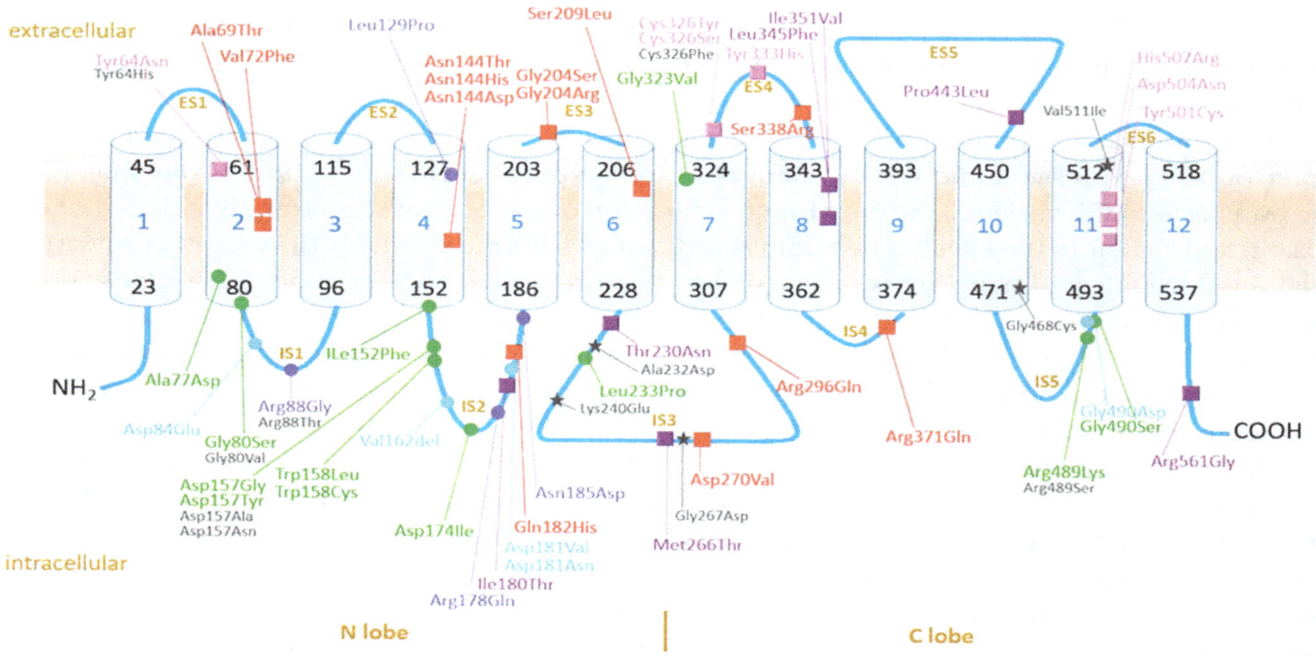

Figure 3. The two-dimensional (2D) structure of ferroportin protein adapted from Liu and Wallace [6,56], revealing 12 transmembrane helices and six extracellular and five intracellular segments. All the variants described in this review are shown as hepcidin-resistant (pink), hepcidin-sensitive or neutral (purple) and hepcidin conflicting/uncertain/unknown (red) GOF variants (squares). and hepcidin resistant (light blue), hepcidin sensitive (dark blue), and hepcidin conflicting-uncertain-unknown (green) LOF variants (dots), or non-classified variants (grey asterix).

Since sites containing an Asp, Glu, His, or Tyr residue are reported be involved in iron binding, Asp39, Glu52, Tyr54, Asp181, Tyr318, Asp325, Tyr331, Tyr501, and Glu518 are potential iron binding sites and Arg88, As157, Asn174, and Arg489 are involved in the intracellular gate interaction [46,115]. Functional studies revealed cation binding at Ser35, Asp39, Asn212, and Ser215 and site mutagenesis studies suggest that Asp39 and Asp181 are essential iron binding sites [46,115]. The residues Arg88, Ile152, and Asn174 are thought to be directly involved in iron egress [39].

Ferroportin-mediated cellular iron export is systemically regulated by the hepatocyte-derived peptide hormone hepcidin. The way hepcidin binding inhibits iron efflux is not fully elucidated [117–119]. Functional studies reveal the internalization of ferroportin upon hepcidin binding with subsequent endosomal and lysosomal degradation resulting in the diminution of cellular iron export, while three-dimensional (3D) structural studies suggest that hepcidin binding disrupts the conformational transition into the intracellular gate with the subsequent inhibition of the access of cytoplasmatic iron to the substrate binding-sites [115,120,121]. Site mutagenesis studies and the exploration of various three dimensional models suggests that the Phe324, Cys326, Tyr333, Asp504, and His507 residues are important binding and docking sites for hepcidin [32,39,46,115]. Recent structural models indicate that these hepcidin binding residues are clustered in the extracellular gate in the open-outward structure. Residues found to be involved in internalization include Tyr64, Gly80, andAsn144, and the residues Lys229, Lys253, and Lys269 are present in the large intracellular loop, and seem to be involved in the degradation of ferroportin [39,114,122].

In an effort to unravel the pathogenicity of ferroportin variants, we depicted the various variants in the structure of ferroportin molecule. For the two-dimensional (2D) model (Figure 3), we adapted the structure constructed by Liu and Wallace [6,56] and for three-dimensional (3D) model (Figure 4), we used the recently developed model (Bacterial ferroportin, PDB file 5AYN) and homology modeling in the Yet Another Scientific Artificial Reality Application (YASARA) [123] and WHAT IF Twinset [124] programs.

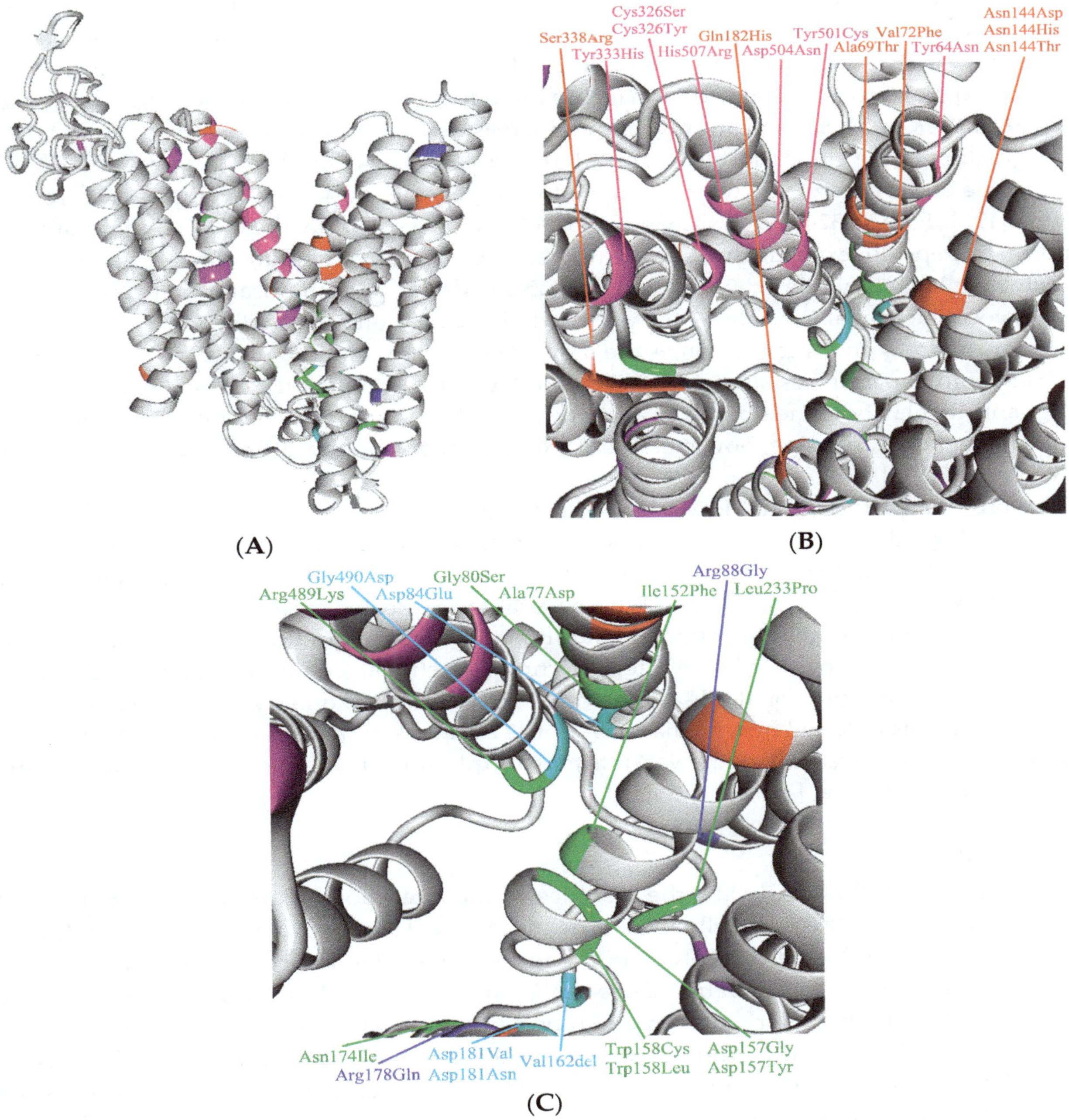

Figure 4. 3D model of ferroportin. **(A)**. Overview. Ferroportin facing outward position. Top: extracellular; Bottom: intracellular. **(B)**. Localization of hepcidin-resistant GOF variants. View inside the "channel" from extracellular to intracellular. Six (Cys326Tyr, Cys326Ser, Tyr333His, Tyr501Cys, Asp504Asn, and His507Arg) of the seven residues of GOF hepcidin-resistant variants are located inside the channel. The Ala69, Val72, Asn144, Gln182, and Ser338 residues are also located inside the channel. However, these variants have conflicting or no data on hepcidin sensitivity. **(C)**. Clustering of LOF variants at the intracellular side of ferroportin. View inside the channel from extracellular to intracellular. Red: GOF without or conflicting data about hepcidin sensitivity; Pink: GOF hepcidin-resistant variants; Purple: GOF hepcidin-sensitive or neutral variants; Green: LOF without or conflicting data about hepcidin sensitivity; Light blue: LOF hepcidin-resistant variants; Blue: LOF hepcidin-sensitive variants. We used bacterial ferroportin for the 3D model (PDB file 5AYN).

4.3.2. GOF Variants

We identified Tyr64Asn, Cys326Tyr, Cys326Ser, Tyr501Cys, Asp504Asn, and His507Arg as definitely hepcidin-resistant GOF variants, and a co-culture of hepcidin with cells transfected with these variants does not lead to the internalization of the ferroportin variant with maintained iron export capacity and variant membrane expression [8,11,31–35,39–42,46]. Consequently, there is increased iron export from enterocytes and macrophages leading to hepatocellular iron overload. Observations in mice with the Cys326Ser variant reveal that increased dietary iron absorption is maintained by the upregulation of the Duodenal cytochrome b (Dcytb) and Divalent Metal Transporter 1 (DMT1) at the apical site of the enterocyte, which is likely to compensate for the pending intraenterocytic iron depletion [125]. For Cys326Tyr, Cys326Ser, Tyr501Cys and Asp504Asn, the blocked internalization of ferroportin on hepcidin exposure has been attributed to the impaired binding of hepcidin to ferroportin in the extracellular gate, while for Tyr64Asn and His507Arg—of which the location in relation to this gate varies between the available models—the impaired ubiquitination of hepcidin, which was most likely due to interference with conformation, is the most likely mechanism (Figure 4B) [30]. The Tyr333Ala, Tyr333His (both hepcidin-resistant variants in a functional test) and Tyr333Phe (hepcidin-sensitive) GOF variants display both membrane localization and intact iron export, but impaired ubiquitination after normal hepcidin binding; however, there are no data on configural changes due to presence of these variants [30,45].

The Ile180Thr, Thr230Asn, Met266Thr, Leu345Phe, Ile351Val, Pro443Leu, and Arg561Gly were designated as hepcidin-sensitive GOF variants. In functional studies, the iron export capacity, hepcidin uptake, and hepcidin-induced reduction of the cell surface expression of these variants were comparable with WT ferroportin [8,11,31,35]. None of these variants are located at residues that are known to be involved in hepcidin binding, ferroportin ubiquitination, or iron binding/egress. Notwithstanding that these seven variants behaved as WT ferroportin in functional studies and are located at residues without an established functional role, the reported 16 patients had otherwise unexplained mild iron overload, which was reflected by a median TSAT of 42.5% and serum ferritin concentration of 980 μg/l. Nevertheless, the pathogenicity of the variants may be questioned, and therefore, the variants may as well be classified as neutral [8].

4.3.3. LOF Variants

Except for Leu129 and Gly323, the residues of the alterations that are associated with LOF variants are located at the intracellular site of the molecule, especially in the IS1, IS2, and IS5 (Figure 3) structures, which are involved in the formation of the intracellular gate responsible for iron transport (Figure 4C) [115]. In transfected cells, the majority of LOF variants are reported to be located intracellularly or have reduced membrane expression, although the data are not consistent for some variants (Table 2). Alteration in these residues may lead to conformational changes due to improper folding with mislocalization and disrupted intracellular gate formation. The substitution of Arg by Gly at residue 88 may lead to direct impaired iron handling with disrupted iron egress. That four hepcidin-sensitive variants display more or less intact membrane expression suggests intact extracellular gate formation enabling hepcidin binding. It was recently demonstrated that the hepcidin-sensitive LOF variant Arg178Gln, which is properly localized on the cellular membrane with disappearance after hepcidin exposure, is likely to form a non-covalent interaction between Arg178 and Asp473, which are located on the N and C lobe, respectively. This interaction may lead to a loss of stabilization of the open-outward conformation that is needed to preserve iron egress [84]. Residues of the four hepcidin-resistant LOF variants are not involved in hepcidin binding, so hepcidin resistance is likely to result from conformational changes in the extracellular gate, even though these variants have demonstrable but reduced membrane expression.

Overall, we conclude from that for most variants, clinical, functional, molecular, and in silico assessments of pathogenicity are not fully concordant, complicating the assessment of their likelihood of being the disease-causing variant (Table 4). For instance, the hepcidin-resistant GOF variants

Tyr64Asn Cys326Ser, Cys326Tyr, Asp504Asn, and His507Arg are benign in two of the predicting in silico models, while clearly damaging variants in the three applied prediction models such as Leu129Pro and Ile180Thr were clinically likely to be benign. On the other hand, six out of the seven hepcidin-sensitive GOF variants had a low likelihood for pathogenicity both on clinical and molecular ground as well as in the predicting models.

4.4. Is the Mode of Iron Overload in LOF Variants Related to a Difference in Ferroportin Expression and Activation between Enterocytes and Macrophages?

Despite clear differences in iron distribution between patients with GOF and LOF variants, hepatic iron content and iron that is needed to be removed by phlebotomy to obtain a normalized iron phenotype are not found to differ, which might suggest that the total amount of absorbed iron in GOF and LOF patients is similar. Therefore, we hypothesize that in enterocytes, all the pathogenic ferroportin variants are associated with increased iron transport, irrespective of the (in vitro) function of the variant, while iron transport in macrophages and thereby the mode of systemic iron distribution is dependent on variant function. For patients with LOF variants, this hypothesis includes iron export being relatively decreased in macrophages, and being increased in enterocytes.

Ferroportin knock-out mice are not viable [110]. Mice with mono-allelic expression of wild-type (WT) ferroportin [111] and *TMPRSS6* knock-out mice with subsequent reduced ferroportin expression on enterocytic membrane, develop iron deficiency anemia with intra-enterocytic iron retention [126] and patients with *TMPRSS6* variants develop Iron Refractory Iron Deficiency Anemia (IRIDA) due to impaired intestinal iron absorption [127–129]. In contrast, patients heterozygous for LOF variants, which fail to export iron in functional tests, do not develop iron deficiency anemia; instead, they develop systemic, predominantly reticuloendothelial iron overload with limited but consistent proof for iron depletion in the enterocytes [79,88].

It has been recently suggested that differences in amount of intracellular iron turnover between enterocytes and macrophages may influence iron export capacity of these cells in patients with ferroportin disease due to LOF variants [130]. The monoallelic-expressed WT ferroportin protein would be sufficient to preserve iron export in cells with low iron turnover, such as enterocytes, but insufficient to maintain iron export capacity in cells with high iron turnover, such as splenic and hepatic macrophages, with subsequent intracellular iron retention in these cells. However, this hypothesis is insufficient to explain the state of iron overload. Functional consequences of a variant leading to the designation LOF is foremost established in HEK293T, which is a human embryonic kidney cell line, and are in accordance with events as observed in macrophages but fail to elucidate events that must be present in the enterocytes. So, HEK293T cells might not be the most appropriate experimental cell line to predict the functional consequences of at least LOF variants.

Experimental data provide evidence for differences in ferroportin expression and the activation between enterocytes and macrophages. Ferroportin is expressed on the enterocytic basolateral membrane and predominantly in intramacrophagic vesicles [108,131], and there are indications that the mode of hepcidin-induced internalization differs in macrophages [120,132].

Intracellular transcription and the translation of *SLC40A1* is primarily regulated by iron and oxygen in enterocytes and heme and iron in macrophages, [113,131,133]; also, the modulatory capacity by the iron-regulatory protein-iron-responsive element (IRP-IRE) system may differ between both cell types [134–138]. After iron egress from enterocytes, ferrous iron is oxidized by membrane-bound hephaestin, co-located with ferroportin, while ferrous iron release from macrophages is oxidized by circulating ceruloplasmin [139,140].

Ferroportin expression differs between enterocytes and macrophages in response to systemic regulatory stimuli such as erythropoietin and hepcidin, changes in iron state, and inflammation (hepcidin independent) in experimental animals, as well as in isolated cell cultures [132,141–152].

Taken together, these experimental data suggest a regulation difference of ferroportin production and activation, between enterocytes and macrophages [153]. However, the extrapolation of results obtained from experimental models to physiology must be done with caution.

5. Conclusions

We analyzed 60 low-frequency missense variants in the coding sequence of the ferroportin gene reported over the past 20 years, which has been assumed to be responsible for iron overload in individual patients reported in the English literature with or without subsequent evaluation of the relatives. The clinical and laboratory features of the patients (phenotype) with these ferroportin variants were correlated with data on variant properties in functional in vitro tests, which were available for 80% of the variants. However, the reported clinical features are often incomplete and functional tests are artificial, not standardized, or unvalidated, which impedes the interpretation of the correlation between the functional properties and phenotype. The establishment of variant pathogenicity is hampered by a lack of sufficiently reported data regarding the presence of iron-modifying confounders and because the outcomes of available in silico prediction models is limited in the absence of a fully elucidated structure and function. Therefore, it is likely that not all reported variants are indeed pathogenic, but from the available data, it is nearly impossible to accurately establish the pathogenicity of individual variants. Notwithstanding these limitations, we can conclude that ferroportin disease is a heterogeneous iron overload disorder. Clinical symptoms are non-specific, and mostly consist of fatigue and arthralgia. At presentation, patients are generally middle aged with strongly elevated ferritin concentrations and mildly elevated TSAT and iron concentrations. Iron parameters and the severity of iron overload show considerable inter-individual variation and are also related to gender, age, and type of variant. The mode of organ iron distribution is primarily determined by the effect of ferroportin variants on macrophage iron export, which is comparable with that observed in functional in vitro studies. LOF variants are associated with macrophage iron retention with a high serum ferritin and low to normal TSAT, in contrast to GOF variants, which are associated with high TSAT and hepatocellular iron deposition. These distinct phenotypes are typically present in patients with hepcidin-resistant variants. Patients with GOF variants had a higher prevalence and higher grade of hepatic fibrosis, indicating that parenchymal iron deposition is more toxic than macrophage iron overload. This corroborates the notion that high TSAT facilitates parenchymal iron deposition, which is considered to be more toxic than macrophage iron overload [154]. On the other hand, with regard to toxicity in macrophages, it has been stated that macrophage iron overload is resistant to iron withdrawal, and that iron-loaded Kupffer cells may contribute to the development of hepatic fibrosis and even carcinogenesis [106].

Since iron distribution patterns and clinical features of patients with hepcidin-resistant GOF variants are indistinguishable from patients with other types of HH, we support the proposition to categorize these variants as ferroportin-associated HH, and to confine the entity ferroportin disease to patients with LOF variants [116]. For both entities, repeated phlebotomies to normalize the iron parameters in order to prevent organ damage remain the mainstay of treatment. Although we found no increased intolerance to phlebotomy in patients with LOF variants, we advocate for the regular determination of Hb levels during the phlebotomy program, especially in patients with hepcidin-resistant LOF variants, to avoid the occurrence of early anemia.

The pathophysiology, especially of the LOF variants, is only partially understood. The iron handling within the various human cell types is not fully clarified, and the mechanisms by which ferroportin transports iron and is degraded are still not fully elucidated. To improve patient management, there is an unmet need for a better understanding of yet unresolved issues on the pathophysiology. A global registry, with a standardized diagnostic work-up and evaluation of the clinical, biochemical, radiological, and histological features of the liver and spleen, is needed, such as the registry sponsored by the European Association for the Study of the Liver (EASL) (http://non-hfe.com/) [155], a collaboration between various European Expert centers, or registries launched by the European Reference Network (ERN) of rare Hematological Disorders

(EUROBLOODNET). Also, the histologic and molecular examination of enterocytes in duodenal biopsies of these patients by assessing iron content, as well as the expression of iron storage and transport proteins, will add to a better understanding of the iron handling. The secondary and tertiary structure of ferroportin as well as the identification of residues that are involved in hepcidin binding, ferroportin ubiquitination, and iron transport need to be further elucidated. Finally, the standardization of validated functional tests, which are preferably performed in human-derived enterocytic and macrophagic cell lines, will enable exploring iron transport and the modulating effect of hepcidin of known and yet unclassified variants, and will improve our insights of the pathophysiology of ferroportin disease.

Figure 1S: Relation between age and serum iron/TSAT/ferritin, Table 1S: Characteristics and iron parameters of probands versus probands' relatives, Table 2S: Phenotypical features by the reported presence of hereditary HFE and non-HFE iron overload conditions, Table 3S: Phenotypical features by the reported current use of alcohol, Table 4S: Phenotypical features of patients with functional LOF ferroportin variant by hepcidin sensitivity, Table 5S: Phenotypical features by hepcidin resistant GOF and LOF ferroportin variants.

Author Contributions: L.T.V. and D.W.S. designed the study, L.T.V. and R.J. wrote the manuscript, prepared the tables and figures, and performed and interpreted the statistical analysis, H.V. constructed the 3D model, all the authors contributed to the interpretation of tables and figures, D.W.S., H.D., H.V., E.B.-J., and H.H.-R. critically read and revised the manuscript. All the authors approved the final version of the manuscript.

Acknowledgments: We thank Heinz Zoller for his critical revision on earlier versions of this work.

References

1. Pietrangelo, A.; Montosi, G.; Totaro, A.; Garuti, C.; Fraquelli, M.; Sardini, C.; Vasta, F.; Pietrangelo, A.; Conte, D.; Cassanelli, S.; et al. Hereditary hemochromatosis in adults without pathogenic mutations in the hemochromatosis gene. *N. Engl. J. Med.* **1999**, *341*, 725–732. [CrossRef] [PubMed]
2. Montosi, G.; Donovan, A.; Totaro, A.; Garuti, C.; Pignatti, E.; Cassanelli, S.; Trenor, C.C.; Gasparini, P.; Andrews, N.C.; Pietrangelo, A. Autosomal-dominant hemochromatosis is associated with a mutation in the ferroportin (SLC11A3) gene. *J. Clin. Investig.* **2001**, *108*, 619–623. [CrossRef] [PubMed]
3. Njajou, O.T.; Vaessen, N.; Joosse, M.; Berghuis, B.; Van Dongen, J.W.; Breuning, M.H.; Snijders, P.J.; Rutten, W.P.; Sandkuijl, L.A.; Oostra, B.A.; et al. A mutation in SLC11A3 is associated with autosomal dominant hemochromatosis. *Nat. Genet.* **2001**, *28*, 213–214. [CrossRef] [PubMed]
4. Nemeth, E. Ferroportin mutations: A tale of two phenotypes. *Blood* **2005**, *105*, 3763–3764. [CrossRef]
5. Fleming, R.E.; Sly, W.S. Ferroportin mutation in autosomal dominant hemochromatosis: Loss of function, gain in understanding. *J. Clin. Investig.* **2001**, *108*, 521–522. [CrossRef]
6. Wallace, D.F.; Harris, J.M.; Subramaniam, V.N. Functional analysis and theoretical modeling of ferroportin reveals clustering of mutations according to phenotype. *Am. J. Physiol. Cell Physiol.* **2010**, *298*, C75–C84. [CrossRef]
7. Mayr, R.; Janecke, A.R.; Schranz, M.; Griffiths, W.J.; Vogel, W.; Pietrangelo, A.; Zoller, H. Ferroportin disease: A systematic meta-analysis of clinical and molecular findings. *J. Hepatol.* **2010**, *53*, 941–949. [CrossRef]
8. Callebaut, I.; Joubrel, R.; Pissard, S.; Kannengiesser, C.; Gérolami, V.; Ged, C.; Cadet, E.; Cartault, F.; Ka, C.; Gourlaouen, I.; et al. Comprehensive functional annotation of 18 missense mutations found in suspected hemochromatosis type 4 patients. *Hum. Mol. Genet.* **2014**, *23*, 4479–4490. [CrossRef]
9. Le Lan, C.; Mosser, A.; Ropert, M.; Détivaud, L.; Loustaud–Ratti, V.; Vital–Durand, D.; Roget, L.; Bardou–Jacquet, E.; Turlin, B.; David, V.; et al. Sex and acquired cofactors determine phenotypes of ferroportin disease. *Gastroenterology* **2011**, *140*, 1199–1207. [CrossRef]
10. Pietrangelo, A.; Caleffi, A.; Corradini, E. Non-HFE hepatic iron overload. *Semin. Liver Dis.* **2011**, *31*, 302–318. [CrossRef]
11. Detivaud, L.; Island, M.L.; Jouanolle, A.M.; Ropert, M.; Bardou-Jacquet, E.; Le Lan, C.; Mosser, A.; Leroyer, P.; Deugnier, Y.; David, V. Ferroportin diseases: Functional studies, a link between genetic and clinical phenotype. *Hum. Mutat.* **2013**, *34*, 1529–1536. [CrossRef] [PubMed]

12. Hayashi, H.; Yano, M.; Urawa, N.; Mizutani, A.; Hamaoka, S.; Araki, J.; Kojima, Y.; Naito, Y.; Kato, A.; Tatsumi, Y.; et al. A 10-year follow-up study of a Japanese family with ferroportin disease A: Mild iron overload with mild hyperferritinemia co-occurring with hyperhepcidinemia may be benign. *Intern. Med.* **2018**, *57*, 2865–2871. [CrossRef] [PubMed]
13. Altes, A.; Bach, V.; Ruiz, A.; Esteve, A.; Remacha, A.F.; Sarda, M.P.; Felez, J.; Baiget, M. Does the SLC40A1 gene modify HFE-related haemochromatosis phenotypes? *Annu. Hematol.* **2009**, *88*, 341–345. [CrossRef] [PubMed]
14. Zaahl, M.G.; Merryweather-Clarke, A.T.; Kotze, M.J.; van der Merwe, S.; Warnich, L.; Robson, K.J. Analysis of genes implicated in iron regulation in individuals presenting with primary iron overload. *Hum. Genet.* **2004**, *115*, 409–417. [CrossRef] [PubMed]
15. Santos, P.C.; Cancado, R.D.; Pereira, A.C.; Schettert, I.T.; Soares, R.A.; Pagliusi, R.A.; Hirata, R.D.; Hirata, M.H.; Teixeira, A.C.; Figueiredo, M.S.; et al. Hereditary hemochromatosis: Mutations in genes involved in iron homeostasis in Brazilian patients. *Blood Cells Mol. Dis.* **2011**, *46*, 302–307. [CrossRef]
16. Barton, J.C.; LaFreniere, S.A.; Li, H.; Acton, R.T.; Press, R.D.; Eckfeldt, J.H.; Leiendecker-Foster, C.; Leiendecker-Foster, C. HFE, SLC40A1, HAMP, HJV, TFR2, and FTL mutations detected by denaturing high-performance liquid chromatography after iron phenotyping and HFE C282Y and H63D genotyping in 785 HEIRS study participants. *Am. J. Hematol.* **2009**, *84*, 710–714. [CrossRef] [PubMed]
17. Lee, P.L.; Gelbart, T.; West, C.; Halloran, C.; Felitti, V.; Beutler, E. A study of genes that may modulate the expression of hereditary hemochromatosis: Transferrin receptor-1, ferroportin, ceruloplasmin, ferritin light and heavy chains, iron regulatory proteins (IRP)-1 and -2, and hepcidin. *Blood Cells Mol. Dis.* **2001**, *27*, 783–802. [CrossRef]
18. McNamara, L.; Gordeuk, V.R.; MacPhail, A.P. Ferroportin (Q248H) mutations in African families with dietary iron overload. *J. Gastroenterol. Hepatol.* **2005**, *20*, 1855–1858. [CrossRef]
19. Rivers, C.A.; Barton, J.C.; Gordeuk, V.R.; Acton, R.T.; Speechley, M.R.; Snively, B.M.; Leiendecker-Foster, C.; Press, R.D.; Adams, P.C.; McLaren, G.D.; et al. Association of ferroportin Q248H polymorphism with elevated levels of serum ferritin in African Americans in the hemochromatosis and iron overload screening (HEIRS) study. *Blood Cells Mol. Dis.* **2007**, *38*, 247–252. [CrossRef]
20. Albuquerque, D.; Manco, L.; Loua, K.M.; Arez, A.P.; Trovoada, M.D.J.; Relvas, L.; Milimono, T.S.; Rath, S.L.; Lopes, D.; Nogueira, F.; et al. SLC40A1 Q248H allele frequencies and associated SLC40A1 haplotypes in three West African population samples. *Ann. Hum. Biol.* **2011**, *38*, 378–381. [CrossRef]
21. Beutler, E.; Barton, J.C.; Felitti, V.J.; Gelbart, T.; West, C.; Lee, P.L.; Waalen, J.; Vulpe, C. Ferroportin 1 (SCL40A1) variant associated with iron overload in African-Americans. *Blood Cells Mol. Dis.* **2003**, *31*, 305–309. [CrossRef]
22. Jarvik, G.P.; Browning, B.L. Consideration of cosegregation in the pathogenicity classification of Genomic variants. *Am. J. Hum. Gen.* **2016**, *98*, 1077–1781. [CrossRef] [PubMed]
23. Moller, P.; Clark, N.; Maehle, L. A simplified method for segregation analysis (SISA) to determine penetrance and expression of a genetic variant in a family. *Hum. Mutat.* **2011**, *32*, 568–571. [CrossRef] [PubMed]
24. Richards, S.; Aziz, N.; Bale, S.; Bick, D.; Das, S.; Gastier-Foster, J.; Grody, W.W.; Hegde, M.; Lyon, E.; Spector, E.; et al. Standards and guidelines for the interpretation of sequence variants: A joint consensus recommendation of the American college of medical genetics and genomics and the Association for molecular pathology. *Off. J. Am. Coll. Med. Gen.* **2015**, *17*, 405–424. [CrossRef] [PubMed]
25. Broad Institute. Available online: http://gnomad.broadinstitute.org (accessed on 12 July 2019).
26. PolyPhen-2 Prediction of Functional Effects of Human nsSNPs. Available online: http://genetics.bwh.harvard.edu/pph2 (accessed on 12 July 2019).
27. Sorting Intolerant from Tolerant. Available online: http://www.blocks.fhcrc.org/sift/SIFT.html (accessed on 12 July 2019).
28. Align-GVGD. Available online: http://agvgd.hci.utah.edu (accessed on 12 July 2019).
29. Duca, L.; Delbini, P.; Nava, I.; Vaja, V.; Fiorelli, G.; Cappellini, M.D. Mutation analysis of hepcidin and ferroportin genes in Italian prospective blood donors with iron overload. *Am. J. Hematol.* **2009**, *84*, 592–593. [CrossRef] [PubMed]
30. Aschemeyer, S.; Qiao, B.; Stefanova, D.; Valore, E.V.; Sek, A.C.; Ruwe, T.A.; Vieth, K.R.; Jung, G.; Casu, C.; Rivella, S.; et al. Structure-function analysis of ferroportin defines the binding site and an alternative mechanism of action of hepcidin. *Blood* **2018**, *131*, 899–910. [CrossRef] [PubMed]

31. Drakesmith, H.; Schimanski, L.M.; Ormerod, E.; Merryweather-Clarke, A.T.; Viprakasit, V.; Edwards, J.P.; Sweetland, E.; Bastin, J.M.; Cowley, D.; Chinthammitr, Y.; et al. Resistance to hepcidin is conferred by hemochromatosis-associated mutations of ferroportin. *Blood* **2005**, *106*, 1092–1097. [CrossRef] [PubMed]
32. Fernandes, A.; Preza, G.C.; Phung, Y.; De Domenico, I.; Kaplan, J.; Ganz, T.; Nemeth, E. The molecular basis of hepcidin-resistant hereditary hemochromatosis. *Blood* **2009**, *114*, 437–443. [CrossRef]
33. Letocart, E.; Le Gac, G.; Majore, S.; Ka, C.; Radio, F.C.; Gourlaouen, I.; De Bernardo, C.; Ferec, C.; Grammatico, P. A novel missense mutation in SLC40A1 results in resistance to hepcidin and confirms the existence of two ferroportin-associated iron overload diseases. *Br. J. Haematol.* **2009**, *147*, 379–385. [CrossRef]
34. Rice, A.E.; Mendez, M.J.; Hokanson, C.A.; Rees, D.C.; Bjorkman, P.J. Investigation of the biophysical and cell biological properties of ferroportin, a multipass integral membrane protein iron exporter. *J. Mol. Biol.* **2009**, *386*, 717–732. [CrossRef]
35. Schimanski, L.M.; Drakesmith, H.; Merryweather-Clarke, A.T.; Viprakasit, V.; Edwards, J.P.; Sweetland, E.; Bastin, J.M.; Cowley, D.; Chinthammitr, Y.; Robson, K.J.; et al. In vitro functional analysis of human ferroportin (FPN) and hemochromatosis-associated FPN mutations. *Blood* **2005**, *105*, 4096–4102. [CrossRef] [PubMed]
36. Rivard, S.R.; Lanzara, C.; Grimard, D.; Carella, M.; Simard, H.; Ficarella, R.; Simard, R.; D'Adamo, A.P.; De Braekeleer, M.; Gasparini, P. Autosomal dominant reticuloendothelial iron overload (HFE type 4) due to a new missense mutation in the FERROPORTIN 1 gene (SLC11A3) in a large French-Canadian family. *Haematologica* **2003**, *88*, 824–826. [PubMed]
37. Sham, R.L.; Phatak, P.D.; Nemeth, E.; Ganz, T. Hereditary hemochromatosis due to resistance to hepcidin: high hepcidin concentrations in a family with C326S ferroportin mutation. *Blood* **2009**, *114*, 493–494. [CrossRef] [PubMed]
38. Sham, R.L.; Phatak, P.D.; West, C.; Lee, P.; Andrews, C.; Beutler, E. Autosomal dominant hereditary hemochromatosis associated with a novel ferroportin mutation and unique clinical features. *Blood Cells Mol. Dis.* **2005**, *34*, 157–161. [CrossRef] [PubMed]
39. Le Gac, G.; Ka, C.; Joubrel, R.; Gourlaouen, I.; Lehn, P.; Mornon, J.P.; Ferec, C.; Callebaut, I. Structure-function analysis of the human ferroportin iron exporter (SLC40A1): Effect of hemochromatosis type 4 disease mutations and identification of critical residues. *Hum. Mutat.* **2013**, *34*, 1371–1380. [CrossRef] [PubMed]
40. Griffiths, W.J.; Mayr, R.; McFarlane, I.; Hermann, M.; Halsall, D.J.; Zoller, H.; Cox, T.M. Clinical presentation and molecular pathophysiology of autosomal dominant hemochromatosis caused by a novel ferroportin mutation. *Hepatology* **2010**, *51*, 788–795. [CrossRef] [PubMed]
41. Mayr, R.; Griffiths, W.J.; Hermann, M.; McFarlane, I.; Halsall, D.J.; Finkenstedt, A.; Douds, A.; Davies, S.E.; Janecke, A.R.; Vogel, W.; et al. Identification of mutations in SLC40A1 that affect ferroportin function and phenotype of human ferroportin iron overload. *Gastroenterology* **2011**, *140*, 2056–2063.e1. [CrossRef]
42. Praschberger, R.; Schranz, M.; Griffiths, W.J.; Baumgartner, N.; Hermann, M.; Lomas, D.J.; Pietrangelo, A.; Cox, T.M.; Vogel, W.; Zoller, H. Impact of D181V and A69T on the function of ferroportin as an iron export pump and hepcidin receptor. *Biochimica et Biophysica Acta* **2014**, *1842*, 1406–1412. [CrossRef]
43. Wallace, D.F.; McDonald, C.J.; Ostini, L.; Iser, D.; Tuckfield, A.; Subramaniam, V.N. The dynamics of hepcidin-ferroportin internalization and consequences of a novel ferroportin disease mutation. *Am. J. Hematol.* **2017**, *92*, 1052–1061. [CrossRef]
44. Lok, C.Y.; Merryweather-Clarke, A.T.; Viprakasit, V.; Chinthammitr, Y.; Srichairatanakool, S.; Limwongse, C.; Oleesky, D.; Robins, A.J.; Hudson, J.; Wai, P.; et al. Iron overload in the Asian community. *Blood* **2009**, *114*, 20–25. [CrossRef]
45. Zhang, W.; Xu, A.; Li, Y.; Zhao, S.; Zhou, D.; Wu, L.; Zhang, B.; Zhao, X.; Wang, Y.; Wang, X.; et al. A novel SLC40A1 p.Y333H mutation with gain of function of ferroportin: A recurrent cause of haemochromatosis in China. *Liver Int. Off. J. Int. Assoc. Study Liver* **2019**, *39*, 1120–1127. [CrossRef] [PubMed]
46. Bonaccorsi di Patti, M.C.; Polticelli, F.; Cece, G.; Cutone, A.; Felici, F.; Persichini, T.; Musci, G. A structural model of human ferroportin and of its iron binding site. *FEBS J.* **2014**, *281*, 2851–2860. [CrossRef]
47. Yamakawa, N.; Oe, K.; Yukawa, N.; Murakami, K.; Nakashima, R.; Imura, Y.; Yoshifuji, H.; Ohmura, K.; Miura, Y.; Tomosugi, N.; et al. A Novel Phenotype of a Hereditary Hemochromatosis Type 4 with Ferroportin-1 Mutation, Presenting with Juvenile Cataracts. *Intern. Med.* **2016**, *55*, 2697–2701. [CrossRef] [PubMed]

48. Bach, V.; Remacha, A.; Altes, A.; Barcelo, M.J.; Molina, M.A.; Baiget, M. Autosomal dominant hereditary hemochromatosis associated with two novel Ferroportin 1 mutations in Spain. *Blood Cells Mol. Dis.* **2006**, *36*, 41–45. [CrossRef] [PubMed]
49. Del-Castillo-Rueda, A.; Moreno-Carralero, M.I.; Cuadrado-Grande, N.; Alvarez-Sala-Walther, L.A.; Enriquez-de-Salamanca, R.; Mendez, M.; Moran-Jimenez, M.J. Mutations in the HFE, TFR2, and SLC40A1 genes in patients with hemochromatosis. *Gene* **2012**, *508*, 15–20. [CrossRef] [PubMed]
50. Sussman, N.L.; Lee, P.L.; Dries, A.M.; Schwartz, M.R.; Barton, J.C. Multi-organ iron overload in an African-American man with ALAS2 R452S and SLC40A1 R561G. *Acta Haematol.* **2008**, *120*, 168–173. [CrossRef] [PubMed]
51. Majore, S.; Bonaccorsi di Patti, M.C.; Valiante, M.; Polticelli, F.; Cortese, A.; Di Bartolomeo, S.; De Bernardo, C.; De Muro, M.; Faienza, F.; Radio, F.C.; et al. Characterization of three novel pathogenic SLC40A1 mutations and genotype/phenotype correlations in 7 Italian families with type 4 hereditary hemochromatosis. *Biochim. Biophys. Acta. Mol. Basis Dis.* **2018**, *1864*, 464–470. [CrossRef]
52. Ferbo, L.; Manzini, P.M.; Badar, S.; Campostrini, N.; Ferrarini, A.; Delledonne, M.; Francisci, T.; Tassi, V.; Valfre, A.; Dall'omo, A.M.; et al. Detection of a rare mutation in the ferroportin gene through targeted next generation sequencing. *Blood Transfus.* **2016**, 1–4.
53. Pelucchi, S.; Mariani, R.; Salvioni, A.; Bonfadini, S.; Riva, A.; Bertola, F.; Trombini, P.; Piperno, A. Novel mutations of the ferroportin gene (SLC40A1): analysis of 56 consecutive patients with unexplained iron overload. *Clin Genet* **2008**, *73*, 171–178. [CrossRef]
54. Wallace, D.F.; Clark, R.M.; Harley, H.A.; Subramaniam, V.N. Autosomal dominant iron overload due to a novel mutation of ferroportin1 associated with parenchymal iron loading and cirrhosis. *J. Hepatol.* **2004**, *40*, 710–713. [CrossRef]
55. De Domenico, I.; Ward, D.M.; Nemeth, E.; Vaughn, M.B.; Musci, G.; Ganz, T.; Kaplan, J. The molecular basis of ferroportin-linked hemochromatosis. *Proc. Natl. Acad. Sci. USA* **2005**, *102*, 8955–8960. [CrossRef] [PubMed]
56. Liu, X.B.; Yang, F.; Haile, D.J. Functional consequences of ferroportin 1 mutations. *Blood Cells Mol. Dis.* **2005**, *35*, 33–46. [CrossRef] [PubMed]
57. McDonald, C.J.; Wallace, D.F.; Ostini, L.; Bell, S.J.; Demediuk, B.; Subramaniam, V.N. G80S-linked ferroportin disease: classical ferroportin disease in an Asian family and reclassification of the mutant as iron transport defective. *J. Hepatol.* **2011**, *54*, 538–544. [CrossRef] [PubMed]
58. Njajou, O.T.; de Jong, G.; Berghuis, B.; Vaessen, N.; Snijders, P.J.; Goossens, J.P.; Wilson, J.H.; Breuning, M.H.; Oostra, B.A.; Heutink, P.; et al. Dominant hemochromatosis due to N144H mutation of SLC11A3: Clinical and biological characteristics. *Blood Cells Mol. Dis.* **2002**, *29*, 439–443. [CrossRef] [PubMed]
59. Rosmorduc, O.; Wendum, D.; Arrive, L.; Elnaggar, A.; Ennibi, K.; Hannoun, L.; Charlotte, F.; Grange, J.D.; Poupon, R. Phenotypic expression of ferroportin disease in a family with the N144H mutation. *Gastroenterol. Clin. Biol.* **2008**, *32*, 321–327. [CrossRef] [PubMed]
60. Arden, K.E.; Wallace, D.F.; Dixon, J.L.; Summerville, L.; Searle, J.W.; Anderson, G.J.; Ramm, G.A.; Powell, L.W.; Subramaniam, V.N. A novel mutation in ferroportin1 is associated with haemochromatosis in a Solomon Islands patient. *Gut* **2003**, *52*, 1215–1217. [CrossRef] [PubMed]
61. Hetet, G.; Devaux, I.; Soufir, N.; Grandchamp, B.; Beaumont, C. Molecular analyses of patients with hyperferritinemia and normal serum iron values reveal both L ferritin IRE and 3 new ferroportin (slc11A3) mutations. *Blood* **2003**, *102*, 1904–1910. [CrossRef]
62. An, P.; Jiang, L.; Guan, Y.; Wang, H.; Wang, J.; Tian, Y.; Yang, W.; Shi, Y.; Xue, J.; Min, J.; et al. Identification of hereditary hemochromatosis pedigrees and a novel SLC40A1 mutation in Chinese population. *Blood Cells Mol. Dis.* **2017**, *63*, 34–36. [CrossRef]
63. Wang, Y.; Du, Y.; Liu, G.; Guo, S.; Hou, B.; Jiang, X.; Han, B.; Chang, Y.; Nie, G. Identification of novel mutations in HFE, HFE2, TfR2, and SLC40A1 genes in Chinese patients affected by hereditary hemochromatosis. *Int. J. Hematol.* **2016**, *105*, 521–525. [CrossRef]
64. Lee, P.L.; Gaasterland, T.; Barton, J.C. Mild iron overload in an African American man with SLC40A1 D270V. *Acta Haematol.* **2012**, *128*, 28–32. [CrossRef]
65. Wallace, D.F.; Dixon, J.L.; Ramm, G.A.; Anderson, G.J.; Powell, L.W.; Subramaniam, V.N. A novel mutation in ferroportin implicated in iron overload. *J. Hepatol.* **2007**, *46*, 921–926. [CrossRef] [PubMed]

66. McGregor, J.A.; Shayeghi, M.; Vulpe, C.D.; Anderson, G.J.; Pietrangelo, A.; Simpson, R.J.; McKie, A.T. Impaired iron transport activity of ferroportin 1 in hereditary iron overload. *J. Membr. Biol.* **2005**, *206*, 3–7. [CrossRef] [PubMed]
67. Akoum, R. Point mutations in ferroportin disease: genotype/phenotype correlation. In *Point Mutation*; Logie, C., Ed.; InTech: London, UK, 2012; pp. 285–300.
68. Cazzola, M.; Cremonesi, L.; Papaioannou, M.; Soriani, N.; Kioumi, A.; Charalambidou, A.; Paroni, R.; Romtsou, K.; Levi, S.; Ferrari, M.; et al. Genetic hyperferritinaemia and reticuloendothelial iron overload associated with a three base pair deletion in the coding region of the ferroportin gene (SLC11A3). *Br. J. Haematol.* **2002**, *119*, 539–546. [CrossRef] [PubMed]
69. Galicia-Poblet, G.; Cid-Paris, E.; Lopez-Andres, N.; Losada-Pajares, A.; Jurado-Lopez, J.C.; Moreno-Carralero, M.I.; Moran-Jimenez, M.J. A Pediatric Case Report of Ferroportin Disease. *J. Pediatr. Gastroenterol. Nutr.* **2015**, *63*, e205–e207. [CrossRef]
70. Ikuta, K.; Hatayama, M.; Addo, L.; Toki, Y.; Sasaki, K.; Tatsumi, Y.; Hattori, A.; Kato, A.; Kato, K.; Hayashi, H.; et al. Iron overload patients with unknown etiology from national survey in Japan. *Int. J. Hematol.* **2017**, *105*, 353–360. [CrossRef] [PubMed]
71. Lim, F.L.; Dooley, J.S.; Roques, A.W.; Grellier, L.; Dhillon, A.P.; Walker, A.P. Hepatic iron concentration, fibrosis and response to venesection associated with the A77D and V162del "loss of function" mutations in ferroportin disease. *Blood Cells Mol. Dis.* **2008**, *40*, 328–333. [CrossRef] [PubMed]
72. Papanikolaou, G.; Tzilianos, M.; Christakis, J.I.; Bogdanos, D.; Tsimirika, K.; MacFarlane, J.; Goldberg, Y.P.; Sakellaropoulos, N.; Ganz, T.; Nemeth, E. Hepcidin in iron overload disorders. *Blood* **2005**, *105*, 4103–4105. [CrossRef] [PubMed]
73. Pietrangelo, A.; Corradini, E.; Ferrara, F.; Vegetti, A.; De Jong, G.; Luca Abbati, G.; Paolo Arcuri, P.; Martinelli, S.; Cerofolini, E. Magnetic resonance imaging to identify classic and nonclassic forms of ferroportin disease. *Blood Cells Mol. Dis.* **2006**, *37*, 192–196. [CrossRef]
74. Roetto, A.; Merryweather-Clarke, A.T.; Daraio, F.; Livesey, K.; Pointon, J.J.; Barbabietola, G.; Piga, A.; Mackie, P.H.; Robson, K.J.; Camaschella, C. A valine deletion of ferroportin 1: A common mutation in hemochromastosis type 4. *Blood* **2002**, *100*, 733–734. [CrossRef]
75. Speletas, M.; Kioumi, A.; Loules, G.; Hytiroglou, P.; Tsitouridis, J.; Christakis, J.; Germenis, A.E. Analysis of SLC40A1 gene at the mRNA level reveals rapidly the causative mutations in patients with hereditary hemochromatosis type IV. *Blood Cells Mol. Dis.* **2008**, *40*, 353–359. [CrossRef]
76. Unal, S.; Piperno, A.; Gumruk, F. Iron chelation with deferasirox in a patient with de-novo ferroportin mutation. *J. Trace Elem. Med. Biol.* **2015**, *30*, 1–3. [CrossRef] [PubMed]
77. Wallace, D.F.; Browett, P.; Wong, P.; Kua, H.; Ameratunga, R.; Subramaniam, V.N. Identification of ferroportin disease in the Indian subcontinent. *Gut* **2005**, *54*, 567–568. [CrossRef] [PubMed]
78. Wallace, D.F.; Pedersen, P.; Dixon, J.L.; Stephenson, P.; Searle, J.W.; Powell, L.W.; Subramaniam, V.N. Novel mutation in ferroportin1 is associated with autosomal dominant hemochromatosis. *Blood* **2002**, *100*, 692–694. [CrossRef] [PubMed]
79. Zoller, H.; McFarlane, I.; Theurl, I.; Stadlmann, S.; Nemeth, E.; Oxley, D.; Ganz, T.; Halsall, D.J.; Cox, T.M.; Vogel, W. Primary iron overload with inappropriate hepcidin expression in V162del ferroportin disease. *Hepatology* **2005**, *42*, 466–472. [CrossRef] [PubMed]
80. Cremonesi, L.; Forni, G.L.; Soriani, N.; Lamagna, M.; Fermo, I.; Daraio, F.; Galli, A.; Pietra, D.; Malcovati, L.; Ferrari, M.; et al. Genetic and clinical heterogeneity of ferroportin disease. *Br. J. Haematol.* **2005**, *131*, 663–670. [CrossRef] [PubMed]
81. Jouanolle, A.M.; Douabin-Gicquel, V.; Halimi, C.; Loreal, O.; Fergelot, P.; Delacour, T.; de Lajarte-Thirouard, A.S.; Turlin, B.; Le Gall, J.Y.; Cadet, E.; et al. Novel mutation in ferroportin 1 gene is associated with autosomal dominant iron overload. *J. Hepatol.* **2003**, *39*, 286–289. [CrossRef]
82. Cunat, S.; Giansily-Blaizot, M.; Bismuth, M.; Blanc, F.; Dereure, O.; Larrey, D.; Quellec, A.L.; Pouderoux, P.; Rose, C.; Raingeard, I.; et al. Global sequencing approach for characterizing the molecular background of hereditary iron disorders. *Clin. Chem.* **2007**, *53*, 2060–2069. [CrossRef]
83. Moreno-Carralero, M.I.; Munoz-Munoz, J.A.; Cuadrado-Grande, N.; Lopez-Rodriguez, R.; Jose Hernandez-Alfaro, M.; del-Castillo-Rueda, A.; Enriquez-de-Salamanca, R.; Mendez, M.; Moran-Jimenez, M.J. A novel mutation in the SLC40A1 gene associated with reduced iron export in vitro. *Am. J. Hematol.* **2014**, *89*, 689–694. [CrossRef]

84. Ka, C.; Guellec, J.; Perpermans, X.; Kannengiesser, C.; Ged, C.; Wuyts, W.; Cassiman, D.; de Ledinghen, V.; Varet, B.; de Kerguenec, C.; et al. The SLC40A1 R178Q mutation is a recurrent cause of hemochromatosis and is associated with a novel pathogenic mechanism. *Haematologica* **2018**, *103*, 1796–1805. [CrossRef]
85. Speletas, M.; Kioumi, A.; Germenis, A.E. Reply to: "SLC40A1-R178G or R178Q and ferroportin disease? A call for vigilance in mutation reporting". *J. Hepatol.* **2013**, *59*, 397. [CrossRef]
86. Morris, T.J.; Litvinova, M.M.; Ralston, D.; Mattman, A.; Holmes, D.; Lockitch, G. A novel ferroportin mutation in a Canadian family with autosomal dominant hemochromatosis. *Blood Cells Mol. Dis.* **2005**, *35*, 309–314. [CrossRef] [PubMed]
87. De Domenico, I.; McVey Ward, D.; Nemeth, E.; Ganz, T.; Corradini, E.; Ferrara, F.; Musci, G.; Pietrangelo, A.; Kaplan, J. Molecular and clinical correlates in iron overload associated with mutations in ferroportin. *Haematologica* **2006**, *91*, 1092–1095. [PubMed]
88. Corradini, E.; Montosi, G.; Ferrara, F.; Caleffi, A.; Pignatti, E.; Barelli, S.; Garuti, C.; Pietrangelo, A. Lack of enterocyte iron accumulation in the ferroportin disease. *Blood Cells Mol. Dis.* **2005**, *35*, 315–318. [CrossRef] [PubMed]
89. Relvas, L.C.M.; Bento, M.C.; Ribeiro, L. Novel human pathological mutation: Gene Symbol: SLC40A1. Disease: Haemochromatosis, type IV. *Hum. Genet.* **2009**, *125*, 338. [PubMed]
90. Subramaniam, V.N.; Wallace, D.F.; Dixon, J.L.; Fletcher, L.M.; Crawford, D.H. Ferroportin disease due to the A77D mutation in Australia. *Gut* **2005**, *54*, 1048–1049. [CrossRef] [PubMed]
91. Mougiou, A.; Pietrangelo, A.; Caleffi, A.; Kourakli, A.; Karakantza, M.; Zoumbos, N. G80S-linked ferroportin disease: the first clinical description in a Greek family. *Blood Cells Mol. Dis.* **2008**, *41*, 138–139. [CrossRef] [PubMed]
92. Wolff, F.; Bailly, B.; Gulbis, B.; Cotton, F. Monitoring of hepcidin levels in a patient with G80S-linked ferroportin disease undergoing iron depletion by phlebotomy. *Clin. Chim. Acta* **2014**, *430*, 20–21. [CrossRef]
93. Girelli, D.; De Domenico, I.; Bozzini, C.; Campostrini, N.; Busti, F.; Castagna, A.; Soriani, N.; Cremonesi, L.; Ferrari, M.; Colombari, R.; et al. Clinical, pathological, and molecular correlates in ferroportin disease: A study of two novel mutations. *J. Hepatol.* **2008**, *49*, 664–671. [CrossRef]
94. Hattori, A.; Miyajima, H.; Tomosugi, N.; Tatsumi, Y.; Hayashi, H.; Wakusawa, S. Clinicopathological study of Japanese patients with genetic iron overload syndromes. *Pathol. Int.* **2012**, *62*, 612–618. [CrossRef]
95. Raszeja-Wyszomirska, J.; Caleffi, A.; Milkiewicz, P.; Pietrangelo, A. Ferroportin-related haemochromatosis associated with novel Y64H mutation of the SCL40A1 gene. *Prz. Gastroenterol.* **2014**, *9*, 307–309. [CrossRef]
96. Muehlenberg, K.; Faltermeier, N.; Lohse, P.; Tannapfel, A.; Pech, O. [Family with marked hyperferritinemia as a result of hemochromatosis type 4 (ferroportin disease)]. *Z. Gastroenterol.* **2014**, *52*, 1075–1080. [PubMed]
97. Saja, K.; Bignell, P.; Robson, K.; Provan, D. A novel missense mutation c.470 A>C (p.D157A) in the SLC40A1 gene as a cause of ferroportin disease in a family with hyperferritinaemia. *Br. J. Haematol.* **2010**, *149*, 914–916. [CrossRef] [PubMed]
98. Yamashita, T.; Morotomi, N.; Sohda, T.; Hayashi, H.; Yoshida, N.; Ochi, K.; Ohkura, I.; Karita, M.; Fujiwara, H.; Yamashita, H.; et al. A male patient with ferroportin disease B and a female patient with iron overload similar to ferroportin disease B. *Clin. J. Gastroenterol.* **2014**, *7*, 260–264. [CrossRef] [PubMed]
99. Caetano, G.; Relvas, L.; Bento, C.; Silveira, M.P.; Ribeiro, L. Atypical iron deficiency anemia—Association of two new mutations in ferroportin and TMPRSS6 genes. In Proceedings of the International BioIron Society Annual Meeting, Porto, Portugal, 7–11 June 2009.
100. Del-Castillo-Rueda, A.; Moreno-Carralero, M.I.; Alvarez-Sala-Walther, L.A.; Cuadrado-Grande, N.; Enriquez-de-Salamanca, R.; Mendez, M.; Moran-Jimenez, M.J. Two novel mutations in the SLC40A1 and HFE genes implicated in iron overload in a Spanish man. *Eur. J. Haematol.* **2011**, *86*, 260–264. [CrossRef] [PubMed]
101. Chen, S.R.; Yang, L.Q.; Chong, Y.T.; Jie, Y.S.; Wu, Y.K.; Yang, J.; Lin, G.L.; Li, X.H. Novel gain of function mutation in the SLC40A1 gene associated with hereditary haemochromatosis type 4. *Intern. Med. J.* **2015**, *45*, 672–676. [CrossRef] [PubMed]
102. Lee, P.L.; Gelbart, T.; West, C.; Barton, J.C. SLC40A1 c.1402G–>a results in aberrant splicing, ferroportin truncation after glycine 330, and an autosomal dominant hemochromatosis phenotype. *Acta Haematol.* **2007**, *118*, 237–241. [CrossRef] [PubMed]

103. Koyama, C.; Wakusawa, S.; Hayashi, H.; Ueno, T.; Suzuki, R.; Yano, M.; Saito, H.; Okazaki, T. A Japanese family with ferroportin disease caused by a novel mutation of SLC40A1 gene: hyperferritinemia associated with a relatively low transferrin saturation of iron. *Intern. Med.* **2005**, *44*, 990–993. [CrossRef]
104. Nekhai, S.; Xu, M.; Foster, A.; Kasvosve, I.; Diaz, S.; Machado, R.F.; Castro, O.L.; Kato, G.J.; Taylor, J.G.; Gordeuk, V.R. Reduced sensitivity of the ferroportin Q248H mutant to physiological concentrations of hepcidin. *Haematologica* **2013**, *98*, 455–463. [CrossRef] [PubMed]
105. Pietrangelo, A. The ferroportin disease. *Blood Cells Mol. Dis.* **2004**, *32*, 131–138. [CrossRef] [PubMed]
106. Corradini, E.; Ferrara, F.; Pollicino, T.; Vegetti, A.; Abbati, G.L.; Losi, L.; Raimondo, G.; Pietrangelo, A. Disease progression and liver cancer in the ferroportin disease. *Gut* **2007**, *56*, 1030–1032. [CrossRef]
107. Devalia, V.; Carter, K.; Walker, A.P.; Perkins, S.J.; Worwood, M.; May, A.; Dooley, J.S. Autosomal dominant reticuloendothelial iron overload associated with a 3-base pair deletion in the ferroportin 1 gene (SLC11A3). *Blood* **2002**, *100*, 695–697. [CrossRef] [PubMed]
108. Abboud, S.; Haile, D.J. A novel mammalian iron-regulated protein involved in intracellular iron metabolism. *J. Biol. Chem.* **2000**, *275*, 19906–19912. [CrossRef] [PubMed]
109. McKie, A.T.; Marciani, P.; Rolfs, A.; Brennan, K.; Wehr, K.; Barrow, D.; Miret, S.; Bomford, A.; Peters, T.J.; Farzaneh, F.; et al. A novel duodenal iron-regulated transporter, IREG1, implicated in the basolateral transfer of iron to the circulation. *Mol. Cell* **2000**, *5*, 299–309. [CrossRef]
110. Donovan, A.; Brownlie, A.; Zhou, Y.; Shepard, J.; Pratt, S.J.; Moynihan, J.; Paw, B.H.; Drejer, A.; Barut, B.; Zapata, A.; et al. Positional cloning of zebrafish ferroportin1 identifies a conserved vertebrate iron exporter. *Nature* **2000**, *403*, 776–781. [CrossRef] [PubMed]
111. Donovan, A.; Lima, C.A.; Pinkus, J.L.; Pinkus, G.S.; Zon, L.I.; Robine, S.; Andrews, N.C. The iron exporter ferroportin/Slc40a1 is essential for iron homeostasis. *Cell Metab.* **2005**, *1*, 191–200. [CrossRef] [PubMed]
112. Thomas, C.; Oates, P.S. Ferroportin/IREG-1/MTP-1/SLC40A1 modulates the uptake of iron at the apical membrane of enterocytes. *Gut* **2004**, *53*, 44–49. [CrossRef] [PubMed]
113. Drakesmith, H.; Nemeth, E.; Ganz, T. Ironing out Ferroportin. *Cell Metab.* **2015**, *22*, 777–787. [CrossRef] [PubMed]
114. Ward, D.M.; Kaplan, J. Ferroportin-mediated iron transport: expression and regulation. *Biochimica Biophysica Acta* **2012**, *1823*, 1426–1433. [CrossRef] [PubMed]
115. Taniguchi, R.; Kato, H.E.; Font, J.; Deshpande, C.N.; Wada, M.; Ito, K.; Ishitani, R.; Jormakka, M.; Nureki, O. Outward- and inward-facing structures of a putative bacterial transition-metal transporter with homology to ferroportin. *Nat. Commun.* **2015**, *6*, 8545. [CrossRef] [PubMed]
116. Pietrangelo, A. The ferroportin disease: pathogenesis, diagnosis and treatment. *Haematologica* **2017**. [CrossRef] [PubMed]
117. Ross, S.L.; Tran, L.; Winters, A.; Lee, K.J.; Plewa, C.; Foltz, I.; King, C.; Miranda, L.P.; Allen, J.; Beckman, H.; et al. Molecular mechanism of hepcidin-mediated ferroportin internalization requires ferroportin lysines, not tyrosines or JAK-STAT. *Cell Metab.* **2012**, *15*, 905–917. [CrossRef] [PubMed]
118. De Domenico, I.; Lo, E.; Ward, D.M.; Kaplan, J. Hepcidin-induced internalization of ferroportin requires binding and cooperative interaction with Jak2. *Proc. Natl. Acad. Sci. USA* **2009**, *106*, 3800–3805. [CrossRef] [PubMed]
119. Le Tertre, M.; Ka, C.; Guellec, J.; Gourlaouen, I.; Ferec, C.; Callebaut, I.; Le Gac, G. Deciphering the molecular basis of ferroportin resistance to hepcidin: Structure/function analysis of rare SLC40A1 missense mutations found in suspected hemochromatosis type 4 patients. *Transfusion Clinique et Biologique: Journal de la Societe Francaise de Transfusion Sanguine* **2017**, *24*, 462–467. [CrossRef] [PubMed]
120. Nemeth, E.; Tuttle, M.S.; Powelson, J.; Vaughn, M.B.; Donovan, A.; Ward, D.M.; Ganz, T.; Kaplan, J. Hepcidin regulates cellular iron efflux by binding to ferroportin and inducing its internalization. *Science* **2004**, *306*, 2090–2093. [CrossRef] [PubMed]
121. Clark, R.J.; Tan, C.C.; Preza, G.C.; Nemeth, E.; Ganz, T.; Craik, D.J. Understanding the structure/activity relationships of the iron regulatory peptide hepcidin. *Chem. Biol.* **2011**, *18*, 336–343. [CrossRef] [PubMed]
122. Qiao, B.; Sugianto, P.; Fung, E.; Del-Castillo-Rueda, A.; Moran-Jimenez, M.J.; Ganz, T.; Nemeth, E. Hepcidin-induced endocytosis of ferroportin is dependent on ferroportin ubiquitination. *Cell Metab.* **2012**, *15*, 918–924. [CrossRef] [PubMed]
123. Krieger, E.; Koraimann, G.; Vriend, G. Increasing the precision of comparative models with YASARA NOVA–a self-parameterizing force field. *Proteins* **2002**, *47*, 393–402. [CrossRef] [PubMed]

124. Vriend, G. WHAT IF: a molecular modeling and drug design program. *J. Mol. Graph.* **1990**, *8*, 52–56. [CrossRef]
125. Altamura, S.; Kessler, R.; Grone, H.J.; Gretz, N.; Hentze, M.W.; Galy, B.; Muckenthaler, M.U. Resistance of ferroportin to hepcidin binding causes exocrine pancreatic failure and fatal iron overload. *Cell Metab.* **2014**, *20*, 359–367. [CrossRef]
126. Folgueras, A.R.; de Lara, F.M.; Pendas, A.M.; Garabaya, C.; Rodriguez, F.; Astudillo, A.; Bernal, T.; Cabanillas, R.; Lopez-Otin, C.; Velasco, G. Membrane-bound serine protease matriptase-2 (Tmprss6) is an essential regulator of iron homeostasis. *Blood* **2008**, *112*, 2539–2545. [CrossRef]
127. De Falco, L.; Sanchez, M.; Silvestri, L.; Kannengiesser, C.; Muckenthaler, M.U.; Iolascon, A.; Gouya, L.; Camaschella, C.; Beaumont, C. Iron refractory iron deficiency anemia. *Haematologica* **2013**, *98*, 845–853. [CrossRef] [PubMed]
128. McDonald, C.J.; Ostini, L.; Bennett, N.; Subramaniam, N.; Hooper, J.; Velasco, G.; Wallace, D.F.; Subramaniam, V.N. Functional analysis of matriptase-2 mutations and domains: insights into the molecular basis of iron-refractory iron deficiency anemia. *Am. J. Physiol. Cell Physiol.* **2015**, *308*, C539–C547. [CrossRef] [PubMed]
129. Donker, A.E.; Raymakers, R.A.; Vlasveld, L.T.; van Barneveld, T.; Terink, R.; Dors, N.; Brons, P.P.; Knoers, N.V.; Swinkels, D.W. Practice guidelines for the diagnosis and management of microcytic anemias due to genetic disorders of iron metabolism or heme synthesis. *Blood* **2014**, *123*, 3873–3886, quiz 4005. [CrossRef] [PubMed]
130. Sabelli, M.; Montosi, G.; Garuti, C.; Caleffi, A.; Oliveto, S.; Biffo, S.; Pietrangelo, A. Human macrophage ferroportin biology and the basis for the ferroportin disease. *Hepatology* **2017**, *65*, 1512–1525. [CrossRef] [PubMed]
131. Delaby, C.; Pilard, N.; Goncalves, A.S.; Beaumont, C.; Canonne-Hergaux, F. Presence of the iron exporter ferroportin at the plasma membrane of macrophages is enhanced by iron loading and down-regulated by hepcidin. *Blood* **2005**, *106*, 3979–3984. [CrossRef] [PubMed]
132. Nairz, M.; Schroll, A.; Demetz, E.; Tancevski, I.; Theurl, I.; Weiss, G. 'Ride on the ferrous wheel'–the cycle of iron in macrophages in health and disease. *Immunobiology* **2015**, *220*, 280–294. [CrossRef] [PubMed]
133. Taylor, M.; Qu, A.; Anderson, E.R.; Matsubara, T.; Martin, A.; Gonzalez, F.J.; Shah, Y.M. Hypoxia-inducible factor-2alpha mediates the adaptive increase of intestinal ferroportin during iron deficiency in mice. *Gastroenterology* **2011**, *140*, 2044–2055. [CrossRef]
134. Muckenthaler, M.U.; Galy, B.; Hentze, M.W. Systemic iron homeostasis and the iron-responsive element/iron-regulatory protein (IRE/IRP) regulatory network. *Annu. Rev. Nutr.* **2008**, *28*, 197–213. [CrossRef]
135. Wilkinson, N.; Pantopoulos, K. The IRP/IRE system in vivo: insights from mouse models. *Front. Pharmacol.* **2014**, *5*, 176. [CrossRef]
136. Zhang, D.L.; Ghosh, M.C.; Rouault, T.A. The physiological functions of iron regulatory proteins in iron homeostasis—An update. *Front. Pharmacol.* **2014**, *5*, 124. [CrossRef]
137. Lymboussaki, A.; Pignatti, E.; Montosi, G.; Garuti, C.; Haile, D.J.; Pietrangelo, A. The role of the iron responsive element in the control of ferroportin1/IREG1/MTP1 gene expression. *J. Hepatol.* **2003**, *39*, 710–715. [CrossRef]
138. Zhang, D.L.; Hughes, R.M.; Ollivierre-Wilson, H.; Ghosh, M.C.; Rouault, T.A. A ferroportin transcript that lacks an iron-responsive element enables duodenal and erythroid precursor cells to evade translational repression. *Cell Metab.* **2009**, *9*, 461–473. [CrossRef] [PubMed]
139. Han, O.; Kim, E.Y. Colocalization of ferroportin-1 with hephaestin on the basolateral membrane of human intestinal absorptive cells. *J. Cell. Biochem.* **2007**, *101*, 1000–1010. [CrossRef] [PubMed]
140. Musci, G.; Polticelli, F.; Bonaccorsi di Patti, M.C. Ceruloplasmin-ferroportin system of iron traffic in vertebrates. *World J. Biol. Chem.* **2014**, *5*, 204–215. [PubMed]
141. Canonne-Hergaux, F.; Donovan, A.; Delaby, C.; Wang, H.J.; Gros, P. Comparative studies of duodenal and macrophage ferroportin proteins. *Am. J. Physiol. Gastrointest. Liver Physiol.* **2006**, *290*, G156–G163. [CrossRef] [PubMed]
142. Theurl, I.; Aigner, E.; Theurl, M.; Nairz, M.; Seifert, M.; Schroll, A.; Sonnweber, T.; Eberwein, L.; Witcher, D.R.; Murphy, A.T.; et al. Regulation of iron homeostasis in anemia of chronic disease and iron deficiency anemia: Diagnostic and therapeutic implications. *Blood* **2009**, *113*, 5277–5286. [CrossRef]

143. Jacolot, S.; Ferec, C.; Mura, C. Iron responses in hepatic, intestinal and macrophage/monocyte cell lines under different culture conditions. *Blood Cells Mol. Dis.* **2008**, *41*, 100–108. [CrossRef]
144. Mena, N.P.; Esparza, A.; Tapia, V.; Valdes, P.; Nunez, M.T. Hepcidin inhibits apical iron uptake in intestinal cells. *Am. J. Physiol. Gastrointest. Liver Physiol.* **2008**, *294*, G192–G198. [CrossRef]
145. Yamaji, S.; Sharp, P.; Ramesh, B.; Srai, S.K. Inhibition of iron transport across human intestinal epithelial cells by hepcidin. *Blood* **2004**, *104*, 2178–2180. [CrossRef]
146. Chaston, T.; Chung, B.; Mascarenhas, M.; Marks, J.; Patel, B.; Srai, S.K.; Sharp, P. Evidence for differential effects of hepcidin in macrophages and intestinal epithelial cells. *Gut* **2008**, *57*, 374–382. [CrossRef]
147. Bergamaschi, G.; Di Sabatino, A.; Pasini, A.; Ubezio, C.; Costanzo, F.; Grataroli, D.; Masotti, M.; Alvisi, C.; Corazza, G.R. Intestinal expression of genes implicated in iron absorption and their regulation by hepcidin. *Clin. Nutr.* **2016**. [CrossRef] [PubMed]
148. Guida, C.; Altamura, S.; Klein, F.A.; Galy, B.; Boutros, M.; Ulmer, A.J.; Hentze, M.W.; Muckenthaler, M.U. A novel inflammatory pathway mediating rapid hepcidin-independent hypoferremia. *Blood* **2015**, *125*, 2265–2275. [CrossRef] [PubMed]
149. Enculescu, M.; Metzendorf, C.; Sparla, R.; Hahnel, M.; Bode, J.; Muckenthaler, M.U.; Legewie, S. Modelling Systemic Iron Regulation during Dietary Iron Overload and Acute Inflammation: Role of Hepcidin-Independent Mechanisms. *PLoS Comput. Biol.* **2017**, *13*, e1005322. [CrossRef] [PubMed]
150. Deschemin, J.C.; Vaulont, S. Role of hepcidin in the setting of hypoferremia during acute inflammation. *PLoS ONE* **2013**, *8*, e61050. [CrossRef] [PubMed]
151. Agoro, R.; Mura, C. Inflammation-induced up-regulation of hepcidin and down-regulation of ferroportin transcription are dependent on macrophage polarization. *Blood Cells Mol. Dis.* **2016**, *61*, 16–25. [CrossRef] [PubMed]
152. Biswas, S.K.; Mantovani, A. Orchestration of metabolism by macrophages. *Cell Metab.* **2012**, *15*, 432–437. [CrossRef] [PubMed]
153. Vlasveld, L.T.; Swinkels, D.W. Loss-of-function ferroportin disease: novel mechanistic insights and unanswered questions. *Haematologica* **2018**, *103*, 1753–1755. [CrossRef] [PubMed]
154. Wang, W.; Knovich, M.A.; Coffman, L.G.; Torti, F.M.; Torti, S.V. Serum ferritin: Past, present and future. *Biochimica et Biophysica Acta* **2010**, *1800*, 760–769. [CrossRef] [PubMed]
155. NON-HFE Registry. Available online: http://non-hfe.com/ (accessed on 12 July 2019).

11

Mitochondrial Targeting in Neurodegeneration: A Heme Perspective

Veronica Fiorito *,†, Deborah Chiabrando † and Emanuela Tolosano

Department of Molecular Biotechnology and Health Sciences, Molecular Biotechnology Center, University of Torino, 10126 Torino, Italy; deborah.chiabrando@unito.it (D.C.); emanuela.tolosano@unito.it (E.T.)
* Correspondence: veronica.fiorito@unito.it
† These authors equally contributed.

Abstract: Mitochondrial dysfunction has achieved an increasing interest in the field of neurodegeneration as a pathological hallmark for different disorders. The impact of mitochondria is related to a variety of mechanisms and several of them can co-exist in the same disease. The central role of mitochondria in neurodegenerative disorders has stimulated studies intended to implement therapeutic protocols based on the targeting of the distinct mitochondrial processes. The review summarizes the most relevant mechanisms by which mitochondria contribute to neurodegeneration, encompassing therapeutic approaches. Moreover, a new perspective is proposed based on the heme impact on neurodegeneration. The heme metabolism plays a central role in mitochondrial functions, and several evidences indicate that alterations of the heme metabolism are associated with neurodegenerative disorders. By reporting the body of knowledge on this topic, the review intends to stimulate future studies on the role of heme metabolism in neurodegeneration, envisioning innovative strategies in the struggle against neurodegenerative diseases.

Keywords: neurodegeneration; mitochondria; therapy; heme; haem

---

1. Implication of Heme in Neurodegeneration

Heme is a molecule composed by protoporphyrin IX and iron produced by all the cells in the organism, including neurons. Heme mediates a series of functions that encompass oxygen transport, the regulation of gene expression and the modulation of enzyme activity, just to cite the most relevant ones. Moreover, heme can also promote oxidative stress, thus performing as a double-face molecule with both positive and negative properties [1]. This concept is also true for neuronal cells. Indeed, on one hand heme is required for the survival and differentiation of neuronal cells, as demonstrated by the observation that heme deficiency interferes with neurite outgrowth in nerve growth factor (NGF)-induced PC12 cells [2,3] and results in apoptosis in PC12 pheochromocytoma cells, SHSY5Y neuroblastoma cells and U373 astrocytoma cells, as well as in rat primary hippocampal neurons [2–4]. However, on the other hand, an excess of free-heme is associated with neurodegeneration. The large amount of hemoglobin and heme released in the brain during intracerebral or subarachnoid hemorrhages promotes oxidative stress, lipid peroxidation, inflammatory response and finally, neuronal cell death [5–7]. Moreover, loss of the heme scavenger hemopexin (Hx) causes defective myelination in mice [8–10]. Furthermore, impairment of cellular heme export reduces SHSY5Y cells survival [11]. Together, these data indicate that both heme deficiency and excess are deleterious for the survival of neuronal cells (Figure 1), thus suggesting that heme levels must be finely controlled both at the systemic and cellular level. At the systemic level, circulating free-heme is scavenged by the plasma proteins haptoglobin and hemopexin [6–8,10,12–14]. However, at cellular level, the amount of intracellular free-heme (*labile heme* or *heme regulatory pool*) is regulated at multiple steps: heme synthesis, incorporation into hemoproteins, catabolism, import and export [1,15].

Although this tight regulation has been extensively studied in non-neuronal cells, similar mechanisms likely occur in the nervous system. Indeed, the main proteins involved in the control of labile heme are also expressed in the nervous system [16].

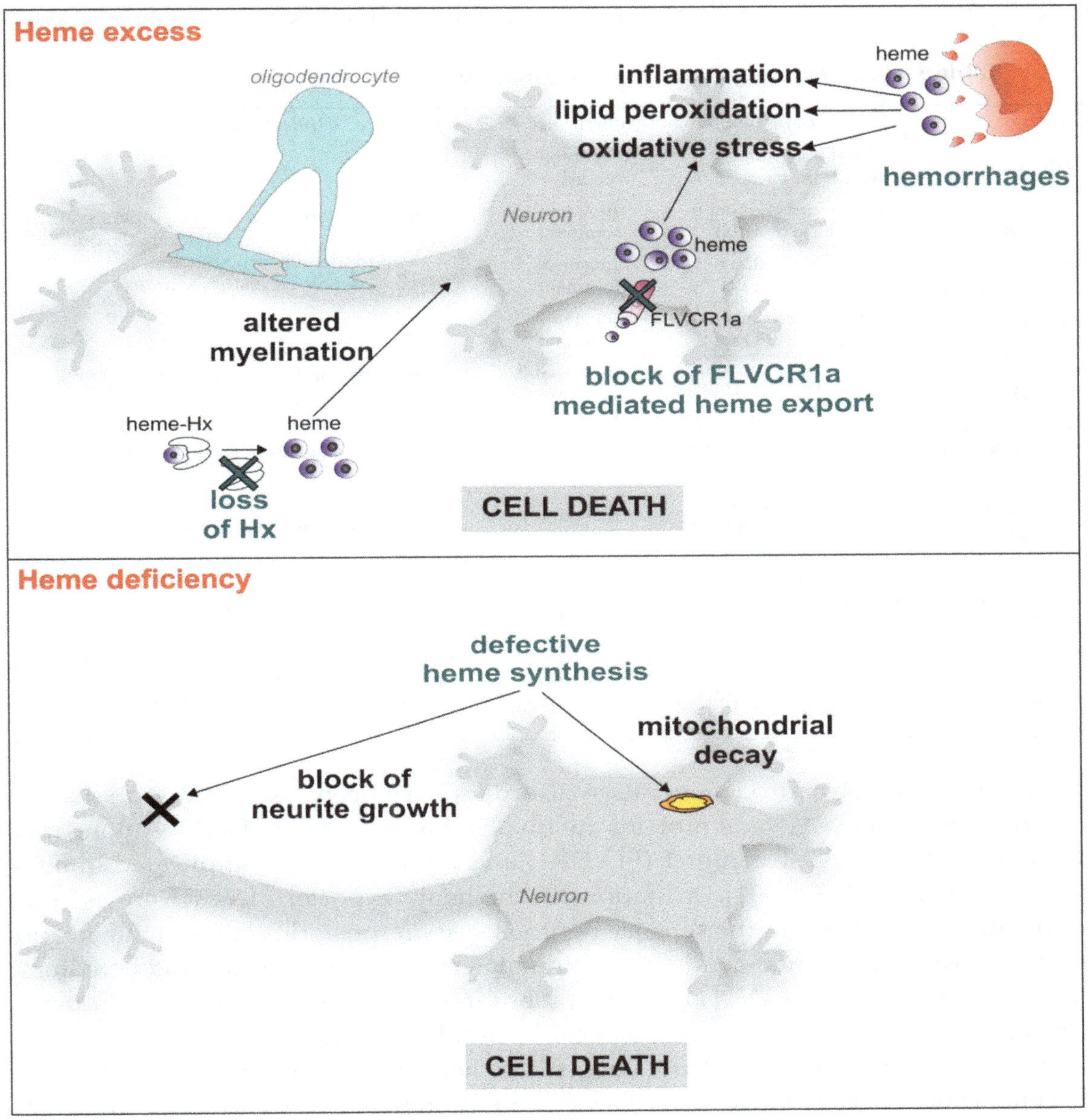

Figure 1. Implication of heme in neurodegeneration. Both heme excess and heme deficiency contribute to neurodegeneration. Heme released during hemorrhages leads to inflammation, lipid peroxidation and oxidative stress; the loss of the heme scavenger Hx causes defective myelination of axons; the impairment of intracellular heme export by FLVCR1a is associated with increased oxidative stress. On the other hand, heme deficiency, due to defective synthesis, leads to mitochondrial decay and the blocking of neurite growth. These events all result in neuronal cell death. In the figure, neurons are represented as the main target for heme-mediated effects; however, other cell types of the nervous system could be affected by the same phenomena.

Neurodegenerative disorders are a common and growing cause of mortality and morbidity worldwide [17]. Recently, a series of rare neurodegenerative disorders have been directly linked to alterations of heme metabolism (see Table 1). Defective heme synthesis causes porphyrias, some of which are associated with a wide array of neurological disturbances involving both the central and peripheral nervous systems (neuropathic porphyria). Neuropathic porphyria includes acute intermittent porphyria (AIP), hereditary coproporphyria (HCP), variegate porphyria (VP) and 5-aminolevulinate dehydratase deficiency (ALAD deficiency) [18–20]. Furthermore, reduced heme synthesis has been observed in Friederich Ataxia (FRDA), an autosomal recessive disorder caused by mutations in Frataxin (FXN), a mitochondrial iron chaperone involved in iron-sulfur (Fe-S) clusters and heme biosynthesis [21–24]. Finally, reduced heme synthesis has been observed during aging [4,25].

Table 1. Rare neurodegenerative disorders linked to defective heme metabolism.

Disease	*Gene*	*Inheritance*	*Clinical Features*	OMIM
ALAD deficiency	5-aminolevulinate dehydratase (ALAD)	autosomal recessive	Neuropathic Porphyria: acute neurovisceral attacks involving severe abdominal pain, peripheral neuropathies and psychiatric disturbances	612740
Acute intermittent porphyria (AIP)	Hydroxymethylbilane synthase (*HMBS*)	autosomal dominant		176000
Hereditary coproporphyria (HCP)	Coproporphyrinogen oxidase (*CPOX*)	autosomal dominant		121300
Variegate porphyria (VP)	Protoporphyrinogen oxidase (PPOX)	autosomal dominant		176200
Friederich Ataxia (FRDA)	Frataxin (FXN)	autosomal recessive	Progressive gait and limb ataxia associated with cardiomyopathy and diabetes	229300
Posterior Column Ataxia and Retinitis Pigmentosa (PCARP)	Feline Leukemia Virus Subgroup C Receptor 1 (FLVCR1)	autosomal recessive	Sensory ataxia and retinitis pigmentosa	609033
Non syndromic Retinitis pigmentosa (RP)	Feline Leukemia Virus Subgroup C Receptor 1 (FLVCR1)	autosomal recessive	Retinitis pigmentosa	268000
Hereditary Sensory and Autonomic Neuropathy (HSAN)	Feline Leukemia Virus Subgroup C Receptor 1 (FLVCR1)	autosomal recessive	Loss of pain perception	201300
Fowler syndrome (PVHH)	Feline Leukemia Virus Subgroup C Receptor 2 (FLVCR2)	autosomal recessive	Proliferative glomerular vasculopathy in the central nervous system associated with severe hydrocephaly, ventriculomegaly, cortical thinning and hypoplastic cerebellum.	225790

In addition, other rare neurodegenerative disorders have been associated with defective heme transport across membranes. Several proteins are involved in this process [1,15]. Among them, Feline Leukemia Virus Subgroup C Receptor 1 (FLVCR1) and 2 (FLVCR2) are implicated in heme export and import, respectively [11,26–31]. Mutations in the heme exporter FLVCR1 are associated with three distinct disorders affecting the sensory nervous system: posterior column ataxia and retinitis pigmentosa (PCARP) [32–34], non-syndromic retinitis pigmentosa (RP) [35,36] and hereditary sensory and autonomic neuropathy (HSAN) [11,37]. Mutations in the heme importer *FLVCR2* are responsible for the Fowler syndrome, a proliferative glomerular vasculopathy [30,38,39].

Furthermore, several lines of evidence suggest that heme may also contribute to the pathogenesis of common neurodegenerative disorders. The deregulation of enzymes critically involved in heme synthesis has been reported in both Alzheimer's disease (AD) and Parkinson's disease (PD). Reduced 5-aminolevulinate synthase 1 (ALAS1) and porphobilinogen deaminase (PBGD) mRNA were observed in AD brains [40], suggesting decreased heme synthesis rates in AD. Moreover, heme deficiency has been reported in the brain of patients with AD [41]. It has been proposed that heme deficiency may arise from either decreased heme synthesis rates or heme depletion as a consequence of heme binding to amyloid-β [41–43]. However, increased Ferrochelatase (FECH) levels were reported in another study [41].

Heme binding to α-Synuclein has also been reported [44], suggesting that heme depletion may also occur in PD. In addition, blood transcriptomic meta-analysis showed downregulation of 5-aminolevulinate synthase 2 (ALAS2) and FECH in PD [45]. However, within PD erythroid cells, α-synuclein gene (SNCA) was co-expressed with crucial enzymes involved in heme metabolism, including ALAS2, FECH and biliverdin reductase B (BLVRB) [46]. Moreover, increased striatal 5-aminolevulinate dehydratase (ALAD) activity was observed in the MPTP-induced mouse model of PD, indicative of increased heme synthesis rates [47]. It is difficult to conclude from these studies whether heme synthesis is increased or reduced in AD and PD. Data are still controversial due to the low amount of human samples analyzed and the different experimental approaches adopted. Further studies are required to definitively determine heme synthesis rates in these pathological conditions. Mouse models of AD and PD will be extremely useful to analyze in detail the role of heme metabolism in these disorders.

A role for heme derived from extracellular sources in the pathogenesis of neurodegenerative disorders has also been proposed. The heme scavenger Hx has been found strongly increased in the cerebrospinal fluid of AD patients [48–50]. Similarly, altered expression of the hemoglobin scavenger haptoglobin was shown in AD [51,52], PD [53,54] and Huntington's disease (HD) [55]. The induction of heme oxygenase 1 (HO1), the enzyme responsible for heme degradation, is common in patients affected by neurodegenerative conditions. Although HO1 is induced by a plethora of stimuli, it has been proposed that HO1 overexpression in AD and PD may be a consequence of increased brain-blood barrier permeability and hemoglobin-derived heme levels in AD and PD [16]. Moreover, increased expression of HO1 was reported in a mouse model of amyotrophic lateral sclerosis (ALS) [56] and ALS patients [57].

All the reported examples highlight the importance of the maintenance of heme homeostasis in the context of neurodegeneration. However, the molecular mechanisms underlying these disorders and the precise mechanism through which heme participates to them remains elusive and requires further investigations.

2. Role of Mitochondria in Neurodegenerative Diseases

Neurodegeneration can be elicited by several systems. Among them, mitochondrial-dependent processes have become increasingly relevant [58–63]. Several mechanisms account for mitochondria-dependent neurodegeneration (see Figure 2 for a graphic list of them) and below we attempt to summarize the most important ones.

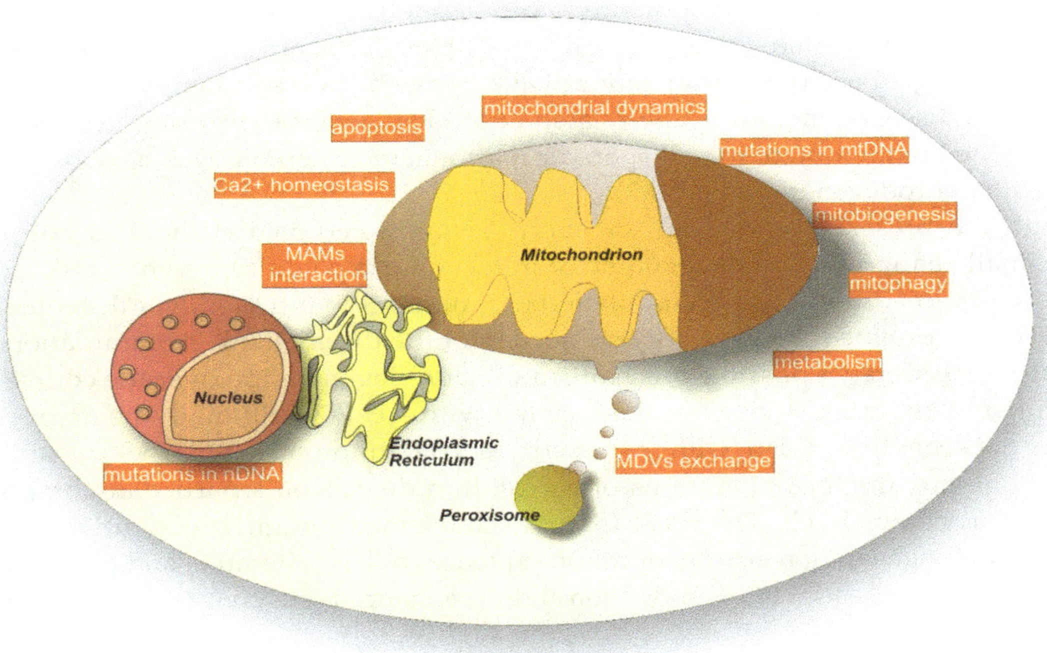

Figure 2. Mitochondrial dependent mechanisms in neurodegeneration. Mitochondria contribute to neurodegeneration by several mechanisms, including alterations in calcium homeostasis, mitochondrial

biogenesis (mitobiogenesis), mitochondrial dynamics, metabolism and mitophagy. Moreover, mutations in mitochondrial DNA (mtDNA) and inappropriate activation of apoptosis can be alternative mechanisms. Finally, additional systems include mutations in nuclear DNA (nDNA) at the level of genes encoding for mitochondrial proteins, the compromised exchange of mitochondria-derived vesicles (MDVs) among mitochondria and peroxisomes and the inefficient interaction among mitochondria and the endoplasmic reticulum at the level of mitochondrial associated membranes (MAMs).

2.1. *Mutations on Mitochondrial DNA (mtDNA) Genes*

Mitochondria contain their own genome, which is made of multiple copies of a circular double stranded molecule, which is 16.6 kb long in humans. It comprises 37 genes, 13 encoding for proteins involved in adenosine triphosphate (ATP) production and the other 24 encoding for two rRNAs and 22 tRNAs. Cells contain thousands of molecules of mtDNA and the majority of them have the same sequence, a condition known as homoplasmy. Inefficient mtDNA repair, localized oxidative environment and increased replication, however, can promote mtDNA mutations that, due to the polyploidy nature of mtDNA, often co-exist with their wildtype counterpart in various proportions (a condition termed heteroplasmy). mtDNA mutations are usually responsible for defects in the respiratory chain functions, but only if they are present above a certain threshold level.

The replication of mtDNA occurs independently on cell cycle, and a particular mtDNA molecule may be strongly replicated (or not at all) during cell division. Moreover, replication occurs also in postmitotic cells. These phenomena account for the clonal expansion of mutated mtDNA molecules and in association with heteroplasmy, result in mosaicism, with the levels of mutated mtDNA varying dramatically between tissues in the same organism and in different regions of the same tissue.

Somatic mtDNA mutations accumulate during a person's lifetime and undergo clonal expansion, so aging is typically associated with mosaic occurrence of respiratory chain-deficient cells in tissues [64].

Mitochondrial reactive oxygen species (ROS) production is the major cause for the higher mtDNA nucleotide instability when compared with nDNA.

Mitochondrial DNA mutations potently affect tissue that require a large amount of ATP to function, such as heart and brain. Some haplogroups [65] (evolutionary selected population subgroups carrying neutral single-base pair variants of mtDNA) have been associated with susceptibility to a variety of human diseases, including age-related neurodegenerative disorders such as PD and AD. Moreover, inherited point mutations and sporadic rearrangements on mtDNA have been described in association with neurodegeneration [65–69].

Although the presence of mtDNA deletions below a certain threshold is not sufficient to induce PD, small changes inside the genome of mitochondria could represent a risk factor for this pathology [70–74]. In addition, the accumulation of mutations in mtDNA over the course of PD has been observed to correlate with severity and burden of the disease [75]. Accumulation of mtDNA damage is also considered a possible mechanism of neurodegeneration over the course of HD [76]. Moreover, mtDNA mutations have been associated with AD [77], although the degree of mtDNA damage does not seem to correlate with the severity of AD symptoms [78].

As stated before, mtDNA alterations often result in defects on a particular component of the electron transport chain (ETC). The three main mechanisms through which mtDNA damage can contribute to neurodegeneration are therefore consequences of ETC alteration and include the decrease of ATP synthesis, the increase of ROS production and the enhanced sensitivity to neurotoxins associated to ETC disruption.

2.2. *Mutations on Nuclear DNA Genes Encoding Proteins Crucial for Mitochondrial Functionality*

Besides mutations on mitochondrial DNA, mutations in nuclear DNA (nDNA) at the level of genes encoding for mitochondrial proteins have also been associated with neurodegenerative disorders. For example, many of the identified ALS genes have a role in mitochondrial-associated functions (see [79] for a comprehensive description on this topic). In addition, mitochondrial dysfunction and oxidative stress in PD have been linked to mutations in genes encoding for parkin RBR E3 ubiquitin protein ligase (PRKN, commonly referred to as parkin), PTEN induced putative kinase 1 (PINK1, a protein that acts in the same pathway of parkin) and parkinsonism associated deglycase (DJ-1) [80], just to cite some of them. Parkin promotes autophagy of damaged mitochondria [81] and its deficiency is associated with defects in mitochondria morphology [82] and low levels of proteins involved in mitochondrial functions, thus resulting in decreased mitochondrial respiration [83]. Similarly, mutations in *PINK1* gene lead to decreased mitochondrial respiration [84] and alterations in mitochondria functions [85–88]. Regarding DJ-1, this protein localizes into mitochondria [89] and exerts crucial antioxidant functions [80,90–92]. Mutations in DJ-1 impair mitochondrial respiration, reduce mitochondrial membrane potential, increase ROS within the mitochondria and alter mitochondrial morphology [93]. Also, nDNA encoded proteins implicated in AD, like presenilin-1 and presenilin 2 (PSEN1 and 2) are related to mitochondria [94,95].

2.3. *Alterations of Mitochondrial Dynamics (Fusion, Fission, Motility)*

Mitochondria are not rigidly structured. They form a complex reticulum that undergoes regulated processes of fusion (the combination of two smaller mitochondria into a single organelle) and fission (the division of one large mitochondrion into two smaller fragments). Fusion allows mitochondria to mix their contents, enabling protein complementation, mtDNA repair and equal distribution of metabolites. Fission facilitates equal segregation of mitochondria into daughter cells during cellular division, enhances the distribution of mitochondria along cytoskeletal tracts and participates in the targeting of damaged segments of mitochondria to the autophagic process. Fusion and fission also contribute to the movement of mitochondria necessary for mitochondria distribution along neuronal axons and dendrites. Mitochondrial dynamics are crucial for neurotransmission, synaptic maintenance and neuronal survival. Proper mitochondrial trafficking is particularly important in neurons compared to other cell types, due to their exceptional cellular morphology. Indeed, neurons extend their axons and dendrites for very long distances that, in the case of human peripheral nerves or corticospinal tracts, extend up to a meter. Thus, the neuron represents an extreme case of mitochondrial distribution: dysfunctions in mitochondrial distribution that are not dangerous for other cells could be fatal for neuronal survival [96].

Alterations in mitochondria motility have been reported in several neurodegenerative disorders and neuropathies [97,98]. Aberrant activity of the fission-fusion machinery contributes to the pathogenesis of PD [99–102]. Moreover, alterations of mitochondrial dynamics have been observed in AD [61,102] and HD [100,103]. Particularly in HD, mitochondrial fission is promoted and mitochondrial fusion proteins are downregulated as the severity of the pathology increases [104]. Finally, defects in mitochondrial dynamics and disruption of the axonal transport of mitochondria have been reported in ALS [60,105–107].

2.4. *Inappropriate Activation of Cell Apoptosis by Mitochondria*

Mitochondria are pivotal organelles for the execution of apoptosis. The inappropriate activation of apoptosis leads to the disruption of the cellular proliferation-death balance. Neurodegenerative disorders are believed to partly depend on alterations of this equilibrium. *PINK1* loss-of-function mutations lead to early signals for apoptosis, promoting neurodegeneration in the context of PD [108]. Moreover, the low levels of *PTPA* (phosphotyrosyl phosphatase activator) observed in AD affected-people contribute to induce cell apoptosis in the brain of these patients [109]. Furthermore, caspase-6, an effector of the caspase-dependent apoptotic pathway, is known to be involved in the cleavage of mutant huntingtin resulting in neurodegeneration in HD patients [110]. Finally, in ALS the mutant SOD1 can trigger cytochrome c release from mitochondria to operate apoptosis [111].

2.5. Alteration of Mitochondria-Dependent Ca^{2+} Homeostasis

An additional neurodegenerative mechanism related to dysfunctions of mitochondria concerns the modulation of calcium. Mitochondria are involved in Ca^{2+} homeostasis as they are able to both accumulate and release Ca^{2+}. Mitochondrial Ca^{2+} concentration is fundamental for the regulation of specific mitochondrial key functions, such as the apoptotic process and the activity of several mitochondrial enzymes. The deregulation of Ca^{2+} homeostasis is a hallmark of different neurodegenerative diseases including PD, AD, HD and ALS [112,113]. Moreover, alterations of calcium levels have been observed in neuropathies. Neuropathic pain phenotypes include chemotherapy induced neuropathy, diabetic neuropathy, human immunodeficiency virus (HIV)-associated neuropathy and Charcot-Marie-Tooth neuropathy. Neuropathies have been associated with mitochondrial dysfunctions [63], and particularly in diabetic neuropathy, impaired cellular calcium homeostasis, including alterations in mitochondrial Ca^{2+} concentration, has been reported. Indeed, in the context of diabetes, sensory neurons, above all the lumbar dorsal root ganglia neurons (which have the longest axons), show an increased intracellular Ca^{2+} concentration that triggers elevated mitochondrial Ca^{2+} levels. This condition induces mitochondrial membrane depolarization and can favor the generation of reactive oxygen species (ROS) and oxidative stress, as well as alterations in mitochondrial functionality that can ultimately lead to neuronal damage [114].

2.6. Additional Alterations of Mitochondrial-Related Processes: Biogenesis, Mitophagy, Mdvs Exchange, Interaction with Mams, Control of Cellular Metabolism

Besides the mechanisms reported above, a series of additional mechanisms involving mitochondria have been described. Among them, neurodegeneration has been associated with the impairment of mitochondrial biogenesis. Particularly, the deficit of peroxisome proliferator-activated receptor gamma coactivator-1α (PGC-1α), a key regulator of mitochondrial biogenesis, has been associated with HD, PD and AD [115–120].

Mitophagy is also linked to neurodegenerative disorders [121–123]. Mitophagy is the selective autophagic process responsible for the elimination of damaged or excess mitochondria. In this process, a peculiar role is played by PINK1, that recruits parkin to dysfunctional mitochondria, where it induces their degradation by mitophagy [124]. Thus, it is not surprising that in addition to other neurodegenerative disorders, defective mitophagy is highly implicated in PD and is considered one of the major pathological mechanisms of mitochondrial dysfunction in autosomal recessive forms of PD [125].

Mitophagy is a cellular process that eliminates whole mitochondria, but other mechanisms exist to partially eliminate portions or components of mitochondria [122]. Mitochondria-derived vesicles (MDVs) exchange between mitochondria and peroxisomes represent one of these possible mechanisms. MDVs are crucial for the transport of cargo from mitochondria to peroxisomes. This process is regulated by the retromer complex. Studies on vacuolar protein sorting 35 (VPS35), a component of the retromer complex, indicate that mutations or alterations in VPS35 expression are associated to PD [126,127]. Moreover, it has been demonstrated that Parkin and PINK1, two genes highly implicated in PD, play crucial roles in the control of this process [128,129].

Other than with peroxisomes, mitochondria also physically interact with other subcellular organelles to ensure efficient and rapid metabolism and signaling. For example, the interaction between mitochondria and the endoplasmic reticulum (ER) occurs at the level of MAMs (mitochondrial associated membranes), a subdomain of the ER. The proteins involved in neurodegenerative diseases such as DRP1 (dynamin related protein 1) and MFN2 (mitofusin 2) are enriched in MAMs [130,131] and the perturbation of mitochondria-ER contacts has been described in neurodegenerative disorders, including PD, AD and ALS [132].

A further mitochondrial-dependent mechanism has been highlighted in neurodegeneration. This is the impairment of cell metabolism [133]. Mitochondria are the main energy-producing organelles of the cell, thus any process impairing mitochondrial functionality may lead to metabolic switching aimed to compensate for their decreased ATP production. Among the different neurodegenerative disorders, many lines of evidence suggest that mitochondria-dependent mechanisms are responsible for the metabolic changes observed in dopaminergic neurons in the context of PD. Mitochondrial ROS are particularly abundant in dopaminergic neurons due to dopamine oxidative metabolism, enhanced Fenton's reaction initiated by the high iron content of these cells, and the high rate of ATP production required to sustain the activity of a particular L-type voltage dependent Ca^{2+} channel expressed by these neurons. An excess of mitochondrial ROS can induce a series of cellular modifications, including hypoxia inducible factor 1α (HIF1α)-dependent up-regulation of glucose transporters [134], favoring the switch of energy metabolism towards glycolysis. When sustained for a long period, this metabolic change can be deleterious for dopaminergic neurons. Indeed, neurons need to deliver glucose in the pentose phosphate pathway (PPP), a process that produces NADPH (nicotinamide adenine dinucleotide phosphate), crucial for the recycling of the antioxidant glutathione. PPP is especially important in neurons as these cells show less robust antioxidant systems and are more vulnerable to oxidative stress than other cell types. Switching from PPP to glycolysis promotes oxidative stress and, consequently, neurodegeneration [135].

3. Heme and Mitochondrial Dysfunction Related to Neurodegenerative Diseases

The examples reported above sustain the notion that mitochondrial dysfunctions play a critical role in neurodegenerative disorders. The mitochondrion is a critical organelle for cells, representing a crossroad for a plethora of reactions contributing to a variety of metabolic processes, including heme metabolism. Considering the impact of impaired heme homeostasis in several neurodegenerative disorders and the interesting potential that heme takes on for the research in the context of neurodegeneration, it is curious to notice that heme is an under-investigated molecule in the field. This discrepancy could be due to the lack of knowledge on the possible systems through which heme can influence pivotal processes implicated in neurodegeneration. Among the possible ways, it is tempting to speculate that heme could directly or indirectly affect many of the mitochondrial-dependent mechanisms of neurodegeneration described in the previous paragraphs. Indeed, the relationship between heme and mitochondria is based on several elements (Figure 3): heme is produced through a series of reactions that occur partly in the mitochondria and partly in the cytosol [136]; heme acts as a cofactor for cytochromes c and cytochromes in complexes II-III-IV of the mitochondrial ETC [137]; heme has been reported to directly or indirectly influence ATP translocation between mitochondria and cytosol [138–140] mediated by adenine nucleotide translocases (ANTs); finally, heme biosynthesis is considered a cataplerotic pathway for the Kreb's cycle due to the fact that the first step of heme production consumes succynil-CoA [141,142]. Thus, modulation of heme homeostasis can affect mitochondrial functions.

Considering the mechanisms by which mitochondria contribute to neurodegeneration, it is interesting to note that heme levels can influence iron homeostasis, and both iron deficiency and iron excess are reported to cause damage on mitochondria [143,144] and on mitochondrial DNA [145,146]. Moreover, a decrease in heme itself leads to mitochondrial decay [4,147].

Furthermore, a connection exists between heme and nDNA genes encoding mitochondrial proteins typically implicated in neurodegenerative disorders. Indeed, it has been demonstrated that amyloid precursor protein, particularly when mutated, interacts and negatively regulates the heme-degrading enzyme HO1 [148]. Also PINK1 mutation is related to alterations in HO1 expression [149]. Moreover, DJ1 regulates nuclear factor-E2-related factor 2 (NRF2) [150], a key transcription factor for the induction of HO1 expression [151].

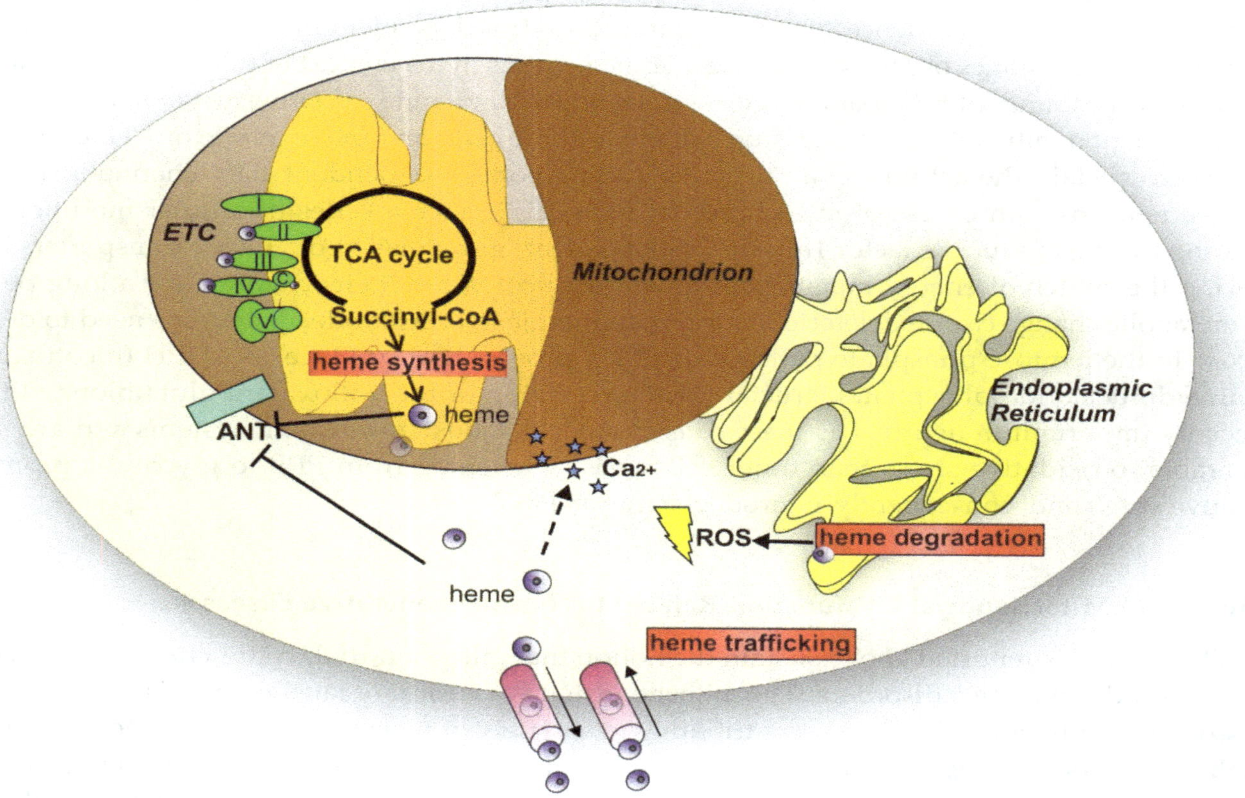

Figure 3. The "heme-mitochondria" relationship and the putative heme-related targets for the therapy of neurodegenerative disorders. Heme and mitochondria share a strong relationship based on several elements: heme synthesis occurs partly in the mitochondrion and acts as a cataplerotic pathway for the Kreb's cycle; heme is a cofactor for cytochromes c and cytochromes in complexes II-III-IV of the mitochondrial ETC [137]; heme influences the ATP translocation between mitochondria and cytosol mediated by adenine nucleotide translocases (ANTs); heme export influences calcium (Ca^{2+}) flux in mitochondria. Therefore, modulation of heme metabolism can lead to modification of mitochondrial functions. The control of intracellular heme levels is achieved by a balance among synthesis, catabolism and proper trafficking of heme. Thus, all these processes (highlighted with red boxes in the figure) represent putative good targets for the therapy of neurodegenerative disorder.

In addition, heme and the heme-degrading enzyme HO1 are implicated in the regulation of mitophagy, mitochondrial biogenesis and morphology [152–154].

In endothelial cells, it has been demonstrated that alterations in heme metabolism, in addition to promoting lipid peroxidation and activation of autophagy, induce mitophagy and apoptosis, indicating mitochondrial dysfunction [155]. Similarly, FLVCR1 loss is associated with alterations in mitochondrial morphology in human microvascular endothelial cells [26].

Furthermore, FLVCR1-deficient HeLa cells show impaired mitochondrial calcium uptake [156].

These data have been obtained in non-neuronal cells. However, similar mechanisms could also occur in neuronal cells.

Finally, compromised ETC complexes activity has been observed in the brain of a mouse model for acute intermittent porphyria, a type of porphyric neuropathy caused by alterations of heme biosynthesis [157]. Moreover, in three cases of Fowler syndrome it was suggested to be the presence of a defect in complex III and IV of the ETC [158,159].

These examples directly suggest that a connection between heme-mitochondria-neurodegeneration exists and open the possibility that future studies on this topic will further strengthen this notion.

4. Current Therapies and Potential Future Approaches to Face Mitochondrial Dysfunction in Neurodegenerative Diseases

Currently, there is no cure for reversing neurodegeneration and the treatment of neurodegenerative disorders is mainly symptomatic [160]. In order to face neurodegeneration, several pathways could be targeted to improve and/or restore mitochondrial functions, including mitochondrial biogenesis and metabolic flexibility, mitochondrial dynamics and mitophagy [161].

There are several pharmacological approaches to induce mitochondrial biogenesis and metabolic flexibility, that is the ability to switch from one fuel source to another. Several compounds have been generated to target the upstream sensors of energy production, including AMP-activated protein kinase (AMPK), mammalian target of rapamycin (mTOR) and sirtuins, or downstream transcriptional factors and co-factors, such as nuclear receptors, nuclear respiratory factor 1 (NRF1) and mitochondrial transcription factor A (TFAM) [161]. The therapeutic potential of these drugs has been evaluated mostly in the context of metabolic diseases, but also seems promising for neurodegeneration. For example, resveratrol is a natural compound that mimics caloric restriction and activates the sirtuin family of histone deacetylases. In humans, resveratrol improves mitochondrial function in obese patients and type 2 diabetes [162]. Furthermore, resveratrol counteracts neurodegeneration in worms and mice [163].

As described above, the disruption of the balance between mitochondrial fusion and fission contributes to neurodegeneration. Therefore, targeting mitochondrial dynamics represents another important strategy to improve mitochondrial function in neurodegenerative diseases. Strategies aimed at increasing mitochondrial fusion or inhibiting mitochondrial fission might improve mitochondrial function and are therapeutically interesting. The promotion of mitochondrial fusion by the overexpression of key components of the fusion machinery, like MFN2 or OPA1, rescues ATP production and mitochondrial morphology in a cellular model of PD [164]. Similar results were obtained with the inhibition of fission through the genetic deletion of DRP1 [164,165]. Although the understanding of the regulation of mitochondrial dynamics is still in its infancy, novel compounds have been identified to promote fusion or inhibit fission [166]. M1 hydrazone [167] and S3-derivative [168] promote mitochondrial fusion in cells deficient for mitofusin 1 (MFN1) and MFN2. Mdivi-1 (mitochondrial division inhibitor) attenuates fission in yeast and mammalian cells by inhibiting DRP1. In vitro, Mdivi-1 delays apoptosis by inhibiting mitochondrial outer membrane permeabilization and blocking cytochrome c release from mitochondria [169]. The therapeutic potential of Mdivi-1 seems promising for neurodegenerative disorders. Indeed, the administration of Mdivi-1 in mouse and cellular models of PD attenuates disease-associated phenotypes [165,170]. Although initially reported as an inhibitor of fission, Mdivi-1 was recently reported to reversibly inhibit complex I in a DRP1-independent manner [171]. The complete inhibition of complex I in vivo would be expected to cause neurodegeneration. Indeed, rotenone completely inhibits complex I, induces ROS levels and causes parkinsonian neurodegeneration in mice [172]. In contrast, Mdivi-1 lacks neuronal toxicity in vivo and is neuroprotective. This is likely due to the ability of Mdivi-1 to attenuate complex I-dependent reverse electron transfer (RET)-mediated ROS production. Indeed, Mdivi-1 fails to increase ROS levels in intact neurons and in isolated brain mitochondria [171].

The accumulation of dysfunctional mitochondria is another key event in several neurodegenerative conditions [173,174]. In this context, mitophagy is essential for the maintenance of mitochondrial integrity. As stated before in this review, the impairment of autophagy/mitophagy is common in neurodegenerative disorders. Therefore, mitophagy may be an additional pathway amenable for therapeutic intervention to ameliorate mitochondria function and counteract neurodegeneration [161,175]. Interestingly, both genetic and pharmacological induction of the mitochondrial autophagy receptor Nip3-like protein X (NIX) restores mitophagy in patient-derived fibroblasts [176].

Considering the crucial role of heme in maintaining mitochondrial function, it is tempting to speculate that targeting heme metabolism might be a promising strategy for the treatment of neurodegenerative diseases. Multiple approaches can be used to target heme metabolism (Figure 3); theoretically, targeting any of the enzymes involved in the heme biosynthetic pathway or proteins involved in the control of the intracellular heme pool may be a good strategy. Among these methods, HO1 represents a potentially interesting target. Due to its anti-oxidant and anti-inflammatory properties, HO1 plays a well-established neuroprotective role. The improvement of HO1 expression has been initially proposed for neurodegenerative conditions [177]. However, it has been reported that the overexpression of HO1 induces oxidative mitochondrial damage [178,179] and macroautophagy [179] in cultured astroglia. More importantly, HO1 induction has been associated with the later phases of neurodegeneration [180] and the deletion of HO1 has been proposed as a therapeutic option [181]. HO1 activity can be suppressed by synthetic metalloporphyrin compounds that unfortunately present important limitations [182]. However, novel HO1 inhibitors have been synthesized to overcome these side effects. Interestingly, these inhibitors confer neuroprotection in a mouse model of AD [182]. Considering the complex role of HO1 in neurodegeneration and the still controversial data reported in literature [180], further work is needed to fully elucidate the therapeutic potential of HO1 targeting. Recently, long-term 5–aminolevulinic acid (ALA) treatment has been exploited as a therapeutic approach in a mouse model of AD. Omori C. et al. reported that the oral administration of ALA increased cytochrome *c* oxidase (COX) activity and protein expression as well as mitochondrial membrane potential in the brain of treated mice [183]. Additional studies are required to understand more in detail the functional consequences of ALA administration in AD pathogenesis and the translation of this therapeutic approach to other neurodegenerative disorders. Considering that ALA formulations are already used for photodynamic therapy in a variety of cancer types [184], results obtained by Omori C. et al. are extremely encouraging for therapeutic purposes and further research in this direction is desirable.

5. Conclusions

The information reported over the course of the present review showed that mitochondria participate to neurodegenerative disorders by different mechanisms, encompassing DNA mutations, mitobiogenesis, mitophagy, mitochondrial dynamics, metabolism and mitochondrial interactions with other organelles. The literary contributions on the role of mitochondria in neurodegeneration are constantly growing and the present review attempted to make an excursus on the most important mechanisms by which these crucial organelles contribute to neurodegenerative diseases, with the awareness that not all the wide literature on this topic has been covered. Some of these mechanisms are currently considered as strategic targets for pharmacological interventions to counteract neurodegeneration. However, the investigation on additional elements contributing to the control of mitochondrial functions in neuronal cells will offer a wider window of intervention. In this perspective, heme metabolism provides an interesting opportunity. Indeed, as reported above in the review, heme participates to crucial processes occurring in mitochondria, influencing their functions and properties. The tight relationship between heme and the mitochondrion has been curiously underestimated and poorly investigated in the context of neurodegeneration. However, the implication of heme in crucial mitochondrial functions and the involvement of heme in a subset of neurodegenerative diseases strongly suggest an implication of heme in these disorders.

The comprehension of these mechanisms will allow the consideration of possible therapies based on the targeting of heme metabolism as an additional option to promote mitochondrial function. Alternatively, targeting heme metabolism may improve the efficacy of other drugs targeting mitochondria. The hope is that the understanding of the role of heme in mitochondria and its implication in neurodegeneration will open new perspectives in the struggle against neurodegenerative diseases.

References

1. Chiabrando, D.; Vinchi, F.; Fiorito, V.; Mercurio, S.; Tolosano, E. Heme in pathophysiology: A matter of scavenging, metabolism and trafficking across cell membranes. *Front. Pharmacol.* **2014**, *5*, 61. [CrossRef] [PubMed]
2. Zhu, Y.; Hon, T.; Ye, W.; Zhang, L. Heme deficiency interferes with the Ras-mitogen-activated protein kinase signaling pathway and expression of a subset of neuronal genes. *Cell Growth Differ.* **2002**, *13*, 431–439. [PubMed]
3. Sengupta, A.; Hon, T.; Zhang, L. Heme deficiency suppresses the expression of key neuronal genes and causes neuronal cell death. *Brain Res. Mol. Brain Res.* **2005**, *137*, 23–30. [CrossRef] [PubMed]
4. Atamna, H.; Killilea, D.W.; Killilea, A.N.; Ames, B.N. Heme deficiency may be a factor in the mitochondrial and neuronal decay of aging. *Proc. Natl. Acad. Sci. USA* **2002**, *99*, 14807–14812. [CrossRef] [PubMed]
5. Righy, C.; Bozza, M.T.; Oliveira, M.F.; Bozza, F.A. Molecular, Cellular and Clinical Aspects of Intracerebral Hemorrhage: Are the Enemies Within? *Curr. Neuropharmacol.* **2016**, *14*, 392–402. [CrossRef] [PubMed]
6. Ma, B.; Day, J.P.; Phillips, H.; Slootsky, B.; Tolosano, E.; Doré, S. Deletion of the hemopexin or heme oxygenase-2 gene aggravates brain injury following stroma-free hemoglobin-induced intracerebral hemorrhage. *J. Neuroinflamm.* **2016**, *13*, 26. [CrossRef] [PubMed]
7. Hahl, P.; Davis, T.; Washburn, C.; Rogers, J.T.; Smith, A. Mechanisms of neuroprotection by hemopexin: Modeling the control of heme and iron homeostasis in brain neurons in inflammatory states. *J. Neurochem.* **2013**, *125*, 89–101. [CrossRef] [PubMed]
8. Morello, N.; Tonoli, E.; Logrand, F.; Fiorito, V.; Fagoonee, S.; Turco, E.; Silengo, L.; Vercelli, A.; Altruda, F.; Tolosano, E. Haemopexin affects iron distribution and ferritin expression in mouse brain. *J. Cell. Mol. Med.* **2009**, *13*, 4192–4204. [CrossRef] [PubMed]
9. Morello, N.; Bianchi, F.T.; Marmiroli, P.; Tonoli, E.; Rodriguez Menendez, V.; Silengo, L.; Cavaletti, G.; Vercelli, A.; Altruda, F.; Tolosano, E. A role for hemopexin in oligodendrocyte differentiation and myelin formation. *PLoS ONE* **2011**, *6*, e20173. [CrossRef] [PubMed]
10. Tolosano, E.; Fagoonee, S.; Morello, N.; Vinchi, F.; Fiorito, V. Heme scavenging and the other facets of hemopexin. *Antioxid. Redox Signal.* **2010**, *12*, 305–320. [CrossRef] [PubMed]
11. Chiabrando, D.; Castori, M.; di Rocco, M.; Ungelenk, M.; Gießelmann, S.; Di Capua, M.; Madeo, A.; Grammatico, P.; Bartsch, S.; Hübner, C.A.; et al. Mutations in the Heme Exporter FLVCR1 Cause Sensory Neurodegeneration with Loss of Pain Perception. *PLoS Genet.* **2016**, *12*, e1006461. [CrossRef] [PubMed]
12. Chiabrando, D.; Vinchi, F.; Fiorito, V.; Tolosano, E. Haptoglobin and Hemopexin in Heme Detoxification and Iron Recycling. In *Acute Phase Proteins Francisco Veas*; IntechOpen: London, UK, 2011; pp. 262–288.
13. Blackburn, S.L.; Kumar, P.T.; McBride, D.; Zeineddine, H.A.; Leclerc, J.; Choi, H.A.; Dash, P.K.; Grotta, J.; Aronowski, J.; Cardenas, J.C.; et al. Unique Contribution of Haptoglobin and Haptoglobin Genotype in Aneurysmal Subarachnoid Hemorrhage. *Front. Physiol.* **2018**, *9*, 592. [CrossRef] [PubMed]
14. Marro, S.; Barisani, D.; Chiabrando, D.; Fagoonee, S.; Muckenthaler, M.U.; Stolte, J.; Meneveri, R.; Haile, D.; Silengo, L.; Altruda, F.; et al. Lack of haptoglobin affects iron transport across duodenum by modulating ferroportin expression. *Gastroenterology* **2007**, *133*, 1261–1271. [CrossRef] [PubMed]
15. Reddi, A.R.; Hamza, I. Heme Mobilization in Animals: A Metallolipid's Journey. *Acc. Chem. Res.* **2016**, *49*, 1104–1110. [CrossRef] [PubMed]
16. Gozzelino, R. The Pathophysiology of Heme in the Brain. *Curr. Alzheimer Res.* **2016**, *13*, 174–184. [CrossRef] [PubMed]
17. Erkkinen, M.G.; Kim, M.O.; Geschwind, M.D. Clinical Neurology and Epidemiology of the Major Neurodegenerative Diseases. *Cold Spring Harb. Perspect. Biol.* **2018**, *10*, a033118. [CrossRef] [PubMed]
18. Tracy, J.A.; Dyck, P.J. Porphyria and its neurologic manifestations. *Handb. Clin. Neurol.* **2014**, *120*, 839–849. [CrossRef] [PubMed]
19. Albers, J.W.; Fink, J.K. Porphyric neuropathy. *Muscle Nerve* **2004**, *30*, 410–422. [CrossRef] [PubMed]
20. Simon, N.G.; Herkes, G.K. The neurologic manifestations of the acute porphyrias. *J. Clin. Neurosci.* **2011**, *18*, 1147–1153. [CrossRef] [PubMed]
21. Campuzano, V.; Montermini, L.; Moltò, M.D.; Pianese, L.; Cossée, M.; Cavalcanti, F.; Monros, E.; Rodius, F.; Duclos, F.; Monticelli, A.; et al. Friedreich's ataxia: Autosomal recessive disease caused by an intronic GAA triplet repeat expansion. *Science* **1996**, *271*, 1423–1427. [CrossRef] [PubMed]

22. Yoon, T.; Cowan, J.A. Frataxin-mediated iron delivery to ferrochelatase in the final step of heme biosynthesis. *J. Biol. Chem.* **2004**, *279*, 25943–25946. [CrossRef] [PubMed]
23. Lange, H.; Mühlenhoff, U.; Denzel, M.; Kispal, G.; Lill, R. The heme synthesis defect of mutants impaired in mitochondrial iron-sulfur protein biogenesis is caused by reversible inhibition of ferrochelatase. *J. Biol. Chem.* **2004**, *279*, 29101–29108. [CrossRef] [PubMed]
24. Schoenfeld, R.A.; Napoli, E.; Wong, A.; Zhan, S.; Reutenauer, L.; Morin, D.; Buckpitt, A.R.; Taroni, F.; Lonnerdal, B.; Ristow, M.; et al. Frataxin deficiency alters heme pathway transcripts and decreases mitochondrial heme metabolites in mammalian cells. *Hum. Mol. Genet.* **2005**, *14*, 3787–3799. [CrossRef] [PubMed]
25. Chernova, T.; Nicotera, P.; Smith, A.G. Heme deficiency is associated with senescence and causes suppression of *N*-methyl-D-aspartate receptor subunits expression in primary cortical neurons. *Mol. Pharmacol.* **2006**, *69*, 697–705. [CrossRef] [PubMed]
26. Petrillo, S.; Chiabrando, D.; Genova, T.; Fiorito, V.; Ingoglia, G.; Vinchi, F.; Mussano, F.; Carossa, S.; Silengo, L.; Altruda, F.; et al. Heme accumulation in endothelial cells impairs angiogenesis by triggering paraptosis. *Cell Death Differ.* **2018**, *25*, 573–588. [CrossRef] [PubMed]
27. Vinchi, F.; Ingoglia, G.; Chiabrando, D.; Mercurio, S.; Turco, E.; Silengo, L.; Altruda, F.; Tolosano, E. Heme exporter FLVCR1a regulates heme synthesis and degradation and controls activity of cytochromes P450. *Gastroenterology* **2014**, *146*, 1325–1338. [CrossRef] [PubMed]
28. Fiorito, V.; Neri, F.; Pala, V.; Silengo, L.; Oliviero, S.; Altruda, F.; Tolosano, E. Hypoxia controls Flvcr1 gene expression in Caco2 cells through HIF2α and ETS1. *Biochim. Biophys. Acta* **2014**, *1839*, 259–264. [CrossRef] [PubMed]
29. Fiorito, V.; Forni, M.; Silengo, L.; Altruda, F.; Tolosano, E. Crucial Role of FLVCR1a in the Maintenance of Intestinal Heme Homeostasis. *Antioxid. Redox Signal.* **2015**, *23*, 1410–1423. [CrossRef] [PubMed]
30. Duffy, S.P.; Shing, J.; Saraon, P.; Berger, L.C.; Eiden, M.V.; Wilde, A.; Tailor, C.S. The Fowler syndrome-associated protein FLVCR2 is an importer of heme. *Mol. Cell. Biol.* **2010**, *30*, 5318–5324. [CrossRef] [PubMed]
31. Quigley, J.G.; Yang, Z.; Worthington, M.T.; Phillips, J.D.; Sabo, K.M.; Sabath, D.E.; Berg, C.L.; Sassa, S.; Wood, B.L.; Abkowitz, J.L. Identification of a human heme exporter that is essential for erythropoiesis. *Cell* **2004**, *118*, 757–766. [CrossRef] [PubMed]
32. Rajadhyaksha, A.M.; Elemento, O.; Puffenberger, E.G.; Schierberl, K.C.; Xiang, J.Z.; Putorti, M.L.; Berciano, J.; Poulin, C.; Brais, B.; Michaelides, M.; et al. Mutations in FLVCR1 cause posterior column ataxia and retinitis pigmentosa. *Am. J. Hum. Genet.* **2010**, *87*, 643–654. [CrossRef] [PubMed]
33. Ishiura, H.; Fukuda, Y.; Mitsui, J.; Nakahara, Y.; Ahsan, B.; Takahashi, Y.; Ichikawa, Y.; Goto, J.; Sakai, T.; Tsuji, S. Posterior column ataxia with retinitis pigmentosa in a Japanese family with a novel mutation in FLVCR1. *Neurogenetics* **2011**, *12*, 117–121. [CrossRef] [PubMed]
34. Shaibani, A.; Wong, L.J.; Wei Zhang, V.; Lewis, R.A.; Shinawi, M. Autosomal recessive posterior column ataxia with retinitis pigmentosa caused by novel mutations in the FLVCR1 gene. *Int. J. Neurosci.* **2015**, *125*, 43–49. [CrossRef] [PubMed]
35. Tiwari, A.; Bahr, A.; Bähr, L.; Fleischhauer, J.; Zinkernagel, M.S.; Winkler, N.; Barthelmes, D.; Berger, L.; Gerth-Kahlert, C.; Neidhardt, J.; et al. Next generation sequencing based identification of disease-associated mutations in Swiss patients with retinal dystrophies. *Sci. Rep.* **2016**, *6*, 28755. [CrossRef] [PubMed]
36. Yusuf, I.H.; Shanks, M.E.; Clouston, P.; MacLaren, R.E. A splice-site variant in FLVCR1 produces retinitis pigmentosa without posterior column ataxia. *Ophthalmic Genet.* **2018**, *39*, 263–267. [CrossRef] [PubMed]
37. Castori, M.; Morlino, S.; Ungelenk, M.; Pareyson, D.; Salsano, E.; Grammatico, P.; Tolosano, E.; Kurth, I.; Chiabrando, D. Posterior column ataxia with retinitis pigmentosa coexisting with sensory-autonomic neuropathy and leukemia due to the homozygous p.Pro221Ser *FLVCR1* mutation. *Am. J. Med. Genet. B Neuropsychiatr. Genet.* **2017**, *174*, 732–739. [CrossRef] [PubMed]
38. Meyer, E.; Ricketts, C.; Morgan, N.V.; Morris, M.R.; Pasha, S.; Tee, L.J.; Rahman, F.; Bazin, A.; Bessières, B.; Déchelotte, P.; et al. Mutations in FLVCR2 are associated with proliferative vasculopathy and hydranencephaly-hydrocephaly syndrome (Fowler syndrome). *Am. J. Hum. Genet.* **2010**, *86*, 471–478. [CrossRef] [PubMed]
39. Kvarnung, M.; Taylan, F.; Nilsson, D.; Albåge, M.; Nordenskjöld, M.; Anderlid, B.M.; Nordgren, A.; Syk Lundberg, E. Mutations in FLVCR2 associated with Fowler syndrome and survival beyond infancy. *Clin. Genet.* **2016**, *89*, 99–103. [CrossRef] [PubMed]

40. Dwyer, B.E.; Smith, M.A.; Richardson, S.L.; Perry, G.; Zhu, X. Down-regulation of aminolevulinate synthase, the rate-limiting enzyme for heme biosynthesis in Alzheimer's disease. *Neurosci. Lett.* **2009**, *460*, 180–184. [CrossRef] [PubMed]
41. Atamna, H.; Frey, W.H. A role for heme in Alzheimer's disease: Heme binds amyloid beta and has altered metabolism. *Proc. Natl. Acad. Sci. USA* **2004**, *101*, 11153–11158. [CrossRef] [PubMed]
42. Atamna, H. Heme binding to Amyloid-beta peptide: Mechanistic role in Alzheimer's disease. *J. Alzheimers Dis.* **2006**, *10*, 255–266. [CrossRef] [PubMed]
43. Smith, A.G.; Raven, E.L.; Chernova, T. The regulatory role of heme in neurons. *Metallomics* **2011**, *3*, 955–962. [CrossRef] [PubMed]
44. Hayden, E.Y.; Kaur, P.; Williams, T.L.; Matsui, H.; Yeh, S.R.; Rousseau, D.L. Heme Stabilization of α-Synuclein Oligomers during Amyloid Fibril Formation. *Biochemistry* **2015**, *54*, 4599–4610. [CrossRef] [PubMed]
45. Santiago, J.A.; Potashkin, J.A. Blood Transcriptomic Meta-analysis Identifies Dysregulation of Hemoglobin and Iron Metabolism in Parkinson' Disease. *Front. Aging Neurosci.* **2017**, *9*, 73. [CrossRef] [PubMed]
46. Scherzer, C.R.; Grass, J.A.; Liao, Z.; Pepivani, I.; Zheng, B.; Eklund, A.C.; Ney, P.A.; Ng, J.; McGoldrick, M.; Mollenhauer, B.; et al. GATA transcription factors directly regulate the Parkinson's disease-linked gene alpha-synuclein. *Proc. Natl. Acad. Sci. USA* **2008**, *105*, 10907–10912. [CrossRef] [PubMed]
47. Sampaio, T.B.; Marcondes Sari, M.H.; Pesarico, A.P.; Nogueira, C.W. δ-Aminolevulinate Dehydratase Activity is Stimulated in a MPTP Mouse Model of Parkinson's Disease: Correlation with Myeloperoxidase Activity. *Cell. Mol. Neurobiol.* **2017**, *37*, 911–917. [CrossRef] [PubMed]
48. Ringman, J.M.; Schulman, H.; Becker, C.; Jones, T.; Bai, Y.; Immermann, F.; Cole, G.; Sokolow, S.; Gylys, K.; Geschwind, D.H.; et al. Proteomic changes in cerebrospinal fluid of presymptomatic and affected persons carrying familial Alzheimer disease mutations. *Arch. Neurol.* **2012**, *69*, 96–104. [CrossRef] [PubMed]
49. Roher, A.E.; Maarouf, C.L.; Sue, L.I.; Hu, Y.; Wilson, J.; Beach, T.G. Proteomics-derived cerebrospinal fluid markers of autopsy-confirmed Alzheimer's disease. *Biomarkers* **2009**, *14*, 493–501. [CrossRef] [PubMed]
50. Castaño, E.M.; Roher, A.E.; Esh, C.L.; Kokjohn, T.A.; Beach, T. Comparative proteomics of cerebrospinal fluid in neuropathologically-confirmed Alzheimer's disease and non-demented elderly subjects. *Neurol. Res.* **2006**, *28*, 155–163. [CrossRef] [PubMed]
51. Song, I.U.; Kim, Y.D.; Chung, S.W.; Cho, H.J. Association between serum haptoglobin and the pathogenesis of Alzheimer's disease. *Intern. Med.* **2015**, *54*, 453–457. [CrossRef] [PubMed]
52. Cocciolo, A.; Di Domenico, F.; Coccia, R.; Fiorini, A.; Cai, J.; Pierce, W.M.; Mecocci, P.; Butterfield, D.A.; Perluigi, M. Decreased expression and increased oxidation of plasma haptoglobin in Alzheimer disease: Insights from redox proteomics. *Free Radic. Biol. Med.* **2012**, *53*, 1868–1876. [CrossRef] [PubMed]
53. de Farias, C.C.; Maes, M.; Bonifacio, K.L.; Matsumoto, A.K.; Bortolasci, C.C.; Nogueira, A.S.; Brinholi, F.F.; Morimoto, H.K.; de Melo, L.B.; Moreira, E.G.; et al. Parkinson's Disease is Accompanied by Intertwined Alterations in Iron Metabolism and Activated Immune-inflammatory and Oxidative Stress Pathways. *CNS Neurol. Disord. Drug Targets* **2017**, *16*, 484–491. [CrossRef] [PubMed]
54. Argüelles, S.; Venero, J.L.; García-Rodriguez, S.; Tomas-Camardiel, M.; Ayala, A.; Cano, J.; Machado, A. Use of haptoglobin and transthyretin as potential biomarkers for the preclinical diagnosis of Parkinson's disease. *Neurochem. Int.* **2010**, *57*, 227–234. [CrossRef] [PubMed]
55. Huang, Y.C.; Wu, Y.R.; Tseng, M.Y.; Chen, Y.C.; Hsieh, S.Y.; Chen, C.M. Increased prothrombin, apolipoprotein A-IV, and haptoglobin in the cerebrospinal fluid of patients with Huntington's disease. *PLoS ONE* **2011**, *6*, e15809. [CrossRef] [PubMed]
56. Gajowiak, A.; Styś, A.; Starzyński, R.R.; Bednarz, A.; Lenartowicz, M.; Staroń, R.; Lipiński, P. Mice Overexpressing Both Non-Mutated Human SOD1 and Mutated SOD1(G93A) Genes: A Competent Experimental Model for Studying Iron Metabolism in Amyotrophic Lateral Sclerosis. *Front. Mol. Neurosci.* **2015**, *8*, 82. [CrossRef] [PubMed]
57. Calingasan, N.Y.; Chen, J.; Kiaei, M.; Beal, M.F. Beta-amyloid 42 accumulation in the lumbar spinal cord motor neurons of amyotrophic lateral sclerosis patients. *Neurobiol. Dis.* **2005**, *19*, 340–347. [CrossRef] [PubMed]
58. Arun, S.; Liu, L.; Donmez, G. Mitochondrial Biology and Neurological Diseases. *Curr. Neuropharmacol.* **2016**, *14*, 143–154. [CrossRef] [PubMed]
59. Bose, A.; Beal, M.F. Mitochondrial dysfunction in Parkinson's disease. *J. Neurochem.* **2016**, *139* (Suppl. 1), 216–231. [CrossRef]

60. Shi, P.; Gal, J.; Kwinter, D.M.; Liu, X.; Zhu, H. Mitochondrial dysfunction in amyotrophic lateral sclerosis. *Biochim. Biophys. Acta* **2010**, *1802*, 45–51. [CrossRef] [PubMed]
61. Cabezas-Opazo, F.A.; Vergara-Pulgar, K.; Pérez, M.J.; Jara, C.; Osorio-Fuentealba, C.; Quintanilla, R.A. Mitochondrial Dysfunction Contributes to the Pathogenesis of Alzheimer's Disease. *Oxid. Med. Cell. Longev.* **2015**, *2015*, 509654. [CrossRef] [PubMed]
62. Costa, V.; Scorrano, L. Shaping the role of mitochondria in the pathogenesis of Huntington's disease. *EMBO J.* **2012**, *31*, 1853–1864. [CrossRef] [PubMed]
63. Bennett, G.J.; Doyle, T.; Salvemini, D. Mitotoxicity in distal symmetrical sensory peripheral neuropathies. *Nat. Rev. Neurol.* **2014**, *10*, 326–336. [CrossRef] [PubMed]
64. Larsson, N.G. Somatic mitochondrial DNA mutations in mammalian aging. *Annu. Rev. Biochem.* **2010**, *79*, 683–706. [CrossRef] [PubMed]
65. Chinnery, P.F.; Hudson, G. Mitochondrial genetics. *Br. Med. Bull.* **2013**, *106*, 135–159. [CrossRef] [PubMed]
66. Keogh, M.J.; Chinnery, P.F. Mitochondrial DNA mutations in neurodegeneration. *Biochim. Biophys. Acta* **2015**, *1847*, 1401–1411. [CrossRef] [PubMed]
67. Cha, M.Y.; Kim, D.K.; Mook-Jung, I. The role of mitochondrial DNA mutation on neurodegenerative diseases. *Exp. Mol. Med.* **2015**, *47*, e150. [CrossRef] [PubMed]
68. Nissanka, N.; Moraes, C.T. Mitochondrial DNA damage and reactive oxygen species in neurodegenerative disease. *FEBS Lett.* **2018**, *592*, 728–742. [CrossRef] [PubMed]
69. Pinto, M.; Moraes, C.T. Mitochondrial genome changes and neurodegenerative diseases. *Biochim. Biophys. Acta* **2014**, *1842*, 1198–1207. [CrossRef] [PubMed]
70. Kraytsberg, Y.; Kudryavtseva, E.; McKee, A.C.; Geula, C.; Kowall, N.W.; Khrapko, K. Mitochondrial DNA deletions are abundant and cause functional impairment in aged human substantia nigra neurons. *Nat. Genet.* **2006**, *38*, 518–520. [CrossRef] [PubMed]
71. Bender, A.; Krishnan, K.J.; Morris, C.M.; Taylor, G.A.; Reeve, A.K.; Perry, R.H.; Jaros, E.; Hersheson, J.S.; Betts, J.; Klopstock, T.; et al. High levels of mitochondrial DNA deletions in substantia nigra neurons in aging and Parkinson disease. *Nat. Genet.* **2006**, *38*, 515–517. [CrossRef] [PubMed]
72. Ikebe, S.; Tanaka, M.; Ozawa, T. Point mutations of mitochondrial genome in Parkinson's disease. *Brain Res Mol. Brain Res.* **1995**, *28*, 281–295. [CrossRef]
73. Perier, C.; Bender, A.; García-Arumí, E.; Melià, M.J.; Bové, J.; Laub, C.; Klopstock, T.; Elstner, M.; Mounsey, R.B.; Teismann, P.; et al. Accumulation of mitochondrial DNA deletions within dopaminergic neurons triggers neuroprotective mechanisms. *Brain* **2013**, *136*, 2369–2378. [CrossRef] [PubMed]
74. Dai, Y.; Clark, J.; Zheng, K.; Kujoth, G.C.; Prolla, T.A.; Simon, D.K. Somatic mitochondrial DNA mutations do not increase neuronal vulnerability to MPTP in young POLG mutator mice. *Neurotoxicol. Teratol.* **2014**, *46*, 62–67. [CrossRef] [PubMed]
75. Parkinson, G.M.; Dayas, C.V.; Smith, D.W. Increased mitochondrial DNA deletions in substantia nigra dopamine neurons of the aged rat. *Curr. Aging Sci.* **2014**, *7*, 155–160. [CrossRef] [PubMed]
76. Siddiqui, A.; Rivera-Sánchez, S.; Castro, M.E.R.; Acevedo-Torres, K.; Rane, A.; Torres-Ramos, C.A.; Nicholls, D.G.; Andersen, J.K.; Ayala-Torres, S. Mitochondrial DNA damage is associated with reduced mitochondrial bioenergetics in Huntington's disease. *Free Radic. Biol. Med.* **2012**, *53*, 1478–1488. [CrossRef] [PubMed]
77. Phillips, N.R.; Simpkins, J.W.; Roby, R.K. Mitochondrial DNA deletions in Alzheimer's brains: A review. *Alzheimers Dement.* **2014**, *10*, 393–400. [CrossRef] [PubMed]
78. Gerschütz, A.; Heinsen, H.; Grünblatt, E.; Wagner, A.K.; Bartl, J.; Meissner, C.; Fallgatter, A.J.; Al-Sarraj, S.; Troakes, C.; Ferrer, I.; et al. Neuron-specific mitochondrial DNA deletion levels in sporadic Alzheimer's disease. *Curr. Alzheimer Res.* **2013**, *10*, 1041–1046. [CrossRef] [PubMed]
79. Smith, E.F.; Shaw, P.J.; De Vos, K.J. The role of mitochondria in amyotrophic lateral sclerosis. *Neurosci. Lett.* **2017**. [CrossRef] [PubMed]
80. Bekris, L.M.; Mata, I.F.; Zabetian, C.P. The genetics of Parkinson disease. *J. Geriatr. Psychiatry Neurol.* **2010**, *23*, 228–242. [CrossRef] [PubMed]
81. Narendra, D.; Tanaka, A.; Suen, D.F.; Youle, R.J. Parkin is recruited selectively to impaired mitochondria and promotes their autophagy. *J. Cell Biol.* **2008**, *183*, 795–803. [CrossRef] [PubMed]

82. Greene, J.C.; Whitworth, A.J.; Kuo, I.; Andrews, L.A.; Feany, M.B.; Pallanck, L.J. Mitochondrial pathology and apoptotic muscle degeneration in Drosophila parkin mutants. *Proc. Natl. Acad. Sci. USA* **2003**, *100*, 4078–4083. [CrossRef] [PubMed]
83. Palacino, J.J.; Sagi, D.; Goldberg, M.S.; Krauss, S.; Motz, C.; Wacker, M.; Klose, J.; Shen, J. Mitochondrial dysfunction and oxidative damage in parkin-deficient mice. *J. Biol. Chem.* **2004**, *279*, 18614–18622. [CrossRef] [PubMed]
84. Gautier, C.A.; Kitada, T.; Shen, J. Loss of PINK1 causes mitochondrial functional defects and increased sensitivity to oxidative stress. *Proc. Natl. Acad. Sci. USA* **2008**, *105*, 11364–11369. [CrossRef] [PubMed]
85. Heeman, B.; Van den Haute, C.; Aelvoet, S.A.; Valsecchi, F.; Rodenburg, R.J.; Reumers, V.; Debyser, Z.; Callewaert, G.; Koopman, W.J.; Willems, P.H.; et al. Depletion of PINK1 affects mitochondrial metabolism, calcium homeostasis and energy maintenance. *J. Cell Sci.* **2011**, *124*, 1115–1125. [CrossRef] [PubMed]
86. Clark, I.E.; Dodson, M.W.; Jiang, C.; Cao, J.H.; Huh, J.R.; Seol, J.H.; Yoo, S.J.; Hay, B.A.; Guo, M. Drosophila pink1 is required for mitochondrial function and interacts genetically with parkin. *Nature* **2006**, *441*, 1162–1166. [CrossRef] [PubMed]
87. Park, J.; Lee, S.B.; Lee, S.; Kim, Y.; Song, S.; Kim, S.; Bae, E.; Kim, J.; Shong, M.; Kim, J.M.; et al. Mitochondrial dysfunction in Drosophila PINK1 mutants is complemented by parkin. *Nature* **2006**, *441*, 1157–1161. [CrossRef] [PubMed]
88. Truban, D.; Hou, X.; Caulfield, T.R.; Fiesel, F.C.; Springer, W. PINK1, Parkin, and Mitochondrial Quality Control: What can we Learn about Parkinson's Disease Pathobiology? *J. Parkinsons Dis.* **2017**, *7*, 13–29. [CrossRef] [PubMed]
89. Zhang, L.; Shimoji, M.; Thomas, B.; Moore, D.J.; Yu, S.W.; Marupudi, N.I.; Torp, R.; Torgner, I.A.; Ottersen, O.P.; Dawson, T.M.; et al. Mitochondrial localization of the Parkinson's disease related protein DJ-1: Implications for pathogenesis. *Hum. Mol. Genet.* **2005**, *14*, 2063–2073. [CrossRef] [PubMed]
90. Taira, T.; Saito, Y.; Niki, T.; Iguchi-Ariga, S.M.; Takahashi, K.; Ariga, H. DJ-1 has a role in antioxidative stress to prevent cell death. *EMBO Rep.* **2004**, *5*, 213–218. [CrossRef] [PubMed]
91. Zhou, W.; Freed, C.R. DJ-1 up-regulates glutathione synthesis during oxidative stress and inhibits A53T alpha-synuclein toxicity. *J. Biol. Chem.* **2005**, *280*, 43150–43158. [CrossRef] [PubMed]
92. Yokota, T.; Sugawara, K.; Ito, K.; Takahashi, R.; Ariga, H.; Mizusawa, H. Down regulation of DJ-1 enhances cell death by oxidative stress, ER stress, and proteasome inhibition. *Biochem. Biophys. Res. Commun.* **2003**, *312*, 1342–1348. [CrossRef] [PubMed]
93. Krebiehl, G.; Ruckerbauer, S.; Burbulla, L.F.; Kieper, N.; Maurer, B.; Waak, J.; Wolburg, H.; Gizatullina, Z.; Gellerich, F.N.; Woitalla, D.; et al. Reduced basal autophagy and impaired mitochondrial dynamics due to loss of Parkinson's disease-associated protein DJ-1. *PLoS ONE* **2010**, *5*, e9367. [CrossRef] [PubMed]
94. Ankarcrona, M.; Hultenby, K. Presenilin-1 is located in rat mitochondria. *Biochem. Biophys. Res. Commun.* **2002**, *295*, 766–770. [CrossRef]
95. Area-Gomez, E.; de Groof, A.J.; Boldogh, I.; Bird, T.D.; Gibson, G.E.; Koehler, C.M.; Yu, W.H.; Duff, K.E.; Yaffe, M.P.; Pon, L.A.; et al. Presenilins are enriched in endoplasmic reticulum membranes associated with mitochondria. *Am. J. Pathol.* **2009**, *175*, 1810–1816. [CrossRef] [PubMed]
96. Schwarz, T.L. Mitochondrial trafficking in neurons. *Cold Spring Harb. Perspect. Biol.* **2013**, *5*, a011304. [CrossRef] [PubMed]
97. Burté, F.; Carelli, V.; Chinnery, P.F.; Yu-Wai-Man, P. Disturbed mitochondrial dynamics and neurodegenerative disorders. *Nat. Rev. Neurol.* **2015**, *11*, 11–24. [CrossRef] [PubMed]
98. Dupuis, L. Mitochondrial quality control in neurodegenerative diseases. *Biochimie* **2014**, *100*, 177–183. [CrossRef] [PubMed]
99. Ryan, B.J.; Hoek, S.; Fon, E.A.; Wade-Martins, R. Mitochondrial dysfunction and mitophagy in Parkinson's: From familial to sporadic disease. *Trends Biochem. Sci.* **2015**, *40*, 200–210. [CrossRef] [PubMed]
100. Franco-Iborra, S.; Vila, M.; Perier, C. Mitochondrial Quality Control in Neurodegenerative Diseases: Focus on Parkinson's Disease and Huntington's Disease. *Front. Neurosci.* **2018**, *12*, 342. [CrossRef] [PubMed]
101. Van Laar, V.S.; Berman, S.B. The interplay of neuronal mitochondrial dynamics and bioenergetics: Implications for Parkinson's disease. *Neurobiol. Dis.* **2013**, *51*, 43–55. [CrossRef] [PubMed]
102. Yan, M.H.; Wang, X.; Zhu, X. Mitochondrial defects and oxidative stress in Alzheimer disease and Parkinson disease. *Free Radic. Biol. Med.* **2013**, *62*, 90–101. [CrossRef] [PubMed]

103. Carmo, C.; Naia, L.; Lopes, C.; Rego, A.C. Mitochondrial Dysfunction in Huntington's Disease. *Adv. Exp. Med. Biol.* **2018**, *1049*, 59–83. [CrossRef] [PubMed]
104. Shirendeb, U.; Reddy, A.P.; Manczak, M.; Calkins, M.J.; Mao, P.; Tagle, D.A.; Reddy, P.H. Abnormal mitochondrial dynamics, mitochondrial loss and mutant huntingtin oligomers in Huntington's disease: Implications for selective neuronal damage. *Hum. Mol. Genet.* **2011**, *20*, 1438–1455. [CrossRef] [PubMed]
105. De Vos, K.J.; Chapman, A.L.; Tennant, M.E.; Manser, C.; Tudor, E.L.; Lau, K.F.; Brownlees, J.; Ackerley, S.; Shaw, P.J.; McLoughlin, D.M.; et al. Familial amyotrophic lateral sclerosis-linked SOD1 mutants perturb fast axonal transport to reduce axonal mitochondria content. *Hum. Mol. Genet.* **2007**, *16*, 2720–2728. [CrossRef] [PubMed]
106. Gao, J.; Wang, L.; Liu, J.; Xie, F.; Su, B.; Wang, X. Abnormalities of Mitochondrial Dynamics in Neurodegenerative Diseases. *Antioxidants* **2017**, *6*, 25. [CrossRef] [PubMed]
107. Carrì, M.T.; Cozzolino, M. SOD1 and mitochondria in ALS: A dangerous liaison. *J. Bioenerg. Biomembr.* **2011**, *43*, 593–599. [CrossRef] [PubMed]
108. Wood-Kaczmar, A.; Gandhi, S.; Yao, Z.; Abramov, A.Y.; Abramov, A.S.; Miljan, E.A.; Keen, G.; Stanyer, L.; Hargreaves, I.; Klupsch, K.; et al. PINK1 is necessary for long term survival and mitochondrial function in human dopaminergic neurons. *PLoS ONE* **2008**, *3*, e2455. [CrossRef]
109. Luo, D.J.; Feng, Q.; Wang, Z.H.; Sun, D.S.; Wang, Q.; Wang, J.Z.; Liu, G.P. Knockdown of phosphotyrosyl phosphatase activator induces apoptosis via mitochondrial pathway and the attenuation by simultaneous tau hyperphosphorylation. *J. Neurochem.* **2014**, *130*, 816–825. [CrossRef] [PubMed]
110. Wang, X.J.; Cao, Q.; Zhang, Y.; Su, X.D. Activation and regulation of caspase-6 and its role in neurodegenerative diseases. *Annu. Rev. Pharmacol. Toxicol.* **2015**, *55*, 553–572. [CrossRef] [PubMed]
111. Takeuchi, H.; Kobayashi, Y.; Ishigaki, S.; Doyu, M.; Sobue, G. Mitochondrial localization of mutant superoxide dismutase 1 triggers caspase-dependent cell death in a cellular model of familial amyotrophic lateral sclerosis. *J. Biol. Chem.* **2002**, *277*, 50966–50972. [CrossRef] [PubMed]
112. Calì, T.; Ottolini, D.; Brini, M. Mitochondrial Ca^{2+} and neurodegeneration. *Cell Calcium* **2012**, *52*, 73–85 [CrossRef] [PubMed]
113. Pelizzoni, I.; Macco, R.; Zacchetti, D.; Grohovaz, F.; Codazzi, F. Iron and calcium in the central nervous system: A close relationship in health and sickness. *Biochem. Soc. Trans.* **2008**, *36*, 1309–1312. [CrossRef] [PubMed]
114. Fernyhough, P.; Roy Chowdhury, S.K.; Schmidt, R.E. Mitochondrial stress and the pathogenesis of diabetic neuropathy. *Expert Rev. Endocrinol. Metab.* **2010**, *5*, 39–49. [CrossRef] [PubMed]
115. Jones, A.W.; Yao, Z.; Vicencio, J.M.; Karkucinska-Wieckowska, A.; Szabadkai, G. PGC-1 family coactivators and cell fate: Roles in cancer, neurodegeneration, cardiovascular disease and retrograde mitochondria-nucleus signalling. *Mitochondrion* **2012**, *12*, 86–99. [CrossRef] [PubMed]
116. Weydt, P.; Pineda, V.V.; Torrence, A.E.; Libby, R.T.; Satterfield, T.F.; Lazarowski, E.R.; Gilbert, M.L.; Morton, G.J.; Bammler, T.K.; Strand, A.D.; et al. Thermoregulatory and metabolic defects in Huntington's disease transgenic mice implicate PGC-1alpha in Huntington's disease neurodegeneration. *Cell Metab.* **2006**, *4*, 349–362. [CrossRef] [PubMed]
117. Cui, L.; Jeong, H.; Borovecki, F.; Parkhurst, C.N.; Tanese, N.; Krainc, D. Transcriptional repression of PGC-1alpha by mutant huntingtin leads to mitochondrial dysfunction and neurodegeneration. *Cell* **2006**, *127*, 59–69. [CrossRef] [PubMed]
118. Qin, W.; Haroutunian, V.; Katsel, P.; Cardozo, C.P.; Ho, L.; Buxbaum, J.D.; Pasinetti, G.M. PGC-1alpha expression decreases in the Alzheimer disease brain as a function of dementia. *Arch. Neurol.* **2009**, *66*, 352–361. [CrossRef] [PubMed]
119. St-Pierre, J.; Drori, S.; Uldry, M.; Silvaggi, J.M.; Rhee, J.; Jäger, S.; Handschin, C.; Zheng, K.; Lin, J.; Yang, W.; et al. Suppression of reactive oxygen species and neurodegeneration by the PGC-1 transcriptional coactivators. *Cell* **2006**, *127*, 397–408. [CrossRef] [PubMed]
120. Zheng, B.; Liao, Z.; Locascio, J.J.; Lesniak, K.A.; Roderick, S.S.; Watt, M.L.; Eklund, A.C.; Zhang-James, Y.; Kim, P.D.; Hauser, M.A.; et al. PGC-1α, a potential therapeutic target for early intervention in Parkinson's disease. *Sci. Transl. Med.* **2010**, *2*, 52ra73. [CrossRef] [PubMed]
121. Chu, C.T. Mechanisms of selective autophagy and mitophagy: Implications for neurodegenerative diseases. *Neurobiol. Dis.* **2018**. [CrossRef] [PubMed]

122. Martinez-Vicente, M. Neuronal Mitophagy in Neurodegenerative Diseases. *Front. Mol. Neurosci.* **2017**, *10*, 64. [CrossRef] [PubMed]
123. Rodolfo, C.; Campello, S.; Cecconi, F. Mitophagy in neurodegenerative diseases. *Neurochem. Int.* **2018**, *117*, 156–166. [CrossRef] [PubMed]
124. Kondapalli, C.; Kazlauskaite, A.; Zhang, N.; Woodroof, H.I.; Campbell, D.G.; Gourlay, R.; Burchell, L.; Walden, H.; Macartney, T.J.; Deak, M.; et al. PINK1 is activated by mitochondrial membrane potential depolarization and stimulates Parkin E3 ligase activity by phosphorylating Serine 65. *Open Biol.* **2012**, *2*, 120080. [CrossRef] [PubMed]
125. Moon, H.E.; Paek, S.H. Mitochondrial Dysfunction in Parkinson's Disease. *Exp. Neurobiol.* **2015**, *24*, 103–116. [CrossRef] [PubMed]
126. Vilariño-Güell, C.; Wider, C.; Ross, O.A.; Dachsel, J.C.; Kachergus, J.M.; Lincoln, S.J.; Soto-Ortolaza, A.I.; Cobb, S.A.; Wilhoite, G.J.; Bacon, J.A.; et al. VPS35 mutations in Parkinson disease. *Am. J. Hum. Genet.* **2011**, *89*, 162–167. [CrossRef] [PubMed]
127. Zimprich, A.; Benet-Pagès, A.; Struhal, W.; Graf, E.; Eck, S.H.; Offman, M.N.; Haubenberger, D.; Spielberger, S.; Schulte, E.C.; Lichtner, P.; et al. A mutation in VPS35, encoding a subunit of the retromer complex, causes late-onset Parkinson disease. *Am. J. Hum. Genet.* **2011**, *89*, 168–175. [CrossRef] [PubMed]
128. McLelland, G.L.; Soubannier, V.; Chen, C.X.; McBride, H.M.; Fon, E.A. Parkin and PINK1 function in a vesicular trafficking pathway regulating mitochondrial quality control. *EMBO J.* **2014**, *33*, 282–295. [CrossRef] [PubMed]
129. Shlevkov, E.; Schwarz, T.L. Have you seen? For parkin, it's not all or nothing. *EMBO J.* **2014**, *33*, 277–279. [CrossRef] [PubMed]
130. Friedman, J.R.; Lackner, L.L.; West, M.; DiBenedetto, J.R.; Nunnari, J.; Voeltz, G.K. ER tubules mark sites of mitochondrial division. *Science* **2011**, *334*, 358–362. [CrossRef] [PubMed]
131. de Brito, O.M.; Scorrano, L. Mitofusin 2 tethers endoplasmic reticulum to mitochondria. *Nature* **2008**, *456*, 605–610. [CrossRef] [PubMed]
132. Liu, Y.; Zhu, X. Endoplasmic reticulum-mitochondria tethering in neurodegenerative diseases. *Transl. Neurodegener.* **2017**, *6*, 21. [CrossRef] [PubMed]
133. Camandola, S.; Mattson, M.P. Brain metabolism in health, aging, and neurodegeneration. *EMBO J.* **2017**, *36*, 1474–1492. [CrossRef] [PubMed]
134. Requejo-Aguilar, R.; Lopez-Fabuel, I.; Fernandez, E.; Martins, L.M.; Almeida, A.; Bolaños, J.P. PINK1 deficiency sustains cell proliferation by reprogramming glucose metabolism through HIF1. *Nat. Commun.* **2014**, *5*, 4514. [CrossRef] [PubMed]
135. Herrero-Mendez, A.; Almeida, A.; Fernández, E.; Maestre, C.; Moncada, S.; Bolaños, J.P. The bioenergetic and antioxidant status of neurons is controlled by continuous degradation of a key glycolytic enzyme by APC/C-Cdh1. *Nat. Cell Biol.* **2009**, *11*, 747–752. [CrossRef] [PubMed]
136. Chiabrando, D.; Mercurio, S.; Tolosano, E. Heme and erythropoieis: More than a structural role. *Haematologica* **2014**, *99*, 973–983. [CrossRef] [PubMed]
137. Kim, H.J.; Khalimonchuk, O.; Smith, P.M.; Winge, D.R. Structure, function, and assembly of heme centers in mitochondrial respiratory complexes. *Biochim. Biophys. Acta* **2012**, *1823*, 1604–1616. [CrossRef] [PubMed]
138. Sabová, L.; Zeman, I.; Supek, F.; Kolarov, J. Transcriptional control of AAC3 gene encoding mitochondrial ADP/ATP translocator in Saccharomyces cerevisiae by oxygen, heme and ROX1 factor. *Eur. J. Biochem.* **1993**, *213*, 547–553. [CrossRef] [PubMed]
139. Giraud, S.; Bonod-Bidaud, C.; Wesolowski-Louvel, M.; Stepien, G. Expression of human ANT2 gene in highly proliferative cells: GRBOX, a new transcriptional element, is involved in the regulation of glycolytic ATP import into mitochondria. *J. Mol. Biol.* **1998**, *281*, 409–418. [CrossRef] [PubMed]
140. Azuma, M.; Kabe, Y.; Kuramori, C.; Kondo, M.; Yamaguchi, Y.; Handa, H. Adenine nucleotide translocator transports haem precursors into mitochondria. *PLoS ONE* **2008**, *3*, e3070. [CrossRef] [PubMed]
141. Frezza, C.; Zheng, L.; Folger, O.; Rajagopalan, K.N.; MacKenzie, E.D.; Jerby, L.; Micaroni, M.; Chaneton, B.; Adam, J.; Hedley, A.; et al. Haem oxygenase is synthetically lethal with the tumour suppressor fumarate hydratase. *Nature* **2011**, *477*, 225–228. [CrossRef] [PubMed]
142. Fukuda, Y.; Wang, Y.; Lian, S.; Lynch, J.; Nagai, S.; Fanshawe, B.; Kandilci, A.; Janke, L.J.; Neale, G.; Fan, Y.; et al. Upregulated heme biosynthesis, an exploitable vulnerability in MYCN-driven leukemogenesis. *JCI Insight* **2017**, *2*. [CrossRef] [PubMed]

143. Paul, B.T.; Manz, D.H.; Torti, F.M.; Torti, S.V. Mitochondria and Iron: Current questions. *Expert Rev. Hematol.* **2017**, *10*, 65–79. [CrossRef] [PubMed]
144. Horowitz, M.P.; Greenamyre, J.T. Mitochondrial iron metabolism and its role in neurodegeneration. *J. Alzheimers Dis.* **2010**, *20* (Suppl. 2), S551–S568. [CrossRef] [PubMed]
145. Walter, P.B.; Knutson, M.D.; Paler-Martinez, A.; Lee, S.; Xu, Y.; Viteri, F.E.; Ames, B.N. Iron deficiency and iron excess damage mitochondria and mitochondrial DNA in rats. *Proc. Natl. Acad. Sci. USA* **2002**, *99*, 2264–2269. [CrossRef] [PubMed]
146. Gao, X.; Campian, J.L.; Qian, M.; Sun, X.F.; Eaton, J.W. Mitochondrial DNA damage in iron overload. *J. Biol. Chem.* **2009**, *284*, 4767–4775. [CrossRef] [PubMed]
147. Atamna, H.; Newberry, J.; Erlitzki, R.; Schultz, C.S.; Ames, B.N. Biotin deficiency inhibits heme synthesis and impairs mitochondria in human lung fibroblasts. *J. Nutr.* **2007**, *137*, 25–30. [CrossRef] [PubMed]
148. Takahashi, M.; Doré, S.; Ferris, C.D.; Tomita, T.; Sawa, A.; Wolosker, H.; Borchelt, D.R.; Iwatsubo, T.; Kim, S.H.; Thinakaran, G.; et al. Amyloid precursor proteins inhibit heme oxygenase activity and augment neurotoxicity in Alzheimer's disease. *Neuron* **2000**, *28*, 461–473. [CrossRef]
149. Sheng, X.J.; Tu, H.J.; Chien, W.L.; Kang, K.H.; Lu, D.H.; Liou, H.H.; Lee, M.J.; Fu, W.M. Antagonism of proteasome inhibitor-induced heme oxygenase-1 expression by PINK1 mutation. *PLoS ONE* **2017**, *12*, e0183076. [CrossRef] [PubMed]
150. Clements, C.M.; McNally, R.S.; Conti, B.J.; Mak, T.W.; Ting, J.P. DJ-1, a cancer- and Parkinson's disease-associated protein, stabilizes the antioxidant transcriptional master regulator Nrf2. *Proc. Natl. Acad. Sci. USA* **2006**, *103*, 15091–15096. [CrossRef] [PubMed]
151. Alam, J.; Stewart, D.; Touchard, C.; Boinapally, S.; Choi, A.M.; Cook, J.L. Nrf2, a Cap'n'Collar transcription factor, regulates induction of the heme oxygenase-1 gene. *J. Biol. Chem.* **1999**, *274*, 26071–26078. [CrossRef] [PubMed]
152. Hull, T.D.; Boddu, R.; Guo, L.; Tisher, C.C.; Traylor, A.M.; Patel, B.; Joseph, R.; Prabhu, S.D.; Suliman, H.B.; Piantadosi, C.A.; et al. Heme oxygenase-1 regulates mitochondrial quality control in the heart. *JCI Insight* **2016**, *1*, e85817. [CrossRef] [PubMed]
153. Atamna, H.; Walter, P.B.; Ames, B.N. The role of heme and iron-sulfur clusters in mitochondrial biogenesis, maintenance, and decay with age. *Arch. Biochem. Biophys.* **2002**, *397*, 345–353. [CrossRef] [PubMed]
154. Suliman, H.B.; Keenan, J.E.; Piantadosi, C.A. Mitochondrial quality-control dysregulation in conditional HO-1. *JCI Insight* **2017**, *2*, e89676. [CrossRef] [PubMed]
155. Higdon, A.N.; Benavides, G.A.; Chacko, B.K.; Ouyang, X.; Johnson, M.S.; Landar, A.; Zhang, J.; Darley-Usmar, V.M. Hemin causes mitochondrial dysfunction in endothelial cells through promoting lipid peroxidation: The protective role of autophagy. *Am. J. Physiol. Heart Circ. Physiol.* **2012**, *302*, H1394–H1409. [CrossRef] [PubMed]
156. Chiabrando, D.; Marro, S.; Mercurio, S.; Giorgi, C.; Petrillo, S.; Vinchi, F.; Fiorito, V.; Fagoonee, S.; Camporeale, A.; Turco, E.; et al. The mitochondrial heme exporter FLVCR1b mediates erythroid differentiation. *J. Clin. Investig.* **2012**, *122*, 4569–4579. [CrossRef] [PubMed]
157. Homedan, C.; Laafi, J.; Schmitt, C.; Gueguen, N.; Lefebvre, T.; Karim, Z.; Desquiret-Dumas, V.; Wetterwald, C.; Deybach, J.C.; Gouya, L.; et al. Acute intermittent porphyria causes hepatic mitochondrial energetic failure in a mouse model. *Int. J. Biochem. Cell Biol.* **2014**, *51*, 93–101. [CrossRef] [PubMed]
158. Castro-Gago, M.; Alonso, A.; Pintos-Martínez, E.; Beiras-Iglesias, A.; Campos, Y.; Arenas, J.; Novo-Rodríguez, M.I.; Eirís-Puñal, J. Congenital hydranencephalic-hydrocephalic syndrome associated with mitochondrial dysfunction. *J. Child Neurol.* **1999**, *14*, 131–135. [CrossRef] [PubMed]
159. Castro-Gago, M.; Pintos-Martínez, E.; Forteza-Vila, J.; Iglesias-Diz, M.; Ucieda-Somoza, R.; Silva-Villar, I.; Codesido-López, J.; Viso-Lorenzo, A.; Campos, Y.; Arenas, J.; et al. Congenital hydranencephalic-hydrocephalic syndrome with proliferative vasculopathy: A possible relation with mitochondrial dysfunction. *J. Child Neurol.* **2001**, *16*, 858–862. [CrossRef] [PubMed]
160. Kiaei, M. New hopes and challenges for treatment of neurodegenerative disorders: Great opportunities for young neuroscientists. *Basic Clin. Neurosci.* **2013**, *4*, 3–4. [PubMed]
161. Andreux, P.A.; Houtkooper, R.H.; Auwerx, J. Pharmacological approaches to restore mitochondrial function. *Nat. Rev. Drug Discov.* **2013**, *12*, 465–483. [CrossRef] [PubMed]

162. Timmers, S.; Konings, E.; Bilet, L.; Houtkooper, R.H.; van de Weijer, T.; Goossens, G.H.; Hoeks, J.; van der Krieken, S.; Ryu, D.; Kersten, S.; et al. Calorie restriction-like effects of 30 days of resveratrol supplementation on energy metabolism and metabolic profile in obese humans. *Cell Metab.* **2011**, *14*, 612–622. [CrossRef] [PubMed]
163. Douglas, P.M.; Dillin, A. Protein homeostasis and aging in neurodegeneration. *J. Cell Biol.* **2010**, *190*, 719–729. [CrossRef] [PubMed]
164. Lutz, A.K.; Exner, N.; Fett, M.E.; Schlehe, J.S.; Kloos, K.; Lämmermann, K.; Brunner, B.; Kurz-Drexler, A.; Vogel, F.; Reichert, A.S.; et al. Loss of parkin or PINK1 function increases Drp1-dependent mitochondrial fragmentation. *J. Biol. Chem.* **2009**, *284*, 22938–22951. [CrossRef] [PubMed]
165. Rappold, P.M.; Cui, M.; Grima, J.C.; Fan, R.Z.; de Mesy-Bentley, K.L.; Chen, L.; Zhuang, X.; Bowers, W.J.; Tieu, K. Drp1 inhibition attenuates neurotoxicity and dopamine release deficits in vivo. *Nat. Commun.* **2014**, *5*, 5244. [CrossRef] [PubMed]
166. Lackner, L.L.; Nunnari, J. Small molecule inhibitors of mitochondrial division: Tools that translate basic biological research into medicine. *Chem. Biol.* **2010**, *17*, 578–583. [CrossRef] [PubMed]
167. Wang, D.; Wang, J.; Bonamy, G.M.; Meeusen, S.; Brusch, R.G.; Turk, C.; Yang, P.; Schultz, P.G. A small molecule promotes mitochondrial fusion in mammalian cells. *Angew. Chem. Int. Ed. Engl.* **2012**, *51*, 9302–9305. [CrossRef] [PubMed]
168. Yue, W.; Chen, Z.; Liu, H.; Yan, C.; Chen, M.; Feng, D.; Wu, H.; Du, L.; Wang, Y.; Liu, J.; et al. A small natural molecule promotes mitochondrial fusion through inhibition of the deubiquitinase USP30. *Cell Res.* **2014**, *24*, 482–496. [CrossRef] [PubMed]
169. Cassidy-Stone, A.; Chipuk, J.E.; Ingerman, E.; Song, C.; Yoo, C.; Kuwana, T.; Kurth, M.J.; Shaw, J.T.; Hinshaw, J.E.; Green, D.R.; et al. Chemical inhibition of the mitochondrial division dynamin reveals its role in Bax/Bak-dependent mitochondrial outer membrane permeabilization. *Dev. Cell* **2008**, *14*, 193–204. [CrossRef] [PubMed]
170. Cui, M.; Tang, X.; Christian, W.V.; Yoon, Y.; Tieu, K. Perturbations in mitochondrial dynamics induced by human mutant PINK1 can be rescued by the mitochondrial division inhibitor mdivi-1. *J. Biol. Chem.* **2010**, *285*, 11740–11752. [CrossRef] [PubMed]
171. Bordt, E.A.; Clerc, P.; Roelofs, B.A.; Saladino, A.J.; Tretter, L.; Adam-Vizi, V.; Cherok, E.; Khalil, A.; Yadava, N.; Ge, S.X.; et al. The Putative Drp1 Inhibitor mdivi-1 Is a Reversible Mitochondrial Complex I Inhibitor that Modulates Reactive Oxygen Species. *Dev. Cell* **2017**, *40*, 583–594. [CrossRef] [PubMed]
172. Sherer, T.B.; Betarbet, R.; Testa, C.M.; Seo, B.B.; Richardson, J.R.; Kim, J.H.; Miller, G.W.; Yagi, T.; Matsuno-Yagi, A.; Greenamyre, J.T. Mechanism of toxicity in rotenone models of Parkinson's disease. *J. Neurosci.* **2003**, *23*, 10756–10764. [CrossRef] [PubMed]
173. Lezi, E.; Swerdlow, R.H. Mitochondria in neurodegeneration. *Adv. Exp. Med. Biol.* **2012**, *942*, 269–286. [CrossRef] [PubMed]
174. Witte, M.E.; Mahad, D.J.; Lassmann, H.; van Horssen, J. Mitochondrial dysfunction contributes to neurodegeneration in multiple sclerosis. *Trends Mol. Med.* **2014**, *20*, 179–187. [CrossRef] [PubMed]
175. Green, D.R.; Galluzzi, L.; Kroemer, G. Mitochondria and the autophagy-inflammation-cell death axis in organismal aging. *Science* **2011**, *333*, 1109–1112. [CrossRef] [PubMed]
176. Koentjoro, B.; Park, J.S.; Sue, C.M. Nix restores mitophagy and mitochondrial function to protect against PINK1/Parkin-related Parkinson's disease. *Sci. Rep.* **2017**, *7*, 44373. [CrossRef] [PubMed]
177. Chen, J. Heme oxygenase in neuroprotection: From mechanisms to therapeutic implications. *Rev. Neurosci.* **2014**, *25*, 269–280. [CrossRef] [PubMed]
178. Song, W.; Su, H.; Song, S.; Paudel, H.K.; Schipper, H.M. Over-expression of heme oxygenase-1 promotes oxidative mitochondrial damage in rat astroglia. *J. Cell Physiol.* **2006**, *206*, 655–663. [CrossRef] [PubMed]
179. Zukor, H.; Song, W.; Liberman, A.; Mui, J.; Vali, H.; Fillebeen, C.; Pantopoulos, K.; Wu, T.D.; Guerquin-Kern, J.L.; Schipper, H.M. HO-1-mediated macroautophagy: A mechanism for unregulated iron deposition in aging and degenerating neural tissues. *J. Neurochem.* **2009**, *109*, 776–791. [CrossRef] [PubMed]
180. Nitti, M.; Piras, S.; Brondolo, L.; Marinari, U.M.; Pronzato, M.A.; Furfaro, A.L. Heme Oxygenase 1 in the Nervous System: Does It Favor Neuronal Cell Survival or Induce Neurodegeneration? *Int. J. Mol. Sci.* **2018**, *19*, 2260. [CrossRef] [PubMed]
181. Schipper, H.M.; Gupta, A.; Szarek, W.A. Suppression of glial HO-1 activity as a potential neurotherapeutic intervention in AD. *Curr. Alzheimer Res.* **2009**, *6*, 424–430. [CrossRef] [PubMed]

182. Gupta, A.; Lacoste, B.; Pistell, P.J.; Pistel, P.J.; Ingram, D.K.; Hamel, E.; Alaoui-Jamali, M.A.; Szarek, W.A.; Vlahakis, J.Z.; Jie, S.; et al. Neurotherapeutic effects of novel HO-1 inhibitors in vitro and in a transgenic mouse model of Alzheimer's disease. *J. Neurochem.* **2014**, *131*, 778–790. [CrossRef] [PubMed]
183. Omori, C.; Motodate, R.; Shiraki, Y.; Chiba, K.; Sobu, Y.; Kimura, A.; Nakaya, T.; Kondo, H.; Kurumiya, S.; Tanaka, T.; et al. Facilitation of brain mitochondrial activity by 5-aminolevulinic acid in a mouse model of Alzheimer's disease. *Nutr. Neurosci.* **2017**, *20*, 538–546. [CrossRef] [PubMed]
184. Gomes, A.T.P.C.; Neves, M.G.P.M.; Cavaleiro, J.A.S. Cancer, Photodynamic Therapy and Porphyrin-Type Derivatives. *An. Acad. Bras. Cienc.* **2018**, *90*, 993–1026. [CrossRef] [PubMed]

12

Protective Role of Histidine Supplementation Against Oxidative Stress Damage in the Management of Anemia of Chronic Kidney Disease

Mayra Vera-Aviles, Eleni Vantana, Emmy Kardinasari, Ngat L. Koh and Gladys O. Latunde-Dada *

King's College London, Department of Nutritional Sciences, Faculty of Life Sciences and Medicine, Franklin-Wilkins Building, 150 Stamford Street, London SE1 9NH, UK; mayra.vera_aviles@kcl.ac.uk (M.V.-A.); el.vantana@outlook.com (E.V.); ekardinasari@gmail.com (E.K.); lea.koh@gmail.com (N.L.K.)

* Correspondence: yemisi.latunde-dada@kcl.ac.uk

Abstract: Anemia is a major health condition associated with chronic kidney disease (CKD). A key underlying cause of this disorder is iron deficiency. Although intravenous iron treatment can be beneficial in correcting CKD-associated anemia, surplus iron can be detrimental and cause complications. Excessive generation of reactive oxygen species (ROS), particularly by mitochondria, leads to tissue oxidation and damage to DNA, proteins, and lipids. Oxidative stress increase in CKD has been further implicated in the pathogenesis of vascular calcification. Iron supplementation leads to the availability of excess free iron that is toxic and generates ROS that is linked, in turn, to inflammation, endothelial dysfunction, and cardiovascular disease. Histidine is indispensable to uremic patients because of the tendency toward negative plasma histidine levels. Histidine-deficient diets predispose healthy subjects to anemia and accentuate anemia in chronic uremic patients. Histidine is essential in globin synthesis and erythropoiesis and has also been implicated in the enhancement of iron absorption from human diets. Studies have found that L-histidine exhibits antioxidant capabilities, such as scavenging free radicals and chelating divalent metal ions, hence the advocacy for its use in improving oxidative stress in CKD. The current review advances and discusses evidence for iron-induced toxicity in CKD and the mechanisms by which histidine exerts cytoprotective functions.

Keywords: histidine; iron; anemia; oxidative stress; kidney

---

1. Introduction

Chronic kidney disease (CKD) is a generic term that includes the majority of renal disorders. Anemia, an invariable consequence of CKD, is higher in patients with renal disease compared to the unaffected population (15.4% vs. 7.6%, respectively) globally according to the 2014 outcome of the National Health and Nutrition Examination Survey (NHANES) [1]. Judging by the glomerular filtrate rate, CKD is classified in stages from 1–5, with 5 being the last stage, also known as end-stage renal disease (ESRD) [2]. In the U.K., the prevalence of stages 3–5 CKD is estimated to be 9% of the adult population [3]. Approximately 50% of patients with CKD in the U.S. are reported to be anemic [4]. Observational studies also reported a 13% increased risk of hospitalizations for patients with low hematocrits [5,6], as well as 6% increased risk of cardiovascular events per 10 g/L decrease in hemoglobin (Hb), for patients with anemia in CKD [7]. Data from patients with hemodialysis from five

European countries showed that lower hemoglobin levels are associated with increased morbidity and mortality [8]. This result is of particular public health concern as anemia in CKD has been reported to significantly reduce quality of life compared to the general population, with Hb levels as the predictive factor [9]. Oxidative stress and chronic inflammation are hallmarks of CKD; the magnitude of the resultant adverse consequences ranges across the different stages of the manifestation of the disorder and depends on the nature of the therapy employed. The origin of oxidative stress in CKD is varied and includes toxicity induced by excess iron supplements, uremic toxins, and the burden imposed by the hemodialysis process and the equipment employed. Consequently, the inflammation that ensues is associated with elevated ferritin and hepcidin levels; the latter inhibits ferroportin, which blocks iron efflux into circulation. This results in low iron availability for erythropoiesis and hyporesponsiveness to iron and Erythropoietin Stimulating Agent (ESA) therapy. The complexity inherent in inflammation-induced elevated serum ferritin and hepcidin levels poses complications when setting predictive cut-off values for these biomarkers of iron deficiency anemia in CKD [10]. Hence, inflammatory confounders are a contentious issue attracting debate on consensus values for international guidelines on biomarkers of ferritin and hepcidin levels, as well as for iron and ESA dosage and routes of administration. Untreated anemia triggers several debilitating symptoms, such as lethargy, muscle fatigue, and deterioration of renal function. These culminate consequently in high prevalence of cardiovascular diseases, such as left ventricular hypertrophy and heart failure, which constitute the main causes of death in patients with CKD [11,12].

2. Anemia of Chronic Kidney Disease (ACKD)

Anemia is a common complication in CKD that increases in prevalence as the disease progresses [1]. Anemia is defined as Hb concentrations <13.0 g/dL in men and <12.0 g/dL in women [13]. Suboptimal levels of Hb and hematocrit in CKD patients are associated with declining survival rate [14,15]. This was evident in a population study that reported anemia as a critical factor in the development of cardiovascular disease (CVD) in CKD patients [16]. Consequently, CVDs such as heart failure and stroke have been implicated as major causes of mortality in CKD patients [11,12,17]. Anemia of CKD could also be due to multifactorial causes (Figure 1). Dysfunctional platelets, the shortening life span of red blood cells, iron deficiency, and inflammation are some of the factors that can trigger the onset of anemia [18]. The primary cause of anemia, however, is iron deficiency which may, in turn, be caused by low iron intake, low iron absorption, or disruption of body iron regulation. The damage that is caused to the kidney induces rapid activation of the immune system, and the inflammatory response, which stimulates IL-6 signal enhancement of hepcidin in the liver [19,20]. Inflammation inhibits erythropoiesis, affects erythropoietin (EPO) hyporesponsiveness [21], and reduces systemic circulation of iron levels by the production of hepcidin [22,23]. This response cascade indirectly contributes to the development of iron deficiency anemia (IDA) [24]. Excess hepcidin causes reduced circulation of iron in the plasma by a mechanism that involves the degradation of ferroportin, the iron efflux protein. Subsequently, iron release into the circulation from enterocytes and macrophages decreases [25,26] as shown in Figure 1. Levels of EPO decrease as a result of kidney damage and this culminates in lower erythroid cell production in the bone marrow. Bleeding during CKD causes loss of red blood cells leading to the development of anemia during CKD. Thus, the etiology of ACKD is a spectrum that involves both absolute and functional iron deficiency. The latter is compounded by an interplay of inflammation, tissue iron sequestration, and a hyporesponsiveness to ESA therapy [27]. Hypoxia-Inducible Factors (HIFs) that are secreted in the kidney during hypoxia can induce EPO production, and provide alternative therapy for (ACKD) [28]. Antibodies against hepcidin have been proposed as alternative approaches to increase iron absorption and iron efflux from the tissues [29].

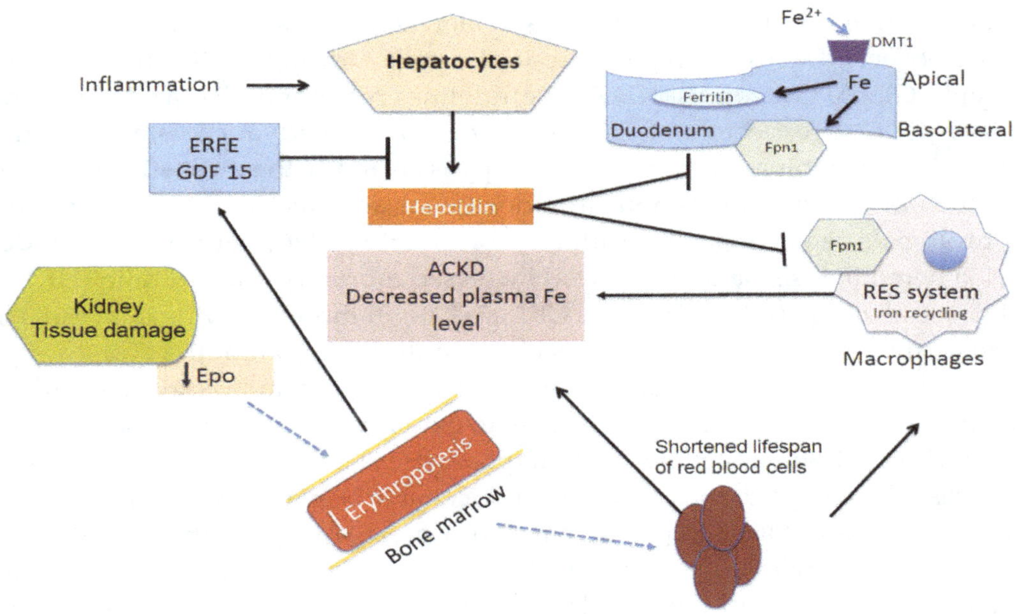

Figure 1. Iron metabolism in anemia of kidney disease. Hepcidin increases during inflammatory conditions and its clearance decreases in dysfunctional kidney cells. Fpn1 is degraded by hepcidin and, as a result, iron transport in the basolateral membrane of enterocytes reduces, as well as the mobilization of iron in macrophages, resulting in lower plasma levels of iron. The hepcidin level decreases during ineffective erythropoiesis and anemia by the actions of erythroid regulators erythroferrone (ERFE) and growth differentiation factor 15 (GDF15). EPO: Erythropoietin; Fpn1: Ferroportin; DMT1: Divalent Metal Transporter; and NTBI: Non-Transferrin Bound Iron.

3. Treatment of ACKD

Reduced production of red blood cell is proposed as the main cause of anemia in CKD patients. This arises from damage to the peritubular cells of the kidney, which produce erythropoietin (EPO), an essential hormone in erythropoiesis [30,31]. Erythropoietin induces the production and proliferation of erythrocytes; hence, a disruption in normal EPO levels causes anemia [32], as shown in Figure 1. Thus, the treatment for ACKD implies the administration of Erythropoiesis Stimulating Agents (ESAs). Recombinant human EPO (rHuEPO) is medically prescribed and several guidelines for promoting its efficacy in alleviating Hb levels have been reported [13,32,33].

The administration of rHuEPO is effective for correcting anemia and increasing hematocrit and reticulocyte count, although a concomitant increase in hypertension among the patients has been reported [34,35]. Currently, a Hb target range of 11.0 to 12.0 g/dL is recommended [36] because full normalization (Hb > 13 g/dL), according to Correction of Hemoglobin and Outcomes in Renal Insufficiency (CHOIR), is not prescribed due to increased cardiovascular events [37]. Additionally, in a post-hoc analysis of the CHOIR trial [38], increased mortality was found to be significantly associated with both the inability to achieve the Hb target and the use of high ESA doses. This was confirmed by a meta-analysis of 24 randomized controlled trials (RCTs), in which higher Hb targets resulted in increased hypertension risk (RR = 1.40, 95% confidence interval (CI) 1.11–1.75), stroke (RR = 1.73; 95% CI 1.31–2.29) and hospitalization (RR = 1.07, 95% CI 1.01–1.14) [6]. It was reported that rHuEPO induces hypo-responsiveness at high doses [39], and causes a greater risk of death due to the oxidative stress that exacerbates cardiovascular risk [40]. Recombinant HuEPO treatment is furthermore associated with increased blood pressure and blood clotting [41,42]. rHuEPO therapy is associated with iron deficiency as iron stores are largely transferred from the bone marrow to the erythroid progenitor cells due to enhanced erythropoiesis. Iron deficiency is observed in most hemodialysis patients arising from recurrent chronic blood losses. Thus, iron supplementation is often required to optimise or complement rHuEPO administration in the treatment of anemia in patients with CKD [18]. Consequently, if iron therapy is used alongside ESAs, significant increases in Hb levels and response are observed without the need to increase ESA dosage [43]. Thus, in practice, Kidney Disease Improving Global Outcomes (KDIGO) guidelines recommended a trial of intravenous iron to treat anemia in CKD, irrespective of ESA treatment [44]. In advanced stages of kidney disease, intravenous (IV) iron in combination with EPO therapy is currently the most effective treatment [44,45]. In light of this, the use of high intravenous iron doses was adopted in the U.S., despite the concerns raised by nephrologists regarding the resultant iron overload [46]. Supporting evidence from an analysis of 32,435 hemodialysis patients showed increased mortality (hazard ratio (HR) = 1.13, 95% CI 1.00–1.27) and hospitalization (HR = 1.12, 95% CI 1.07–1.18) in those receiving above 300 mg/month of intravenous iron compared to other patients receiving only 100 mg/month [47].

Although IV iron and rHuEPO led to improvement of hematological profiles, the risk of toxicity caused by excess iron predisposes patients to oxidative stress, inflammation, and pathogenic consequences [48,49]. Allergic reactions and anaphylactic shock, as well as oxidative stress that is related to cardiovascular complications and tissue injury, have been reported during the administration of IV iron supplementation [46,48,50]. The basis and mechanisms of the oxidative stress are not completely understood; however, excess iron from IV administration could cause iron overload and increase the levels of ROS in patients [12,51]. Also, IV iron supplementation raises levels of malondialdehyde (MDA), a biomarker of lipid peroxidation [52].

Several iron compounds including iron isomaltoside, iron sucrose, iron dextran, iron gluconate, or ferric carboxymaltose [53] are used for the treatment of ACKD. Intravenous iron formulations are colloidal suspensions, composed of a core of iron (iron-oxyhydroxide/oxide) surrounded by a carbohydrate shell [54]. The iron formulation varies in core size, affinity of bound iron to carbohydrate excipient, and electrovalence of iron, all of which influence the reactivity of iron [55].

Exposure of CKD patients to high concentrations of iron supplementation thus poses a potential risk of ROS generation with concomitant damage to DNA, proteins, or lipids [56]. Iron supplementation in patients with ACKD can subsequently result in iron overload, characterized by a "spill over" into hepatocytes if non-transferrin bound iron (NTBI) is present. Clinically relevant concentrations of NTBI would be expected if the iron-carrying capacity of transferrin is saturated [57]. Recommendations for iron management in CKD patient care are currently conflicting and is an ongoing process because of limited research evidence. A number of randomized controlled trials (RCTs) and observational studies have produced varying results on the effectiveness and adverse effects of iron or ESA supplementation. Variability or confounders, mostly associated with study design, have been identified [58] including type, dosage, duration or route of iron administration, population size, and the inherent variability within the baseline hematological status of patients.

4. Iron, Oxidative Stress, and Anemia

Iron (Fe), when supplied in excess, leads to oxidative stress in the mitochondria. Iron molecules trigger the initiation of the Fenton reaction and promote the formation of ROS, such as $O\cdot_2^-$, $OH\cdot$, and H_2O_2, as depicted in the equation: $Fe^{2+} + H_2O_2 \rightarrow Fe^{3+} + OH\cdot + OH^-$ [59]. These reactive species bind to macromolecules, such as lipids, proteins, and nucleic acids, causing lipid peroxidation and oxidative modifications of proteins and DNA [60]. Peroxidation of membrane lipids results in loss of membrane fluidity, elasticity, and disordered cellular functioning. Protein oxidation causes fragmentation of amino acid residues leading to cross-linkage and loss of protein configuration and functions. Oxidative damage of DNA causes mutation in DNA bases. These aberrations play major roles in cell death, ageing, and in degenerative diseases [61]. Observations in clinical trials showed a significant increase in the levels of MDA, a key oxidative stress marker, after IV iron infusion [62], and this is correlated with markers of early atherosclerosis [63]. Patients with CKD have a reduced mitochondrial DNA copy number, reduced energy production, and higher levels of stress markers [64]. Cytochrome c oxidase, an enzyme of the oxidative chain, is reduced in patients suffering from CKD in the final stages [65,66]. In addition, there are increasing concerns regarding the risk of iron therapy in potentially exacerbating oxidative stress, inflammation, and adverse cardiovascular outcomes from excess iron deposition in this population [11]. Atherosclerosis caused by oxidative damage, and evidenced by increased circulating mononuclear superoxide production and vascular cell adhesion molecule-1 (VCAM-1) and triggered by NADPH oxidase (NOx) and NF-kB activation in CKD patients, is associated with IV iron administration [67–70]. Against this evidence, some studies on the role of iron in CKD pathogenesis showed contradictory results [71]. Iron deposition in the liver of both humans [72] and rats [73] did not develop into cirrhosis, possibly because of iron sequestration into innocuous ferritin L and H subunits. Another mechanism that was proposed as a process that prevents iron overload in tissues such as the liver is the secretion of iron-loaded ferritin [74], possibly by an iron-regulated exocytosis efflux process [75] into blood circulation. However, other evidence revealed that high doses of iron were associated with high mortality due to iron-induced oxidative stress [68,71].

CKD patients, apart from a dysregulated iron metabolism, often exhibit hyperphosphatemia, which is associated with vascular calcification [69,76]. Paradoxically, heme iron, rather than being a pro-oxidant, was found to prevent the calcification and osteoblastic differentiation of human aortic smooth muscle cells (HSMCs) [77,78]. Evidence in this study attributed the inhibition of calcification to the upregulation of ferritin in the cells, even in the presence of phosphate. Heme releases Fe, CO, and biliverdin when catabolized. Thereby, iron performs the dual role of chelating phosphate and inducing the transcription of ferritin [79], particularly H-ferritin that exhibits high ferroxidase activity. Although the molecular mechanisms of vascular calcification require further investigation, emerging evidence indicates that ferritin might also function as a transcriptional regulator of gene expression in osteoblastic differentiation and β-globin synthesis [80].

5. Cytoprotective Functions of Histidine against Iron Toxicity during the Treatment of ACKD

L-histidine, a conditionally essential amino acid in adults, was found at significantly lower levels in patients with kidney disease and uremia [81,82]. Histidine, when administered orally or intravenously co-supplemented with iron, showed a positive response as judged by anemia markers, increased levels of plasma iron and Hb during anemia [83–85].

The beneficial effect of histidine is partly mediated by its ability to promote net nitrogen synthesis [84], which prevents negative nitrogen balance and loss of protein in CKD patients. Combined supplementation of IV iron with histidine rather than IV iron alone was more effective in treating anemia in CKD patients [86]. Additional evidence supports the beneficial role of histidine supplementation in uremic and dialysis patients, as a slight increase in Hb levels was triggered. Low histidine levels were shown to be correlated with high mortality (HR = 1.55, 95% CI 1.02, 2.40, $p < 0.05$), even after adjustments for age, sex, cardiovascular disease, inflammation, diabetes mellitus, serum albumin, and amino acid supplementation [81]. Histidine administration was negatively correlated ($p < 0.05$) with levels of 8-OHdG, an oxidative stress biomarker [81]. Histidine is known as an efficient scavenger of ROS [87], and its antioxidant properties have been advocated in the prevention of iron toxicity.

6. Antioxidant Function of Histidine against Oxidative Stress

The management of anemia of CKD presents a conundrum that arises from a role in the treatment of iron deficiency and in improvement of the resultant toxicity of excess iron. Endogenous and dietary antioxidants prevent, neutralize, and terminate chain reactions that produce ROS.

Studies by Halliwell and Wade identified that histidine could serve as an antioxidant as well as a buffer, similar to albumin in the plasma [88,89]. Hence, histidine could function as a buffer regulating free metal ion concentration, thereby providing a safe temporary transport for divalent metals before they are metabolized. In cardiovascular studies, histidine afforded protection to the cardiovascular system because of its ability to scavenge singlet oxygen and hydroxyl radicals in isolated hearts tissues that are predisposed to oxidative stress [90]. The scavenging of singlet oxygen by histidine was found to be significantly higher than that of tryptophan or methionine [89]. Moreover, histidine is suggested to be protective against oxidative stress in a drug model, reflected in its storage stability [91]. Histidine has been shown to have an inhibitory effect on H_2O_2-induced IL-8 secretion in Caco-2 and HT-29 cells [92]. Lipid peroxidation was considerably inhibited when histidine was added to ferric iron in vitro [93], suggesting that histidine formed a complex with ferric iron and prevented the formation of ferrous iron and the Fenton reaction [94]. Histidine quenches and scavenges hydroxyl radicals and singlet oxygen [89]. The intracellular concentration of histidine is higher than found in plasma [89,95], resulting in different cellular responses in the protection against ROS. Histidine and its dipeptides have also been associated with increased expression of catalase and glutathione peroxidase antioxidant enzymes [96,97]. Although histidine exerts a positive effect on the amino acid pool within the cell, the deprivation of histidine could specifically induce a decrease in enzymatic antioxidant defenses [98]. The use of histidine as a scavenger increases the defense of cells against oxidative damage [99]. Histidine supplementation was shown to enhance the expression and the activities of catalase and glutathione peroxidase (GPX), in response to ethanol-induced liver damage in mice [100]. Consequently, the potential resides in histidine to enhance enzymatic antioxidant activity during oxidative stress and inflammatory conditions in the cell [100–102].

A study of the cytoprotective effect of histidine on the nervous system was related to the activity of histidine in the transport of glutamine into mitochondria during edema and inflammatory conditions [97]. As L-histidine readily traverses the blood-brain barrier, supplementations with this amino acid were shown to increase both total nitric oxide synthases (NOS) and total antioxidant capacity, conferring protection against oxidative stress and encephalopathy in rats [103]. Moreover, histidine was reported to be a scavenger of the hydroxyl radical in a study conducted on rabbits [104]. The scavenging of singlet oxygen by histidine was further confirmed in rats [105]. Histidine is, therefore, regarded as an efficient scavenger of the both hydroxyl radical and singlet oxygen based on its antioxidant abilities [87], as well as possessing the capacity to chelate divalent metals such as iron [51,54,63].

Histidine was shown to protect against iron-induced oxidative stress in human embryonic kidney (HEK-293) cells (Figure 2). Cells were pre-treated with histidine at 100, 250, and 500 μM concentrations overnight, and then subjected to iron challenge with 20 μM of 8-hydroquinoline (8-HQ) and 50 μM of ferric ammonium citrate (FAC) for two hours. Histidine significantly protected cell viability in cultured HEK-293 cells at all histidine concentrations [106]. This finding confirms earlier results from the literature on the lowering of inflammation and oxidative stress by histidine in other cell culture models [92]. The molecular mechanisms by which histidine exerts the protective function against iron and oxidative stress require further investigation.

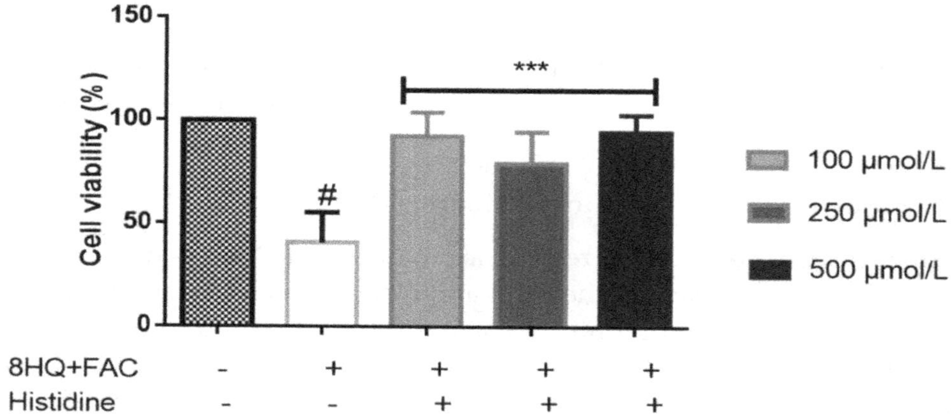

Figure 2. Protective effect of histidine against iron-induced stress in HEK-293 cells. Cells were treated with histidine (100–500 μM) overnight and subjected to 20 μM 8-hydroxyquinoline (8HQ) and 50 μM ferric ammonium citrate (FAC) for two hours, after which cell viability was performed using 3-(4,5-dimethylthiazol-2-yl)-2,5-diphenyltetrazolium bromide (MTT) assay. *** $p < 0.001$ between 8HQ + FAC and the treatments, # $p < 0.001$ between the control and iron treatment.

7. Metal Chelation Capacity of Histidine

Free histidine is an amino acid that is present in cells of the brain, skeletal muscle, and liver [100]. It has an imidazole ring that, in combination with the amino group, facilitates binding and chelation of other compounds. Histidine is also a constituent of some dipeptides such as carnosine, anserine and a precursor of the neurotransmitter histamine [89,96,107,108]. Notably, the iron-chelating property of carnosine has been ascribed to the imidazole ring of histidine [96,102,108]. Histidine is a proximal ligand of heme iron in the Hb molecule [109]. In equimolar solutions, divalent metals can interact with histidine via the amino, imidazole, or carboxyl moiety (Figure 3). This is probably highly specific and selective amongst different divalent metal ions. The formation and stability of most histidine-divalent metal complexes are favored by slightly acidic pH (pH < 5). The histidine molecule thus forms stable strong bonds with iron ions, displaying a bidentate and protonated activity on the primary amino-group at pH 5. Tridentate metal chelate can also form with histidine via the imidazole ring [110–112]. Histidine forms stable bidentate complexes in aqueous systems with Cu^{2+}, Fe^{2+}, and Ni^{2+} [112,113]. Incidentally, complexes of histidine with Zn^{2+}, Cu^{2+}, Ni^{2+}, or Co^{2+} have higher stability constants than with Fe^{2+}, and the binding stability is dependent on the binding moiety, temperature, and pH of the solution [112]. Histidine-divalent metal (Cu^{2+}, Zn^{2+}, and Ni^{2+}) complexes, in aqueous solutions, form with the imidazole and amine group at pH 6 [111]. The iron chelating property of histidine is therefore dependent on pH and the nature of the three possible interacting bonds with ligands (Figure 3). The pKa values of histidine in proteins range between pH 6 and pH 8. Consequently, side chains of histidine contribute to the buffering potentials of proteins such as Hb at the physiological pH of blood. A simulation of the titration curve of histidine reacting with ferrous iron, presented in Figure 4, shows that histidine at 1 mM forms a complex with iron at neutral pH; however, when the concentration of histidine is lowered 10 fold, the formation of the complex decreases and peaks at pH 8. This speciation plot shows that, at neutral pH, histidine, at high concentrations, can bind iron with high affinity; however, this reaction is not at the physiological concentration of histidine in tissues or plasma.

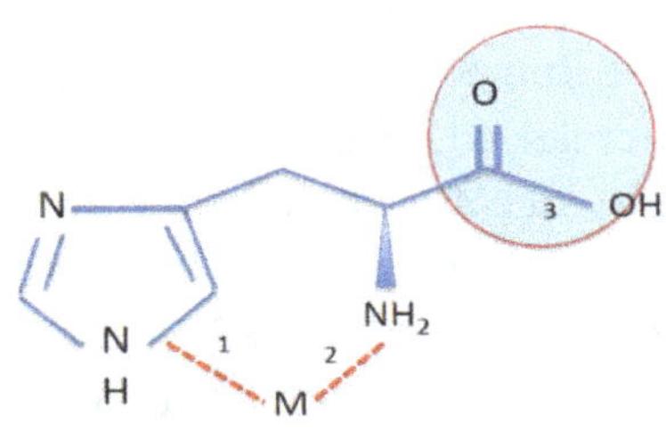

Figure 3. Structure of the histidine molecule showing the imidazole ring, amino, carboxyl groups, and metal ion (M) binding sites.

In vitro studies demonstrated that histidine is the most effective hydroxyl radical scavenger out of the several amino acids that were investigated [114]. The scavenging ability of histidine seems to involve a chelating mechanism that interferes with the redox reaction of metal ions producing hydroxyl radicals [89]. Nair et al. [115] reported that histidine displays a strong binding affinity to Fe^{3+} ions, thereby reducing the amount of ROS generated via the Fenton reaction, and protecting cells from damage due to iron overload [87]. In addition, histidine can interact directly with singlet oxygen through its imidazole ring [89]. Some other studies have shown, in contrast, that histidine may function as a pro-oxidant. Tachon reported that the enhancing effect of histidine on DNA degradation by ferric ions is dependent on the chelator/metal ratio, and is likely mediated by an oxidant such as ferrous-dioxygen-ferric chelate complex or a chelate-ferryl ion [116]. Evidence from studies to support the protective effect of histidine against oxidative stress remains both fragmentary and contradictory. This discrepancy is perhaps due to differences in experimental methodology and design; for example, the types of established cell lines, and histidine dosage employed in the studies.

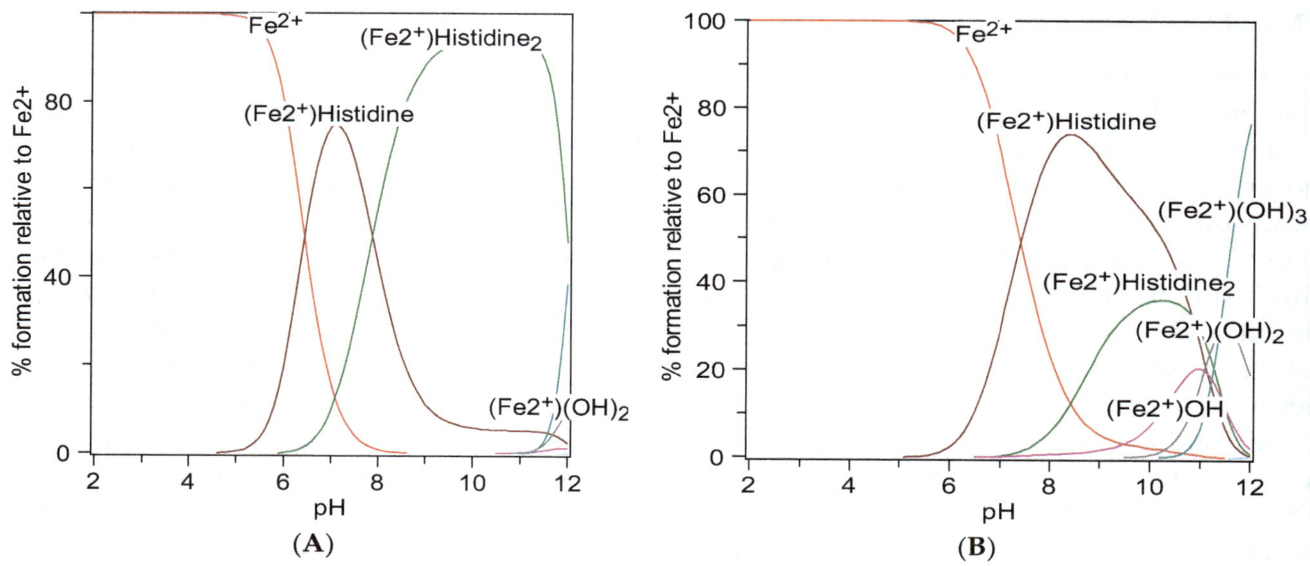

Figure 4. Speciation plots of histidine and ferrous (Fe^{2+}, Fe (II)) iron. Speciation plots with parameters of 50 μM Fe (II) and (**A**) 1 mM histidine or (**B**) 100 μM histidine.

The chelating property of histidine has been correlated with some physiological functions such as the capacity to increase iron uptake [117], as well as its ability to protect against ROS in the nervous system [92]. Histidine has the capacity to bind divalent metal ions (including those of copper, zinc, and iron) and enhance iron absorption [117,118]. The ligand formed by histidine possibly prevents iron precipitation, enhancing iron absorption in the intestine [118,119]. Histidine-containing peptides chelated iron for enhanced iron absorption in the segments of rat intestine [120]. This is, however, in contrast to an earlier finding in a human study in which histidine did not enhance iron absorption [121]. The ratio of histidine content in different peptides has been contradictorily reported regarding either its inorganic iron absorption or enhancing function [117].

Histidine has been associated with the capacity to chelate iron and enhance iron solubility in the duodenum, as ferrous iron is poorly soluble at neutral pH. By binding to histidine and other chelating compounds, the uptake of the metal increases [119]. The role of histidine in binding iron and increasing its uptake is debatable; the positive evidence suggested that the co-supplementation of histidine doses of about 100 mM could increase iron uptake in rats, and in combination with ascorbic acid, this could doubly enhance the positive effect of ascorbic acid [122]. This was also observed in cultured Caco-2 cells [123]. However, another study on intestinal cells and on humans did not report such increases of iron uptake upon histidine supplementation [121,124]. In food extracts, histidine has been found to increase inorganic iron solubility; however, these results arose from vegetables and meat extracts wherein the efficacy of histidine could have been confounded by the presence of other amino acids and peptides [117,125,126]. Histidine undoubtedly has the capacity to bind iron; however, as this reaction is pH-dependent, histidine might serve the important function of maintaining iron in soluble form to enhance iron bioavailability. The presence of other compounds or stronger metal chelators could influence the stability of the histidine-iron complex.

8. Anti-Inflammatory Potential of Histidine

As inflammation promotes iron disorders in anemia of chronic kidney disease, factors that increase or inhibit inflammatory signals are important in the manifestation of the disease symptoms. Inflammatory conditions or responses lead to the secretion of different cytokines, such as interleukin 6 (IL-6), interleukin 8 (IL-8), interleukin-1beta (IL-1b), as well as tumor necrosis factor-alpha (TNF-α) [92]. The physiological effects of histidine as an antioxidant have been associated with the inhibition of the secretion of some of these pro-inflammatory biomarkers, particularly during chronic diseases [89].

Liu et al. [100] reported that mice fed with histidine (at 0.5, 1, or 2 g/L) after the induction of ethanol hepatotoxicity had lower levels of the inflammation markers IL-6, c-reactive protein (CRP), and TNF-a. Histidine suppressed the accumulation of IL-6 and TNF-α mRNA in a dose-dependent manner. This indicates that histidine is not only a scavenger of ROS but could directly affect the regulation of pro-inflammatory cytokines [100]. A similar effect was found in cultured cells, in which histidine protected Caco-2 cells in a dose-dependent manner against hydrogen peroxide-induced damage [89]. Histidine, apart from reducing morphological damage in these cells, suppressed the secretion of IL-8 as well. This outcome is presumably due to the inhibition of signals for TNF-α and NF-kβ to activate transcriptional regulation of IL-8 [92]. Down-regulation of IL-6 and TNF-α by histidine has been reported in a diabetic mouse model [127]. The inhibition of pro-inflammatory cytokines by histidine is linked to its potential to increase the amino acid pool and the antioxidant status of the cells [107]. These changes contribute to the attenuation of ROS in tissues and organs. Histidine was reported to alleviate clinical symptoms and protect mice from intestinal, nervous, and cardiovascular damage [89]. These effects are possibly associated with the anti-inflammatory properties of histidine. Consequently, histidine administration could be an option for reducing and preventing oxidative stress in inflammatory conditions in chronic diseases. Dietary supplementation with histidine could be protective against oxidative damage, arising from the scavenging activity and anti-inflammatory effects of this amino acid in cells and tissues [127].

Arginine is another amino acid that exhibits antioxidant properties as a substrate in nitric oxide (NO) biosynthesis and was shown to be beneficial to kidney functions in both in vivo and in vitro models [128,129]. As well as other histidine dipeptides, carnosine also scavenges ROS and was reported to be beneficial to CKD patients [130].

9. Conclusions

Anemia of chronic kidney disease is a worldwide public health problem, with a constantly-increasing trend in both developed and developing countries. Iron supplementation treatment of ACKD leads to oxidative damage that is associated with iron overload and pro-inflammatory conditions. Co-supplementation with histidine, could have an ameliorating effect against oxidative damage in chronic kidney disease. Histidine can protect against iron overload and oxidative stress caused by CKD, as demonstrated with the Fenton substrate in the HK-2 cell model. The molecular mechanisms of the cytoprotection conferred by histidine are based on its capacity and potential as a metal chelator as well as its ability to scavenge oxygen radicals. Histidine can also function intracellularly to induce enzymatic antioxidant and anti-inflammatory activities in tissues and organs in different disorders [113,114]. The imidazole ring of histidine, as well as binding singlet oxygen molecules, can bind divalent metal ions; however, the effects of pH and histidine concentration that maintains iron in solution have only been clearly demonstrated in cultured cells and in animal models. It remains for these effects to be demonstrated in human subjects. The iron quenching capacity appears to be related to the reactive ability of the imidazole ring of histidine in extracellular solutions. No clear evidence currently exists for the localization of histidine-iron bound complexes or chelates intracellularly.

Further studies are required to clearly delineate the molecular mechanisms by which histidine attenuates oxidative stress damage attendant upon iron toxicity in kidney cells and specific models during the treatment of ACKD.

Author Contributions: G.O.L.-D. and M.V.A. wrote the manuscript, M.V.A. performed the experiments and E.V., E.K., and N.K.L. contributed to the review of literature.

Acknowledgments: We thank Yu-Lin Chen and Robert Hider for their assistance with histidine chemistry.

References

1. Stauffer, M.E.; Fan, T. Prevalence of anemia in chronic kidney disease in the united states. *PLoS ONE* **2014**, *9*, e84943. [CrossRef] [PubMed]
2. Macdougall, I.C.; Bircher, A.J.; Eckardt, K.-U.; Obrador, G.T.; Pollock, C.A.; Stenvinkel, P.; Swinkels, D.W.; Wanner, C.; Weiss, G.; Chertow, G.M. Iron management in chronic kidney disease: Conclusions from a "kidney disease: Improving global outcomes" (KDIGO) controversies conference. *Kidney Int.* **2016**, *89*, 28–39. [CrossRef] [PubMed]
3. National Health System. *Diabetes with Kidney Disease: Key Facts*; Diabetes Kindey Care, Ed.; National Health System England: London, UK, 2011.
4. McClellan, W.; Aronoff, S.L.; Bolton, W.K.; Hood, S.; Lorber, D.L.; Tang, K.L.; Tse, T.F.; Wasserman, B.; Leiserowitz, M. The prevalence of anemia in patients with chronic kidney disease. *Curr. Med. Res. Opin.* **2004**, *20*, 1501–1510. [CrossRef] [PubMed]
5. Khan, S.S.; Kazmi, W.H.; Abichandani, R.; Tighiouart, H.; Pereira, B.J.G.; Kausz, A.T. Health care utilization among patients with chronic kidney disease. *Kidney Int.* **2002**, *62*, 229–236. [CrossRef] [PubMed]
6. Jing, Z.; Wei-jie, Y.; Nan, Z.; Yi, Z.; Ling, W. Hemoglobin targets for chronic kidney disease patients with anemia: A systematic review and meta-analysis. *PLoS ONE* **2012**, *7*, e43655. [CrossRef] [PubMed]
7. Levin, A.; Singer, J.; Thompson, C.R.; Ross, H.; Lewis, M. Prevalent left ventricular hypertrophy in the predialysis population: Identifying opportunities for intervention. *Am. J. Kidney Dis.* **1996**, *27*, 347–354. [CrossRef]
8. Locatelli, F.; Pisoni, R.L.; Combe, C.; Bommer, J.; Andreucci, V.E.; Piera, L.; Greenwood, R.; Feldman, H.I.; Port, F.K.; Held, P.J. Anaemia in haemodialysis patients of five european countries: Association with morbidity and mortality in the dialysis outcomes and practice patterns study (DOPPS). *Nephrol. Dial. Transplant.* **2004**, *19*, 121–132. [CrossRef] [PubMed]
9. Hansen, R.A.; Chin, H.; Blalock, S.; Joy, M.S. Predialysis chronic kidney disease: Evaluation of quality of life in clinic patients receiving comprehensive anemia care. *Res. Soc. Adm. Pharm.* **2009**, *5*, 143–153. [CrossRef] [PubMed]
10. Ueda, N.; Takasawa, K. Impact of inflammation on ferritin, hepcidin and the management of iron deficiency anemia in chronic kidney disease. *Nutrients* **2018**, *10*, 1173. [CrossRef] [PubMed]
11. Macdougall, I.C. Anaemia of chronic kidney disease. *Medicine* **2007**, *35*, 457–460. [CrossRef]
12. Babitt, J.L.; Lin, H.Y. Mechanisms of anemia in CKD. *J. Am. Soc. Nephrol.* **2012**, *23*, 1631–1634. [CrossRef] [PubMed]
13. Locatelli, F.; Bárány, P.; Covic, A.; De Francisco, A.; Del Vecchio, L.; Goldsmith, D.; Hörl, W.; London, G.; Vanholder, R.; Van Biesen, W.; et al. Kidney disease: Improving global outcomes guidelines on anaemia management in chronic kidney disease: A european renal best practice position statement. *Nephrol. Dial. Transplant.* **2013**, *28*, 1346–1359. [CrossRef] [PubMed]
14. Ofsthun, N.; Labrecque, J.; Lacson, E.; Keen, M.; Lazarus, J.M. The effects of higher hemoglobin levels on mortality and hospitalization in hemodialysis patients. *Kidney Int.* **2003**, *63*, 1908–1914. [CrossRef] [PubMed]
15. Phrommintikul, A.; Haas, S.J.; Elsik, M.; Krum, H. Mortality and target haemoglobin concentrations in anaemic patients with chronic kidney disease treated with erythropoietin: A meta-analysis. *Lancet* **2007**, *369*, 381–388. [CrossRef]
16. Abramson, J.L.; Jurkovitz, C.T.; Vaccarino, V.; Weintraub, W.S.; Mcclellan, W. Chronic kidney disease, anemia, and incident stroke in a middle-aged, community-based population: The aric study. *Kidney Int.* **2003**, *64*, 610–615. [CrossRef] [PubMed]
17. Malik, J. Heart disease in chronic kidney disease – Review of the mechanisms and the role of dialysis access. *J. Vasc. Access* **2018**, *19*, 3–11. [CrossRef] [PubMed]
18. Dull, R.B.; Davis, E. Heme iron polypeptide for the management of anaemia of chronic kidney disease. *J. Clin. Pharm. Ther.* **2015**, *40*, 386–390. [CrossRef] [PubMed]
19. Wang, H.; Li, H.; Jiang, X.; Shi, W.; Shen, Z.; Li, M. Hepcidin is directly regulated by insulin and plays an important role in iron overload in streptozotocin-induced diabetic rats. *Diabetes* **2014**, *63*, 1506–1518. [CrossRef] [PubMed]
20. Weiss, G.; Goodnough, L.T. Anemia of chronic disease. *N. Engl. J. Med.* **2005**, *352*, 1011–1023. [CrossRef] [PubMed]

21. De Francisco, A.L.M.; Stenvinkel, P.; Vaulont, S. Inflammation and its impact on anaemia in chronic kidney disease: From haemoglobin variability to hyporesponsiveness. *NDT Plus* **2009**, *2*, i18–i26. [CrossRef] [PubMed]
22. Silverstein, D.M. Inflammation in chronic kidney disease: Role in the progression of renal and cardiovascular disease. *Pediatr. Nephrol.* **2009**, *24*, 1445–1452. [CrossRef] [PubMed]
23. Atkinson, M.A.; White, C.T. Hepcidin in anemia of chronic kidney disease: Review for the pediatric nephrologist. *Pediatr. Nephrol.* **2012**, *27*, 33–40. [CrossRef] [PubMed]
24. Weinstein, D.A.; Roy, C.N.; Fleming, M.D.; Loda, M.F.; Wolfsdorf, J.I.; Andrews, N.C. Inappropriate expression of hepcidin is associated with iron refractory anemia: Implications for the anemia of chronic disease. *Blood* **2002**, *100*, 3776–3781. [CrossRef] [PubMed]
25. Nemeth, E.; Tuttle, M.S.; Powelson, J.; Vaughn, M.B.; Donovan, A.; McVey Ward, D.; Ganz, T.; Kaplan, J. Hepcidin regulates cellular iron efflux by binding to ferroportin and inducing its internalization. *Science* **2004**, *306*, 2090–2093. [CrossRef] [PubMed]
26. Young, B.; Zaritsky, J. Hepcidin for clinicians. *Clin. J. Am. Soc. Nephrol.* **2009**, *4*, 1384–1387. [CrossRef] [PubMed]
27. Goodnough, L.T.; Nemeth, E.; Ganz, T. Detection, evaluation, and management of iron-restricted erythropoiesis. *Blood* **2010**, *116*, 4754–4761. [CrossRef] [PubMed]
28. Locatelli, F.; Fishbane, S.; Block, G.A.; Macdougall, I.C. Targeting hypoxia-inducible factors for the treatment of anemia in chronic kidney disease patients. *Am. J. Nephrol.* **2017**, *45*, 187–199. [CrossRef] [PubMed]
29. Gummer, J.; Trengove, R.; Pascoe, E.M.; Badve, S.V.; Cass, A.; Clarke, P.; McDonald, S.P.; Morrish, A.T.; Pedagogos, E.; Perkovic, V.; et al. Association between serum hepcidin-25 and primary resistance to erythropoiesis-stimulating agents in chronic kidney disease: A secondary analysis of the hero trial. *Nephrology* **2017**, *22*, 548–554. [CrossRef] [PubMed]
30. Lacombe, C.; Da Silva, J.L.; Bruneval, P.; Fournier, J.G.; Wendling, F.; Casadevall, N.; Camilleri, J.P.; Bariety, J.; Varet, B.; Tambourin, P. Peritubular cells are the site of erythropoietin synthesis in the murine hypoxic kidney. *J. Clin. Investig.* **1988**, *81*, 620–623. [CrossRef] [PubMed]
31. Maxwell, P.H.; Osmond, M.K.; Pugh, C.W.; Heryet, A.; Nicholls, L.G.; Tan, C.C.; Doe, B.G.; Ferguson, D.J.P.; Johnson, M.H.; Ratcliffe, P.J. Identification of the renal erythropoietin-producing cells using transgenic mice. *Kidney Int.* **1993**, *44*, 1149–1162. [CrossRef] [PubMed]
32. Koury, M.J.; Haase, V.H. Anaemia in kidney disease: Harnessing hypoxia responses for therapy. *Nat. Rev. Nephrol.* **2015**, *11*, 394–410. [CrossRef] [PubMed]
33. Kopple, J.D. The national kidney foundation k/doqi clinical practice guidelines for dietary protein intake for chronic dialysis patients. *Am. J. Kidney Dis.* **2001**, *38*, S68–S73. [CrossRef] [PubMed]
34. Apsangikar, P.; Chaudhry, S.; Naik, M.; Deoghare, S.; Joseph, J. Comparative efficacy and safety of biosimilar darbepoetin alfa in adults with anemia of chronic kidney disease. *Indian J. Transplant.* **2018**, *12*, 30–34. [CrossRef]
35. Locatelli, F.; Covic, A.; Eckardt, K.-U.; Wiecek, A.; Vanholder, R. Anaemia management in patients with chronic kidney disease: A position statement by the anaemiaworking group of european renal best practice (ERBP). *Nephrol Dial Transplant.* **2009**, *24*, 348–354. [CrossRef] [PubMed]
36. National Clinical Guideline Centre. *Anaemia Management in Chronic Kidney Disease: Partial Update 2015*; NICE Guideline, No. 8. Royal College of Physicians (UK); National Clinical Guideline Centre: London, UK, 2015.
37. Singh, A.K.; Szczech, L.; Tang, K.L.; Barnhart, H.; Sapp, S.; Wolfson, M.; Reddan, D. Correction of anemia with epoetin alfa in chronic kidney disease. *N. Engl. J. Med.* **2006**, *355*, 2085–2098. [CrossRef] [PubMed]
38. Szczech, L.A.; Barnhart, H.X.; Inrig, J.K.; Reddan, D.N.; Sapp, S.; Califf, R.M.; Patel, U.D.; Singh, A.K. Secondary analysis of the choir trial epoetin-alpha dose and achieved hemoglobin outcomes. *Kidney Int.* **2008**, *74*, 791–798. [CrossRef] [PubMed]
39. Singh, A.K. The controversy surrounding hemoglobin and erythropoiesis-stimulating agents: What should we do now? *Am. J. Kidney Dis.* **2008**, *52*, S5–S13. [CrossRef] [PubMed]
40. Vaziri, N.D.; Zhou, X.J. Potential mechanisms of adverse outcomes in trials of anemia correction with erythropoietin in chronic kidney disease. *Nephrol. Dial. Transplant.* **2009**, *24*, 1082–1088. [CrossRef] [PubMed]
41. Krapf, R.; Hulter, H.N. Arterial hypertension induced by erythropoietin and erythropoiesis-stimulating agents (ESA). *Clin. J. Am. Soc. Nephrol.* **2009**, *4*, 470–480. [CrossRef] [PubMed]

42. Pfeffer, M.A.; Burdmann, E.A.; Chen, C.-Y.; Cooper, M.E.; de Zeeuw, D.; Eckardt, K.-U.; Feyzi, J.M.; Ivanovich, P.; Kewalramani, R.; Levey, A.S.; et al. A trial of darbepoetin alfa in type 2 diabetes and chronic kidney disease. *N. Engl. J. Med.* **2009**, *361*, 2019–2032. [CrossRef] [PubMed]
43. Coyne, D.W.; Kapoian, T.; Suki, W.; Singh, A.K.; Moran, J.E.; Dahl, N.V.; Rizkala, A.R. Ferric gluconate is highly efficacious in anemic hemodialysis patients with high serum ferritin and low transferrin saturation: Results of the dialysis patients' response to iv iron with elevated ferritin (drive) study. *J. Am. Soc. Nephrol.* **2007**, *18*, 975–984. [CrossRef] [PubMed]
44. Kidney Disease Improving Global Outcomes (KDIGO). Chapter 2: Use of iron to treat anemia in CKD. *Kidney Int. Suppl.* **2012**, *2*, 292–298. [CrossRef] [PubMed]
45. Ribeiro, S.; Belo, L.; Reis, F.; Santos-Silva, A. Iron therapy in chronic kidney disease: Recent changes, benefits and risks. *Blood Rev.* **2016**, *30*, 65–72. [CrossRef] [PubMed]
46. Del Vecchio, L.; Longhi, S.; Locatelli, F. Safety concerns about intravenous iron therapy in patients with chronic kidney disease. *Clin. Kidney J.* **2016**, *9*, 260–267. [CrossRef] [PubMed]
47. Bailie, G.R.; Larkina, M.; Goodkin, D.A.; Li, Y.; Pisoni, R.L.; Bieber, B.; Mason, N.; Tong, L.; Locatelli, F.; Marshall, M.R.; et al. Data from the dialysis outcomes and practice patterns study validate an association between high intravenous iron doses and mortality. *Kidney Int* **2015**, *87*, 162–168. [CrossRef] [PubMed]
48. Slotki, I.; Cabantchik, Z.I. The labile side of iron supplementation in CKD. *J. Am. Soc. Nephrol.* **2015**, *26*, 2612–2619. [CrossRef] [PubMed]
49. Macdougall, I.C.; Geisser, P. Use of intravenous iron supplementation in chronic kidney disease. An update. *Iran. J. Kidney Dis.* **2013**, *7*, 9–22. [PubMed]
50. Shah, S.V.; Rajapurkar, M.M.; Baliga, R. The role of catalytic iron in acute kidney injury. *Clin. J. Am. Soc. Nephrol.* **2011**, *6*, 2329–2331. [CrossRef] [PubMed]
51. Elliott, S.; Sinclair, A.; Collins, H.; Rice, L.; Jelkmann, W. Progress in detecting cell-surface protein receptors The erythropoietin receptor example. *Ann. Hematol.* **2014**, *93*, 181–192. [CrossRef] [PubMed]
52. Connor, J.R.; Zhang, X.; Nixon, A.M.; Webb, B.; Perno, J.R. Comparative evaluation of nephrotoxicity and management by macrophages of intravenous pharmaceutical iron formulations. *PLoS ONE* **2015**, *10*, e0125272. [CrossRef] [PubMed]
53. Geisser, P.; Burckhardt, S. The pharmacokinetics and pharmacodynamics of iron preparations. *Pharmaceutics* **2011**, *3*, 12. [CrossRef] [PubMed]
54. Kalra, P.A.; Bhandari, S. Efficacy and safety of iron isomaltoside (monofer(®)) in the management of patients with iron deficiency anemia. *Int. J. Nephrol. Renov. Dis.* **2016**, *9*, 53–64. [CrossRef] [PubMed]
55. Gupta, A.; Pratt, R.D.; Crumbliss, A.L. Ferrous iron content of intravenous iron formulations. *BioMetals* **2016**, *29*, 411–415. [CrossRef] [PubMed]
56. Locatelli, F.; Mazzaferro, S.; Yee, J. Iron therapy challenges for the treatment of nondialysis ckd patients. *Clin. J. Am. Soc. Nephrol.* **2016**, *11*, 1269–1280. [CrossRef] [PubMed]
57. Wish, J.B.; Aronoff, G.R.; Bacon, B.R.; Brugnara, C.; Eckardt, K.U.; Ganz, T.; Macdougall, I.C.; Núñez, J.; Perahia, A.J.; Wood, J.C. Positive iron balance in chronic kidney disease: How much is too much and how to tell? *Am. J. Nephrol.* **2018**, *47*, 72–83. [CrossRef] [PubMed]
58. Macdougall, I.C. Intravenous iron therapy in patients with chronic kidney disease: Recent evidence and future directions. *Clin. Kidney J.* **2017**, *10*, i16–i24. [CrossRef] [PubMed]
59. Kruszewski, M. Labile iron pool: The main determinant of cellular response to oxidative stress. *Mutat. Res. Fundam. Mol. Mech. Mutagen.* **2003**, *531*, 81–92. [CrossRef]
60. Meneghini, R. Iron homeostasis, oxidative stress, and DNA damage. *Free Radic. Biol. Med.* **1997**, *23*, 783–792. [CrossRef]
61. Small, D.M.; Coombes, J.S.; Bennett, N.; Johnson, D.W.; Gobe, G.C. Oxidative stress, anti-oxidant therapies and chronic kidney disease. *Nephrology* **2012**, *17*, 311–321. [CrossRef] [PubMed]
62. Lim, P.-S.; Wei, Y.-H.; Yu, Y.L.; Kho, B. Enhanced oxidative stress in haemodialysis patients receiving intravenous iron therapy. *Nephrol. Dial. Transplant.* **1999**, *14*, 2680–2687. [CrossRef] [PubMed]
63. Drueke, T.; Witko-Sarsat, V.; Massy, Z.; Descamps-Latscha, B.; Guerin, A.P.; Marchais, S.J.; Gausson, V.; London, G.M. Iron therapy, advanced oxidation protein products, and carotid artery intima-media thickness in end-stage renal disease. *Circulation* **2002**, *106*, 2212–2217. [CrossRef] [PubMed]
64. Malik, A.N.; Shahni, R.; Iqbal, M.M. Increased peripheral blood mitochondrial DNA in type 2 diabetic patients with nephropathy. *Diabetes Res. Clin. Pract.* **2009**, *86*, e22–e24. [CrossRef] [PubMed]

65. Malik, A.N.; Czajka, A. Is mitochondrial DNA content a potential biomarker of mitochondrial dysfunction? *Mitochondrion* **2013**, *13*, 481–492. [CrossRef] [PubMed]
66. Granata, S.; Dalla Gassa, A.; Tomei, P.; Lupo, A.; Zaza, G. Mitochondria: A new therapeutic target in chronic kidney disease. *Nutr. Metab.* **2015**, *12*, 49. [CrossRef] [PubMed]
67. Kuo, K.-L.; Hung, S.-C.; Lin, Y.-P.; Tang, C.-F.; Lee, T.-S.; Lin, C.-P.; Tarng, D.-C. Intravenous ferric chloride hexahydrate supplementation induced endothelial dysfunction and increased cardiovascular risk among hemodialysis patients. *PLoS ONE* **2012**, *7*, e50295. [CrossRef] [PubMed]
68. Kuo, K.-L.; Hung, S.-C.; Lee, T.-S.; Tarng, D.-C. Iron sucrose accelerates early atherogenesis by increasing superoxide production and upregulating adhesion molecules in ckd. *J. Am. Soc. Nephrol.* **2014**, *25*, 2596–2606. [CrossRef] [PubMed]
69. Neven, E.; De Schutter, T.M.; Behets, G.J.; Gupta, A.; D'Haese, P.C. Iron and vascular calcification. Is there a link? *Nephrol. Dial. Transplant.* **2011**, *26*, 1137–1145. [CrossRef] [PubMed]
70. Nakanishi, T.; Kuragano, T.; Nanami, M.; Nagasawa, Y.; Hasuike, Y. Misdistribution of iron and oxidative stress in chronic kidney disease. *Free Radic. Biol. Med.* **2018**, in press. [CrossRef] [PubMed]
71. Kawada, S.; Nagasawa, Y.; Kawabe, M.; Ohyama, H.; Kida, A.; Kato-Kogoe, N.; Nanami, M.; Hasuike, Y.; Kuragano, T.; Kishimoto, H.; et al. Iron-induced calcification in human aortic vascular smooth muscle cells through interleukin-24 (il-24), with/without tnf-alpha. *Sci. Rep.* **2018**, *8*, 658. [CrossRef] [PubMed]
72. Eschbach, J.W.; Adamson, J.W. Iron overload in renal failure patients: Changes since the introduction of erythropoietin therapy. *Kidney Int.* **1999**, *55*, s-35–S-43. [CrossRef]
73. Malik, I.A.; Wilting, J.; Ramadori, G.; Naz, N. Reabsorption of iron into acutely damaged rat liver: A role for ferritins. *World J. Gastroenterol.* **2017**, *23*, 7347–7358. [CrossRef] [PubMed]
74. Ghosh, S.; Hevi, S.; Chuck, S.L. Regulated secretion of glycosylated human ferritin from hepatocytes. *Blood* **2004**, *103*, 2369–2376. [CrossRef] [PubMed]
75. Tran, T.N.; Eubanks, S.K.; Schaffer, K.J.; Zhou, C.Y.J.; Linder, M.C. Secretion of ferritin by rat hepatoma cells and its regulation by inflammatory cytokines and iron. *Blood* **1997**, *90*, 4979–4986. [PubMed]
76. Giachelli, C.M. Vascular calcification: In vitro evidence for the role of inorganic phosphate. *J. Am. Soc. Nephrol.* **2003**, *14*, S300–S304. [CrossRef] [PubMed]
77. Zarjou, A.; Jeney, V.; Arosio, P.; Poli, M.; Antal-Szalmás, P.; Agarwal, A.; Balla, G.; Balla, J. Ferritin prevents calcification and osteoblastic differentiation of vascular smooth muscle cells. *J. Am. Soc. Nephrol.* **2009**, *20*, 1254–1263. [CrossRef] [PubMed]
78. Zarjou, A.; Jeney, V.; Arosio, P.; Poli, M.; Zavaczki, E.; Balla, G.; Balla, J. Ferritin ferroxidase activity: A potent inhibitor of osteogenesis. *J. Bone Miner. Res.* **2010**, *25*, 164–172. [CrossRef] [PubMed]
79. Arosio, P.; Levi, S. Ferritin, iron homeostasis, and oxidative damage. *Free Radic. Biol. Med.* **2002**, *33*, 457–463. [CrossRef]
80. Broyles, R.H.; Belegu, V.; DeWitt, C.R.; Shah, S.N.; Stewart, C.A.; Pye, Q.N.; Floyd, R.A. Specific repression of β-globin promoter activity by nuclear ferritin. *Proc. Natl. Acad. Sci. USA* **2001**, *98*, 9145–9150. [CrossRef] [PubMed]
81. Watanabe, M.; Suliman, M.E.; Qureshi, A.R.; Garcia-Lopez, E.; Bárány, P.; Heimbürger, O.; Stenvinkel, P.; Lindholm, B. Consequences of low plasma histidine in chronic kidney disease patients: Associations with inflammation, oxidative stress, and mortality. *Am. J. Clin. Nutr.* **2008**, *87*, 1860–1866. [CrossRef] [PubMed]
82. Kopple, J.D.; Swendseid, M.E. Evidence that histidine is an essential amino-acid in normal and chronically uremic man. *J. Clin. Investig.* **1975**, *55*, 881–891. [CrossRef] [PubMed]
83. Jontofsohn, R.; Trivisas, G.; Katz, N.; Kiuthe, I. Amino acid content of erythrocytes in uremia. *Am. J. Clin. Nutr.* **1978**, *31*, 1956–1960. [CrossRef] [PubMed]
84. Bergström, J.; Furst, P.; Josephson, B.; Norée, L.-O. Improvement of nitrogen balance in a uremic patient by the addition of histidine to essential amino acid solutions given intravenously. *Life Sci.* **1970**, *9*, 787–794. [CrossRef]
85. Blumenkrantz, M.J.; Shapiro, D.J.; Swendseid, M.E.; Kopple, J.D. Histidine supplementation for treatment of anaemia of uraemia. *Br. Med. J.* **1975**, *2*, 530–533. [CrossRef] [PubMed]
86. Jontofsohn, R.; Heinze, V.; Katz, N.; Stuber, U.; Wilke, H.; Kluthe, R. Histidine and iron supplementation in dialysis and pre-dialysis patient. *Proc. Eur. Dial. Transpl. Assoc.* **1974**, *11*, 391–397.
87. Kaplan, P.; Matejovicova, M.; Herijgers, P.; Flameng, W. Effect of free radical scavengers on myocardial

function and Na^+, K^+-atpase activity in stunned rabbit myocardium. *Scand. Cardiovasc. J.* **2005**, *39*, 213–219. [CrossRef] [PubMed]

88. Halliwell, B. How to characterize a biological antioxidant. *Free Radic. Res. Commun.* **1990**, *9*, 1–32. [CrossRef] [PubMed]
89. Wade, A.M.; Tucker, H.N. Antioxidant characteristics of L-histidine. *J. Nutr. Biochem.* **1998**, *9*, 308–315. [CrossRef]
90. Pisarenko, O.I. Mechanisms of myocardial protection by amino acids: Facts and hypotheses. *Clin. Exp. Pharmacol. Physiol.* **1996**, *23*, 627–633. [CrossRef] [PubMed]
91. Lim, J.Y.; Kim, N.A.; Lim, D.G.; Kim, K.H.; Hada, S.; Jeong, S.H. Evaluation of etanercept degradation under oxidative stress and potential protective effects of various amino acids. *Int. J. Pharm.* **2015**, *492*, 127–136. [CrossRef] [PubMed]
92. Son, D.O.; Satsu, H.; Shimizu, M. Histidine inhibits oxidative stress- and tnf-a-induced interleukin-8 secretion in intestinal epithelial cells. *FEBS lett.* **2005**, *579*, 4671–4677. [CrossRef] [PubMed]
93. Erickson, M.C.; Hultin, H.O. A unique role of histidine in fe-catalyzed lipid oxidation by fish sarcoplasmic reticulum. In *Oxygen Radicals in Biology and Medicine*; Simic, M.G., Taylor, K.A., Ward, J.F., Sonntag, C., Eds.; Springer: Boston, MA, USA, 1988; pp. 307–312.
94. Erickson, M.C.; Hultin, H.O. Influence of histidine on lipid peroxidation in sarcoplasmic reticulum. *Arch. Biochem. Biophys.* **1992**, *292*, 427–432. [CrossRef]
95. Filho, J.C.D.; Bergström, J.; Stehle, P.; Fürst, P. Simultaneous measurements of free amino acid patternsof plasma, muscle and erythrocytes in healthy human subjects. *Clin. Nutr.* **1997**, *16*, 299–305. [CrossRef]
96. Hobart, L.J.; Seibel, I.; Yeargans, G.S.; Seidler, N.W. Anti-crosslinking properties of carnosine: Significance of histidine. *Life Sci.* **2004**, *75*, 1379–1389. [CrossRef] [PubMed]
97. Rama Rao, K.V.; Reddy, P.V.B.; Tong, X.; Norenberg, M.D. Brain edema in acute liver failure: Inhibition by L-histidine. *Am. J. Pathol.* **2010**, *176*, 1400–1408. [CrossRef] [PubMed]
98. Baldbige, K.C. Effects of thiamine and biboflavin deficiency on histidine metabolism. *J. Nutr.* **1958**, *66*, 29–34.
99. Ruszkiewicz, J.; Albrecht, J. Changes of the thioredoxin system, glutathione peroxidase activity and total antioxidant capacity in rat brain cortex during acute liver failure: Modulation by L-histidine. *Neurochem. Res.* **2015**, *40*, 293–300. [CrossRef] [PubMed]
100. Liu, W.-H.; Liu, T.-C.; Yin, M.-C. Beneficial effects of histidine and carnosine on ethanol-induced chronic liver injury. *Food Chem. Toxicol.* **2008**, *46*, 1503–1509. [CrossRef] [PubMed]
101. Liu, F.; Lu, W.; Fang, Y.; Liu, J. Evolution of oxidation dynamics of histidine: Nonreactivity in the gas phase, peroxides in hydrated clusters, and ph dependence in solution. *Phys. Chem. Chem. Phys.* **2014**, *16*, 22179–22191. [CrossRef] [PubMed]
102. Wu, H.-C.; Shiau, C.-Y.; Chen, H.-M.; Chiou, T.-K. Antioxidant activities of carnosine, anserine, some freeamino acids and their combination. *J. Food Drug Anal.* **2003**, *11*, 148–153.
103. Milewski, K.; Hilgier, W.; Albrecht, J.; Zielinska, M. The dimethylarginine (adma)/nitric oxide pathway in the brain and periphery of rats with thioacetamide-induced acute liver failure: Modulation by histidine. *Neurochem. Int.* **2015**, *88*, 26–31. [CrossRef] [PubMed]
104. Babizhayev, M.A.; Seguin, M.-C.; Gueynej, J.; Evstigneeva, R.P.; Ageyeva, J.E.A.; Zheltukhina, G.A. L-carnosine (beta-alanyl-L-histidine) and carcinine (beta-alanylhistamine) act as natural antioxidants with hydroxyl-radical-scavenging and lipid-peroxidase activities. *Biochem. J.* **1994**, *304*, 509–516. [CrossRef] [PubMed]
105. Lee, J.W.; Miyawaki, H.; Bobst, E.V.; Hester, J.D.; Ashraf, M.; Bobst, A.M. Improved functional recovery of ischemic rat hearts due to singlet oxygen scavengers histidine and carnosine. *J. Mol. Cell Cardiol.* **1999**, *31*, 113–121. [CrossRef] [PubMed]
106. Vera-Aviles, M.; Latunde-Dada, G.O. Protective effect of histidine against iron-induced toxicity in hek-293 cells. *Proc. Nutr. Soc.* **2017**, *76*, E188. [CrossRef]
107. Tyfield, L.A.; Holton, J.B. The effect of high concentrations of histidine on the level of other amino acids in plasma and brain of the mature rat. *J. Neurochem.* **1976**, *26*, 101–105. [PubMed]
108. Kim, N.H.; Kang, J.H. Protective effects of histidine dipeptides on the modification of neurofilament-l by the cytochrome c/hydrogen peroxide system. *J. Biochem. Mol. Biol.* **2007**, *40*, 125–129. [CrossRef] [PubMed]
109. Tabor, H. Metabolic studies on histidine, histamine, and related imidazoles. *Pharmacol. Rev.* **1954**, *6*, 299–343. [PubMed]

110. Sundberg, R.J.; Martin, R.B. Interactions of histidine and other imidazole derivatives with transition metal ions in chemical and biological systems. *Chem. Rev.* **1973**, *74*, 471–516. [CrossRef]
111. Meyer, J.L.; Bauman, J.; John, E. Copper (II) -histidine complexes. *J. Am. Chem. Soc.* **1970**, *92*, 4210–4216. [CrossRef] [PubMed]
112. Leberman, R.; Rabin, B.R. Metal complexes of histidine. *Trans. Faraday Soc.* **1959**, *55*, 1660–1670. [CrossRef]
113. Williams, D.R. Thermodynamic considerations in co-ordination. Part VII. Solubility of the histidine-H^+ system and stability constants, free energies, enthalpies, and entropies of protonation of histidine and tryptophan and of formation of their manganese(II), iron(II), cobalt(II), nickel(II), copper(II), and zinc(II) complexes. *J. Chem. Soc. A* **1970**, 1550–1555.
114. Zs.-Nagy, I.; Floyd, R.A. Hydroxyl free radical reactions with amino acids and proteins studied by electron spin resonance spectroscopy and spin-trapping. *Biochim. Biophys. Acta* **1984**, *790*, 238–250. [CrossRef]
115. Nair, N.G.; Perry, G.; Smithc, M.A.; Reddya, V.P. Nmr studies of zinc, copper, and iron binding to histidine, the principal metal ion complexing site of amyloid-β peptide. *J. Alzheimer's Dis.* **2010**, *20*, 57–66. [CrossRef] [PubMed]
116. Tachon, P. DNA single strand breakage by H_2O_2 and ferric or cupric ions: Its modulation by histidine. *Free Radic. Res. Commun.* **1990**, *9*, 39–47. [CrossRef] [PubMed]
117. Torres-Fuentes, C.; Alaiz, M.; Vioque, J. Iron-chelating activity of chickpea protein hydrolysate peptides. *Food Chem.* **2012**, *134*, 1585–1588. [CrossRef] [PubMed]
118. Sandstrom, B.; Davidsson, L.; Cederblad, A.; Lonnerdal, B. Oral iron, dietary ligands and zinc absorption. *J. Nutr.* **1985**, *115*, 411–414. [CrossRef] [PubMed]
119. Van Campen, D.; Gross, E. Effect of histidine and certain other amino acids on the absorption of iron-59 by rats. *J. Nutr.* **1969**, *99*, 68–74. [CrossRef] [PubMed]
120. Fairbanks, V.F.; Beutler, E. Iron metabolism. In *Hematology*; Beutler, E., Ed.; McGraw-Hill: New York, NY, USA, 1995; pp. 369–380.
121. Layrisse, M.; Martinez-Torres, C.; Leets, I.; Taylor, P.; Ramirez, J. Effect of histidine, cysteine, glutathione or beef on iron absorption in humans. *J. Nutr.* **1984**, *114*, 217–223. [CrossRef] [PubMed]
122. Van Campen, D. Effect of histidine and ascorbic acid on the absorption and retention of ^{59}Fe by iron-depleted rats. *J. Nutr.* **1972**, *102*, 165–170. [CrossRef] [PubMed]
123. Iyengar, V.; Pullakhandam, R.; Nair, K.M. Dietary ligands as determinants of iron–zinc interactions at the absorptive enterocyte. *J. Food Sci.* **2010**, *75*, H260–H264. [CrossRef] [PubMed]
124. Glahn, R.P.; Van Campen, D.R. Iron uptake is enhanced in caco-2 cell monolayers by cysteine and reduced cysteinyl glycine. *J. Nutr.* **1997**, *127*, 642–647. [CrossRef] [PubMed]
125. Swain, J.H.; Tabatabai, L.B.; Reddy, M.B. Histidine content of low-molecular-weight beef proteins influences nonheme iron bioavailability in Caco-2 cells. *Nutr Interact. Toxic.* **2002**, 245–251. [CrossRef] [PubMed]
126. Storcksdieck, S.; Bonsmann, G.; Hurrell, R.F. Iron-binding properties, amino acid composition, and structure of muscle tissue peptides from in vitro digestion of different meat sources. *J. Food Sci.* **2007**, *72*, S019–S029. [CrossRef] [PubMed]
127. Lee, Y.T.; Hsu, C.C.; Lin, M.H.; Liu, K.S.; Yin, M.C. Histidine and carnosine delay diabetic deterioration in mice and protect human low density lipoprotein against oxidation and glycation. *Eur. J. Pharmacol.* **2005**, *513*, 145–150. [CrossRef] [PubMed]
128. Liakopoulos, V.; Roumeliotis, S.; Gorny, X.; Dounousi, E.; Mertens, P.R. Oxidative stress in hemodialysis patients: A review of the literature. *Oxid. Med. Cell. Longev.* **2017**, *2017*, 22. [CrossRef] [PubMed]
129. Baylis, C. Arginine, arginine analogs and nitric oxide production in chronic kidney disease. *Nat. Clin. Pract. Nephrol.* **2006**, *2*, 209. [CrossRef] [PubMed]
130. Coombes, J.S.; Fassett, R.G. Antioxidant therapy in hemodialysis patients: A systematic review. *Kidney Int.* **2012**, *81*, 233–246. [CrossRef] [PubMed]

13

Deregulation of Hepatic Mek1/2–Erk1/2 Signaling Module in Iron Overload Conditions

Naveen Kumar Tangudu [1,†], Nils Buth [1,†], Pavel Strnad [2], Ion C. Cirstea [1] and Maja Vujić Spasić [1,*]

1 Institute of Comparative Molecular Endocrinology, University of Ulm, Ulm 89081, Germany; naveen.tangudu@uni-ulm.de (N.K.T.); nils.buth@uni-ulm.de (N.B.); ion.cirstea@uni-ulm.de (I.C.C.)
2 Department of Medicine III and IZKF, University Hospital Aachen, Aachen 52074, Germany; pstrnad@ukaachen.de
* Correspondence: maja.vujic@uni-ulm.de
† These authors contributed equally to this work.

Abstract: The liver, through the production of iron hormone hepcidin, controls body iron levels. High liver iron levels and deregulated hepcidin expression are commonly observed in many liver diseases including highly prevalent genetic iron overload disorders. In spite of a number of breakthrough investigations into the signals that control hepcidin expression, little progress has been made towards investigations into intracellular signaling in the liver under excess of iron. This study examined hepatic signaling pathways underlying acquired and genetic iron overload conditions. Our data demonstrate that hepatic iron overload associates with a decline in the activation of mitogen-activated protein kinase (MAPK)/extracellular signal-regulated kinase (Erk) kinase (Mek1/2) pathway by selectively affecting the phosphorylation of Erk1/2. We propose that Mek1/2-Erk1/2 signaling is uncoupled from iron-Bmp-Smad-mediated hepcidin induction and that it may contribute to a number of liver pathologies in addition to toxic effects of iron. We believe that our findings will advance the understanding of cellular signaling events in the liver during iron overload of different etiologies.

Keywords: liver; iron; hepcidin; Mek/Erk; Hfe; Bmp/Smad

---

1. Introduction

In vertebrates, the liver is an essential metabolic hub. It hosts numerous biochemical processes and regulates the storage of many essential nutrients, vitamins, and minerals, as well as their release when there is a physiological need for them. The liver is the main parenchymal iron repository and at the same time the principal organ controlling systemic iron fluxes through the production of the iron hormone hepcidin [1]. High hepatic iron levels are commonly observed in many liver diseases including highly prevalent genetic iron overload disorders (i.e., hereditary hemochromatosis), hematologic disorders (i.e., thalassemia and sickle cell disease), chronic hepatitis C, alcoholic liver disease and non-alcoholic fatty liver disease 1 [2,3]. The main pathological effects of hepatic iron overload include liver fibrosis, cirrhosis and hepatocellular carcinoma.

The sensing of plasma iron levels (i.e., transferrin-bound iron) by liver hepatocytes involves a multiprotein membrane-bound complex consisting of transferrin receptors 1 and 2 (TfR1, TfR2), MHC I-like protein Hfe, hemojuvelin, and the bone morphogenetic protein (Bmp) receptors type I such as activin receptor-like kinase 1 (Alk2/Acvr1) and Alk3/Bmpr1a [4–12]. The Bmp-Alk2/3-Smad1/5/8 cascade is currently considered as the central intracellular relay communicating high plasma iron levels to hepcidin, since mice and patients with genetic disruption in the iron-sensing molecules show impaired Bmp/Smad signaling, low hepcidin expression and consequently develop hepatic iron overload [12–15]. Furthermore, the contribution of the extracellular signal-regulated kinases 1 and 2 (Erk1/2) to hepcidin regulation was proposed: studies in erythroleukemia K562 cells, exposed to holo-transferrin, demonstrated activation of ERK1/2 and p38 MAP kinases, a process that was dependent on TfR2 [16]; consequently, silencing of TfR2 and Hfe in HepG2 cells and in mice resulted in decreased ERK1/2 signaling and low hepcidin expression in the liver [8,17]. It was proposed that ERK1/2 might act in concert with Bmp-Smad signaling to control hepcidin expression [18].

The mitogen-activated protein kinases (MAPKs) are among the largest protein families in eukaryotes that transduce a variety of extracellular signals to regulate a plethora of cellular responses [19,20]. MAPKs consist of many protein kinases but three major protein kinases are extensively studied: the ERK1/2, activated by broad spectrum of extracellular ligands such as mitogens/growth factors and differentiation signals [21], and c-Jun amino terminal kinases (JNK1/2/3) and p38 kinases that are activated by stress stimuli [19,20,22]. MAPK-dependent signal transduction is required to maintain physiological metabolic adaptation while inappropriate MAPK signaling has been increasingly associated with the development of metabolic syndrome [23]. In the liver, the MAPKs play an important role in processes that regulate metabolism [23–26]. In particular, activation of stress-responsive p38MAPKs and JNKs was associated with hepatic metabolic dysfunction [20,23,26–28], whereas constitutive Erk1 or liver-specific Erk2 deficiency in mice was proposed to affect hepatic glucose and lipid metabolism, promote insulin resistance and ER stress [27,29,30].

In this study, we examined the association between hepatic iron overload in mice, caused by parenteral, nutritional and genetic iron overload, and the activity of Mek1/2-Erk1/2 signaling. Our data demonstrate decreased Mek1/2-Erk1/2 signaling output in iron overloaded conditions, suggesting that Mek1/2-Erk1/2 signaling is uncoupled from Bmp-Smad1/5/8-mediated hepcidin induction and that it may play an important role in liver diseases characterized by hepatic iron excess.

2. Results and Discussion

2.1. Classical and Stress-Induced MAPKs Activation in Iron-Loaded Livers

The aim of this study was to investigate the activity of intracellular signaling pathways in the livers under excessive iron overload. To this end, we used our previously established mouse model of parenteral iron overload, which is characterized by severe hepatic iron overload, high circulating iron levels, and increased hepcidin mRNA expression [15]. We measured the phosphorylation status of nine intracellular proteins including Mek1 (Ser217/Ser221) and Erk1/2 (Thr202/Tyr204, Thr185/Tyr187), as classical MAPK backbone components, stress-responsive MAPKs, such as JNK (Thr183/Tyr185) and p38 MAPK (Thr180/Tyr182), and effector molecules of MAPKs including p90 RSK (Ser380), Stat3 (Ser727), ATF-2 (Thr71), HSP27 (Ser78), and p53 (Ser15), using Bio-Plex Pro Cell Signaling MAPK Panel 9-plex (BioRad Laboratories, Germany). This analysis revealed a decrease in the phosphorylation levels of Mek1 and p90 RSK in iron-loaded livers, and only marginally in case of Stat3 ($p < 0.0571$); similarly, the levels of pErk1/2 showed a trend towards a decrease however the data were under the level of statistical significance (Figure 1). The levels of pJNK, p38MAPK, pHSP27, p53, and pATF-2 showed no statistically significant differences (Figure 1).

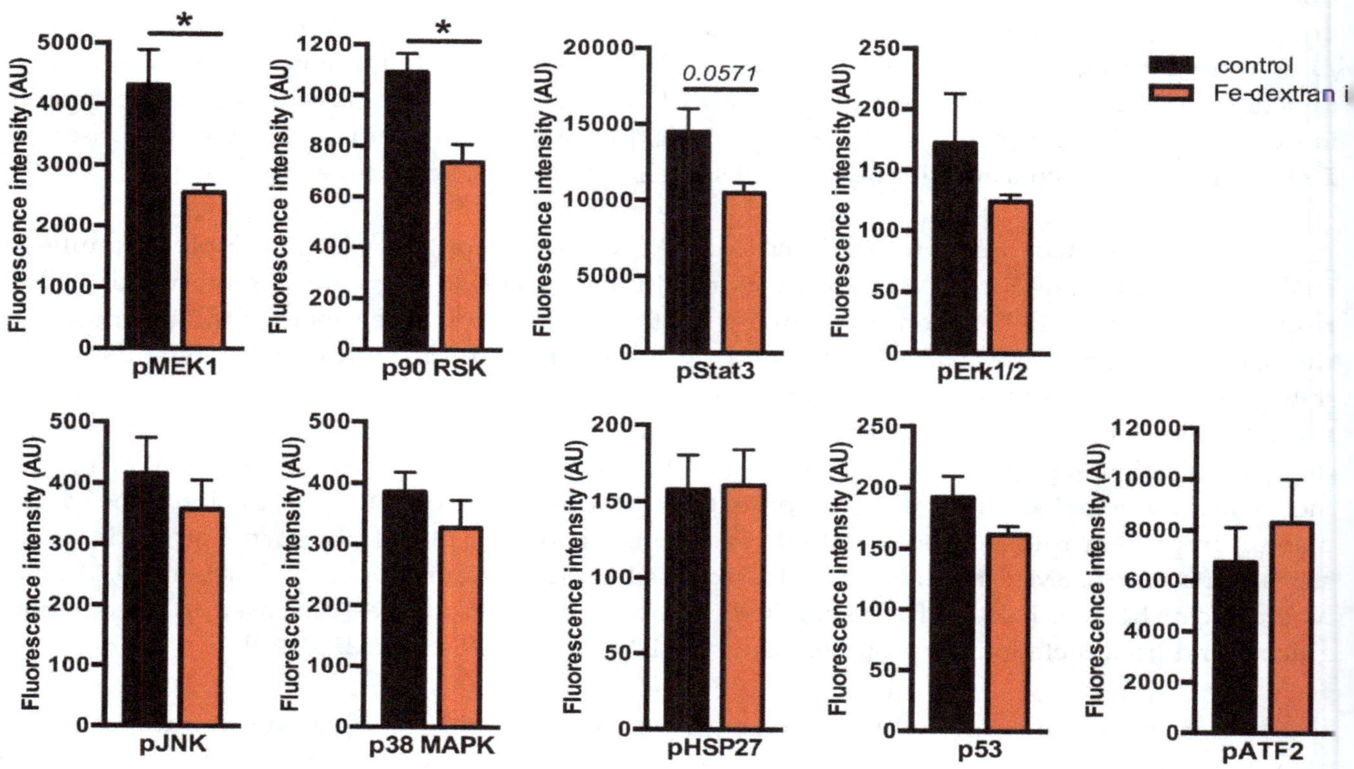

Figure 1. Identification of activated proteins in iron overloaded livers by Bio-Plex Pro Cell Signaling MAPK Panel 9-plex. Phosphorylation status of nine intracellular phosphoproteins was measured in the livers of iron-dextran injected mice and compared to controls. Data were analyzed using GraphPad Prism software and results are shown as mean ± SEM (standard error of mean). For the statistical analysis, a nonparametric distribution and the unpaired Mann–Whitney U Test were used. * p-values < 0.05; AU: arbitrary units; n = 4; 4 per group.

Based on these results, we postulated that the presence of hepatic iron overload might associate with selective impairment of the Mek1/2-Erk1/2 pathway and its downstream pStat3 and pp90 RSK targets. This idea is supported by recent investigations showing selective activation of JNK and the p38 MAPK signaling activity under cellular iron depletion [31]. Moreover, in response to growth factors, Erk1/2, but not JNK or p38, specifically phosphorylate Stat3 at Ser727, which is also stimulated by interleukine-6 cytokine, however, in contrast to growth factors, the latter process occurs independent of Erk1/2 [32].

2.2. *Association of Mitogen-activated Protein Kinases (MAPK) Activity with Hepatic Iron Overload*

To test the above hypothesis we evaluated phosphorylation levels of Mek1/2, Erk1/2, Stat3 and p90 Rsk proteins in iron-loaded livers using immunoblotting analysis. This analysis revealed a significant decrease in the phosphorylation levels of Mek1/2, Erk1/2, and Stat3 (by 3.6-, 4.8-, and 3.8-fold, respectively), while the levels of p90Rsk were increased by 2.1-fold (Figure 2a).

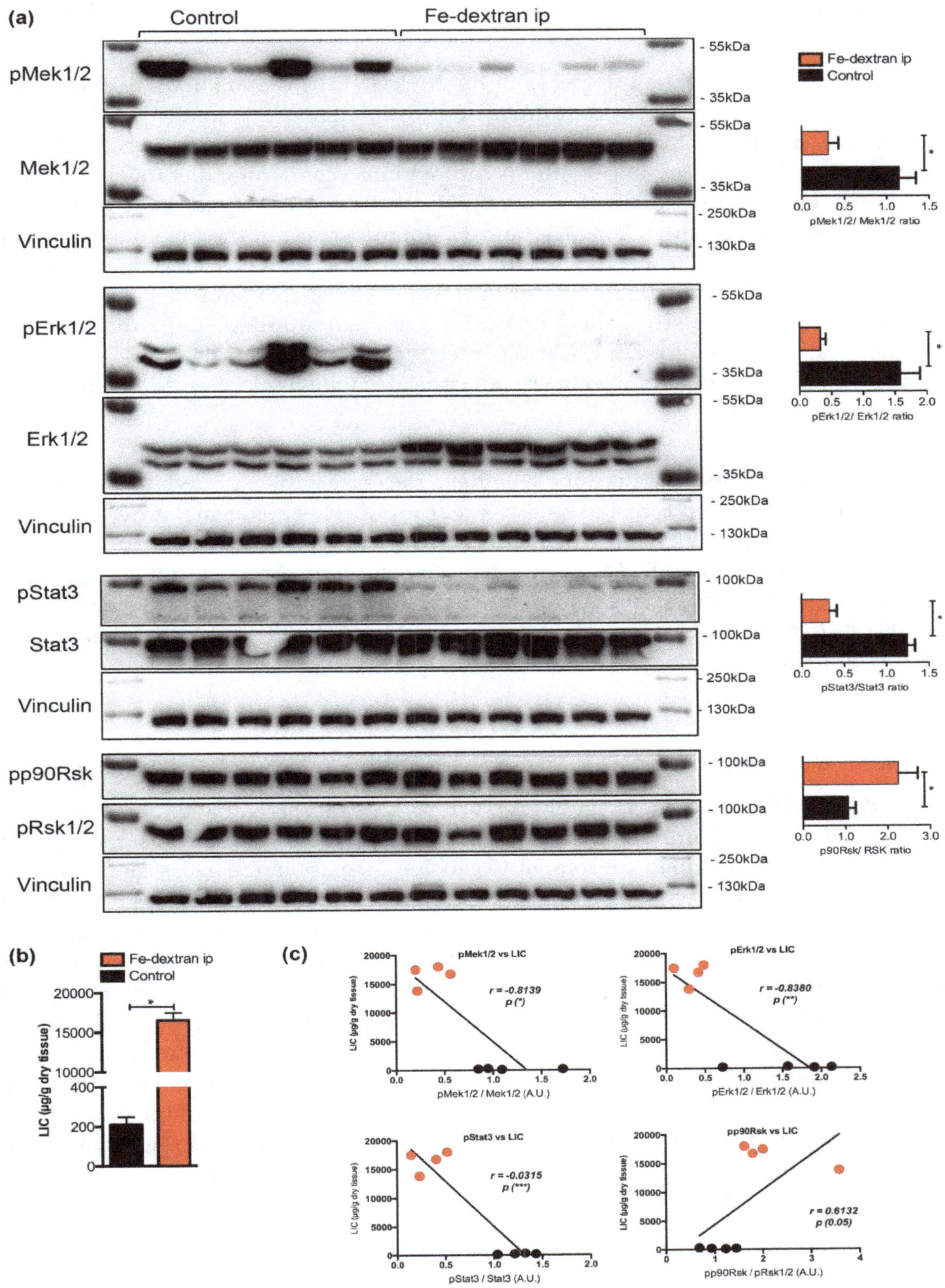

Figure 2. (**a**) Immunoblot analysis and relative quantification (shown in histograms on right) of pMEK1, pERK1/2, pStat3, and pp90Rsk in the livers of iron-dextran injected and control mice (n = 6; 6 mice per group). (**b**) Liver iron content (LIC) of control and iron-dextran injected mice. (**c**) Correlation analysis between LIC and the levels of pMek1/2/Mek1/2, pErk1/2/Erk1/2, pStat3/Stat3, and pp90Rsk/pRsk1/2 in the livers of iron-dextran injected and control mice. M: Page Ruler Plus Prestained Protein Ladder (Thermo Scientific). Data were analyzed using GraphPad Prism software and results are shown as mean ± SEM (standard error of mean). For the statistical analysis, a nonparametric distribution and the unpaired Mann–Whitney U Test were used.

2.3. Nutritional Iron Overload is Characterized by Low Hepatic Mek1/2-Erk1/2-Stat3 Signaling

We next questioned whether a decrease in the Mek1/2-Erk1/2-Stat3 activity, measured during parenteral iron overload, is present in conditions of nutritional iron overload. We thus examined the phosphorylation status of Mek1/2-Erk1/2-Stat3 in the livers of wild type mice undergoing nutritional iron overload, induced by feeding mice with 3% carbonyl iron containing diet for six months starting at one month of age, as we previously described [33]. We show that hepatic iron overload, induced by iron-rich diet, associated with a 2.7-, 3.4-, and 1.7-fold decrease in the phosphorylation levels of Mek1/2-Erk1/2-Stat3 proteins, respectively, while the levels of p90Rsk were unchanged (Figure 3). However the data were only marginally under the level of statistical significance ($p < 0.0571$), which is, in our opinion, caused by stringent statistical analysis we applied (unpaired, nonparametric, Mann–Whitney test; n = 3–4 mice per group). Collectively, our data imply that hepatic response of mice receiving parenteral or dietary iron overload associates with a selective decline in the activity of Mek1/2-Erk1/2-Stat3 branch.

Future studies are needed to determine whether a decrease in phosphorylation of Mek1/2-Erk1/2 might be caused by diminished tyrosine kinase receptors (such as epidermal growth factor receptor, EGFR) mediated signaling activity and whether its activity may correlate with changes in the levels of extracellular ligands that can bind EGFR, such as EGF, transforming growth factor alpha, amphiregulin, heparin-binding EGF, and others. In addition, it will be informative to measure the levels of growth hormone (GH), as defective GH signaling impairs activation of EGFR and ERK signaling and affects liver regeneration [34].

2.4. Low Hepatic Mek1/2-Erk1/2 Signaling is Present in Hfe-/- Mice in Spite of Low Bmp-Smad Signaling

So far, our data indicate a decrease in pMek1/2-pErk1/2-pStat3 signaling under excessive systemic and hepatic iron overload. Contrary to Mek1/2-Erk1/2, the activity of Bmp-Smad signaling was shown to increase following iron overload subsequently causing increase in the expression of hepcidin and genes known to be coregulated with hepcidin [15]. Given that previous studies suggest co-involvement of Erk1/2 and Bmp/Smad signaling for induction of hepcidin in cells [18], it seemed logical to investigate the Mek1/2-Erk1/2 signaling activity in conditions characterized by hepatic iron overload and low hepcidin expression. To this end, we employed *Hfe*-deficient mice, a well-established mouse model of genetic iron-overload, which due to the lack of Hfe, an upstream hepcidin regulator, showed impaired Bmp-Smad signaling, low hepcidin expression, and increased hepatic iron stores [13–15]. We detected that the activation of Mek1/2-Erk1/2, measured by phosphorylation status using immunoblot analysis, was on average 2-fold lower in the livers of *Hfe-/-* mice (with marginal significance of $p = 0.0571$), whereas the levels of pStat3 and pp90Rsk were not significantly changed (Figure 4). These data suggest that a decrease in Mek1/2-Erk1/2 signaling is uncoupled from Bmp-Smad signaling activity and Smad-mediated hepcidin regulation.

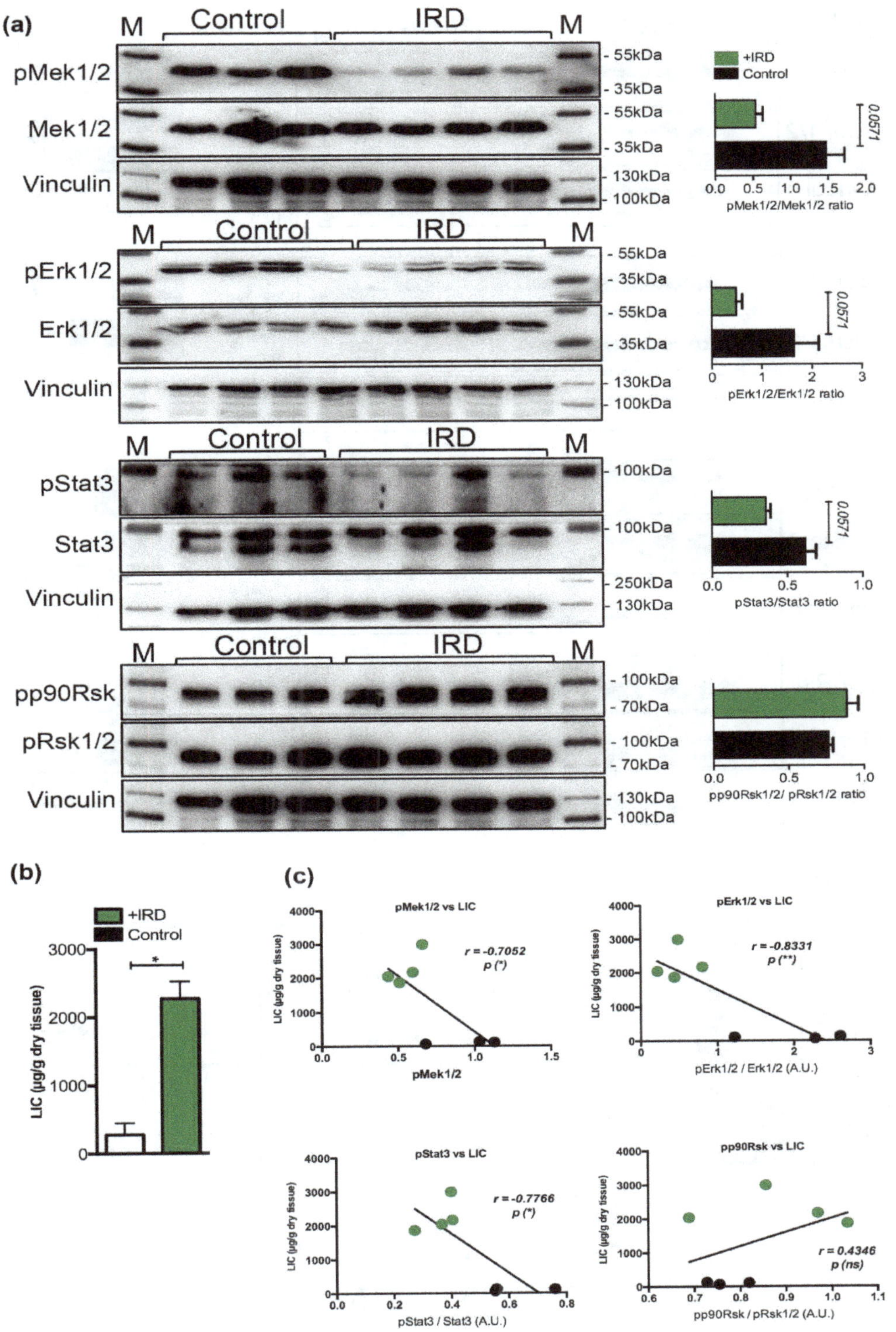

Figure 3. (**a**) Representative immunoblot analysis and relative quantification (shown in histograms on right) of pMek1/2, pErk1/2, pStat3, and pp90Rsk in the livers of mice maintained on an iron rich diet (IRD) and standard diet (control) (n = 3–4 mice per group). (**b**) Liver iron content (LIC) of control and of mice maintained on an iron rich diet (n = 3–4 mice per group). (**c**) Correlation analysis between LIC and the levels of pMek1/2/Mek1/2, pErk1/2/Erk1/2, pStat3/Stat3, and pp90Rsk/pRsk1/2 in the livers of mice maintained on an iron rich diet (IRD) and standard diet (control) (n = 3–4 mice per group). M: Page Ruler Plus Prestained Protein Ladder (Thermo Scientific). Data were analyzed using GraphPad Prism software and results are shown as mean ± SEM (standard error of mean). For the statistical analysis, a nonparametric distribution and the unpaired Mann–Whitney U Test were used. Linear regression and Pearson correlation coefficients were computed for every data set with 95% confidence intervals. * p-values < 0.05.

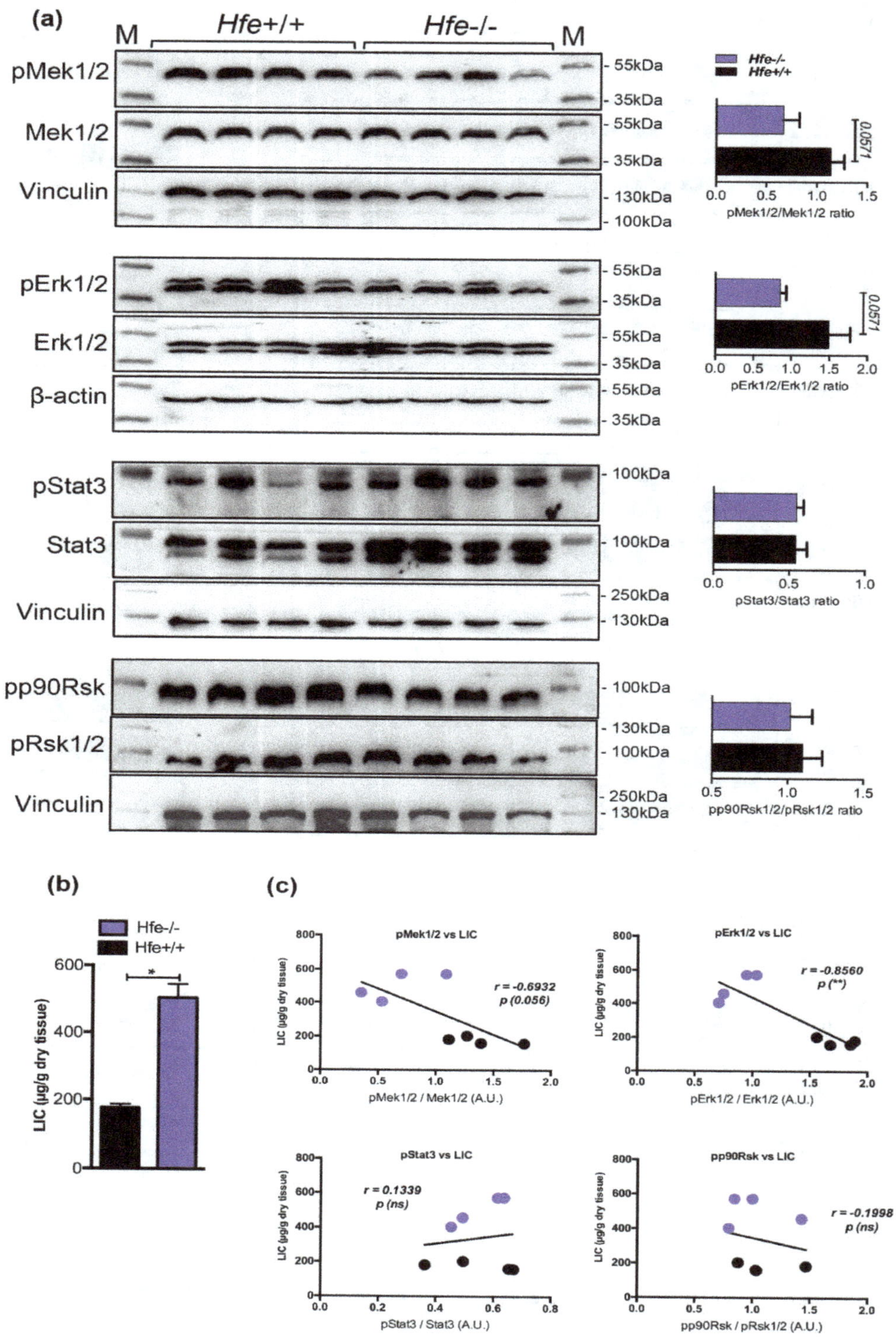

Figure 4. (**a**) Representative immunoblot analysis and relative quantification (shown in histograms on right) of pMek1/2, pErk1/2, pStat3 and pp90Rsk in the livers of Hfe+/+ control and Hfe-/- mutant mice (n = 8;10 mice per group). (**b**) Liver iron content (LIC) of Hfe+/+ and Hfe-/- mice (n = 4;4 mice per group). (**c**) Correlation analysis between LIC and the levels of pMek1/2/Mek1/2, pErk1/2/Erk1/2, pStat3/Stat3, and pp90Rsk/pRsk1/2 in the livers of Hfe+/+ and Hfe-/- mice (n = 4;4 mice per group). M: Page Ruler Plus Prestained Protein Ladder (Thermo Scientific). Data were analyzed using GraphPad Prism software and results are shown as mean ± SEM (standard error of mean). For the statistical analysis, a nonparametric distribution and the unpaired Mann–Whitney U Test were used. Linear regression and Pearson correlation coefficients were computed for every data set with 95% confidence intervals. * p-values <0.05.

2.5. Low Hepatic Mek1/2-Erk1/2 Signaling is Present in Hepcidin-Deficient Mice and is Further Aggravated by Iron Excess

We next investigated Mek1/2-Erk1/2 activation status in the livers of hepcidin knock-out mice (*Hamp-/-*), which are deficient for hepcidin expression but maintain an appropriate Bmp-Smad signaling activity as a response to liver iron overload [15]. Similarly to the observation in the livers of *Hfe-/-* mice, a 2.5- and 3.8-fold decrease in the levels of pMek1/2-pErk1/2 proteins were measured in the livers of *Hamp-/-* mice (with marginal significance of $p = 0.0571$), while the pStat3 and pp90Rsk levels were not significantly changed (Figure 5a–c). Interestingly, the activation of Mek1/2, Erk1/2, and Stat3, measured by their phosphorylated levels, was suppressed by 34-, 7.5-, and 1.5-fold, respectively (with marginal significance of $p = 0.0571$), while the levels of pp90Rsk were unchanged in *Hamp-/-* mice fed an iron-rich diet for six months (Figure 5d–f), which caused the development of chronic liver injury as we previously demonstrated [33].

Interestingly, the initially observed increase in pp90Rsk levels following iron-dextran injections in mice (Figure 2a,c) was not detected in the livers of mice maintained on an iron-rich diet nor in Hfe-/- or Hamp-/- mice. A possible explanation might be the differences in the route of iron application (i.p injections versus nutritional/enteral iron administration) and the duration of iron loading (3-weeks of iron-dextran injections versus six months of iron-rich diet). We suspect that fast influx of iron and excessive liver iron loading following i.p. iron-dextran injections might differentially affect cellular and humoral responses than nutritional iron administration or genetic iron overload.

Taken together, our data reinforce the view that attenuation of Mek1/2-Erk1/2 phosphorylation is a function of hepatic iron overload. Given the variety of iron-overload models used in this study, we speculate that changes in Mek1/2-Erk1/2 signaling may be categorized as initiating mechanism predisposing liver cells to toxic insults. Among them, inflammation, hepatic oxidative stress including the production of highly reactive lipid peroxidation products and iron-catalyzed oxidant stress [35,36] could ultimately lead towards the progression of a chronic liver disease. This hypothesis is supported by recent studies demonstrated that inhibition of ERK1/2 signaling sensitized the cells to chemotaxic stimuli [37].

The collective data let to a working model (Figure 6), in which high hepatic iron burden associates with a decrease in phosphorylation levels of Mek1/2-Erk1/2. This in turn may contribute to a number of liver pathologies in addition to toxic effects of iron.

Data presented in this study raise a number of questions as to whether (i) low Mek1/2-Erk1/2 activity occurs as a selective response to high hepatic iron levels or is triggered by high transferrin and/or non-transferrin-bound iron, (ii) in which hepatic cells (hepatocytes or nonparenchymal cells) and in which cellular compartments does Erk1/2 function, (iii) what is the level of Mek1/2-Erk1/2 cross-talk with parallel pathways such as the PI3K/AKT/mTOR pathway in iron-loaded livers, and (iv) what are the consequences of inhibition of the Erk1/2 pathway in iron-loaded livers on hepatic gene transcription?

Finally, our findings may be of relevance to other conditions where hepatic iron levels are increased such as alcoholic liver disease, characterized by low hepcidin expression, suppressed hepatic Erk1/2 activity and liver injury [27,38–43]. In addition, hepatic iron overload is present in approximately one-third of patients with nonalcoholic fatty liver disease [44–47], which is recognized as the most common chronic liver disease that can progress to non-alcoholic steatohepatitis and liver cancer [48–50]. Hepatic iron overload is also observed in patients with chronic hepatitis C virus infections (and rarely in chronic hepatitis B infections) and in end-stage liver disease [3,46,47,51–54]. Whether hepatic iron overload and the presence of suppressed Mek1/2-Erk1/2 signaling may either accelerate disease progression or whether maintaining low Mek1/2-Erk1/2 signaling may be protective from the induction of *c-Myc* and *c-Jun* as a part of increased proliferation, and therefore reduce the incidence of liver damage, are certainly important questions to address in the future. An equally interesting aspect would be to monitor Mek1/2-Erk1/2 activation from early steps of iron overload until development of liver pathologies and establish whether the activity of MAPK module is accordingly modulated.

Understanding the underlying mechanisms associated with hepatic iron overload and progressive liver failure may provide new modalities for therapeutic interventions. We believe that the data provided here will advance our understanding of cellular signaling events in the liver during iron overload of different etiologies.

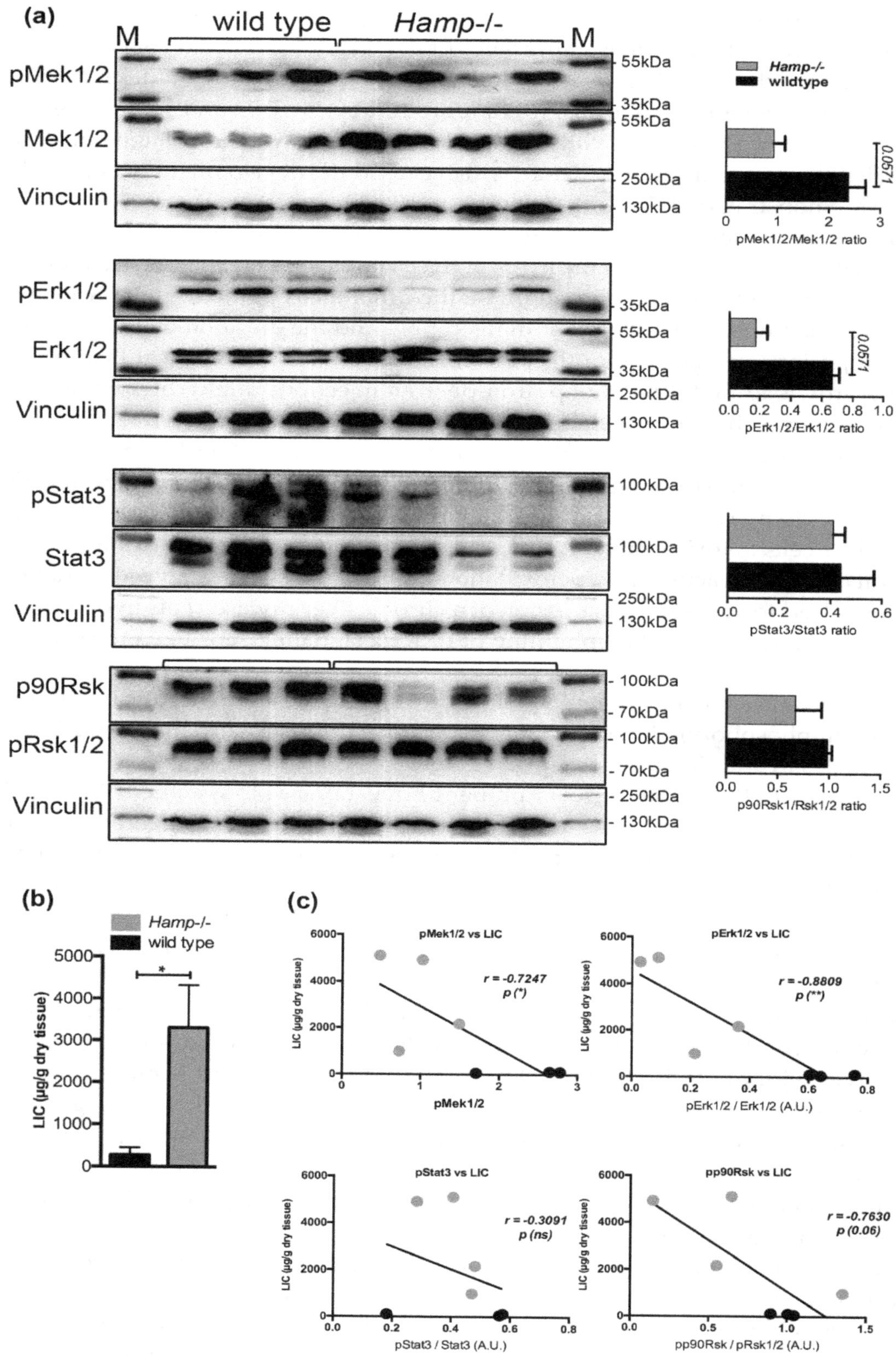

Figure 5. *Cont.*

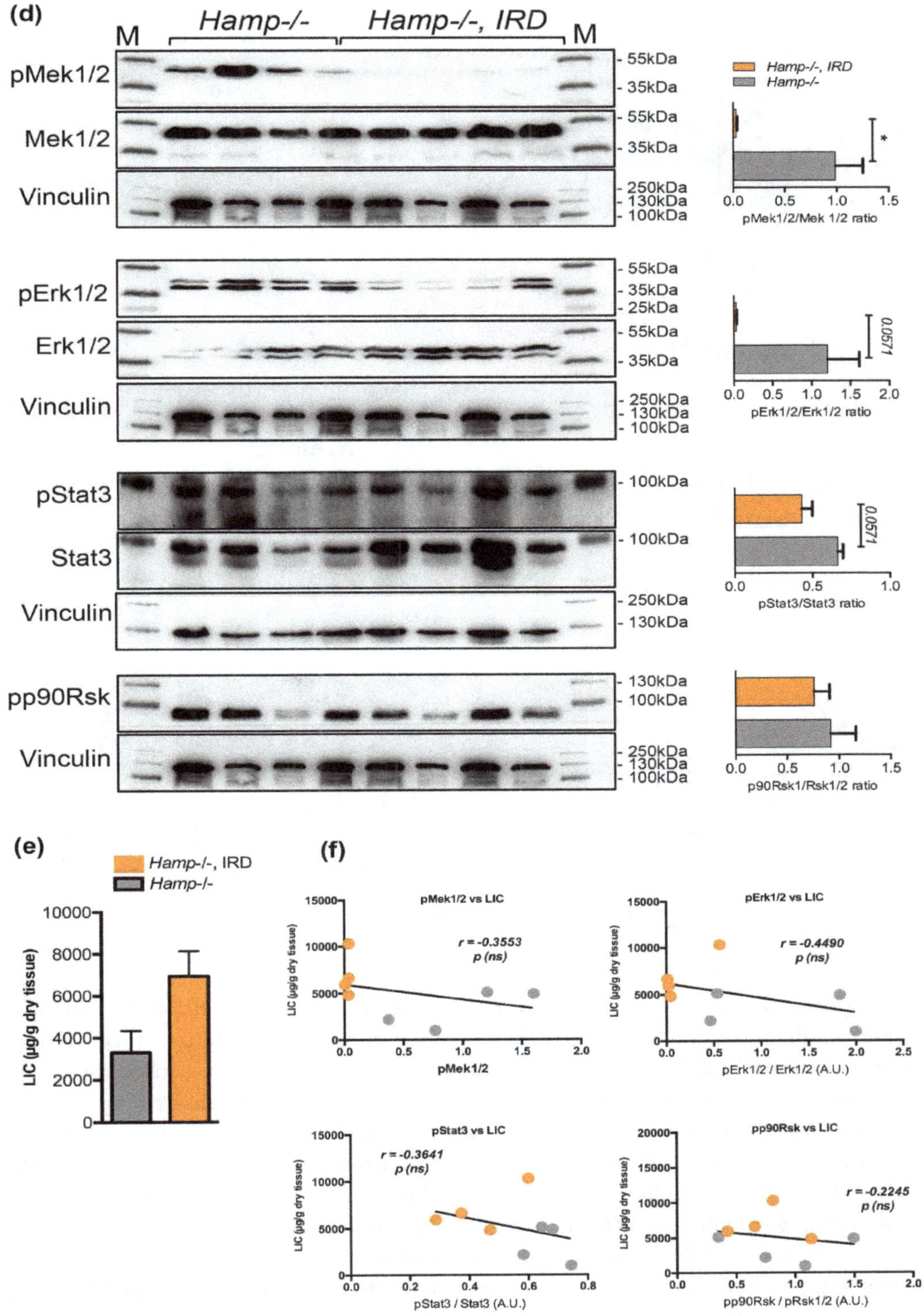

Figure 5. Immunoblot analysis and relative quantification (shown in histograms on right) of pMek1/2, pErk1/2, pStat3 and pp90Rsk in the livers of (**a**) control and Hamp-/- mice and (**d**) Hamp-/- mice maintained on an iron-rich diet (IRD) (n = 3;4;4 mice per group). Liver iron content (LIC) in (**b**) control, Hamp-/- and (**e**) Hamp-/- mice maintained on an iron-rich diet (n = 3;4;4 mice per group). Correlation analysis between LIC and the levels of pMek1/2/Mek1/2, pErk1/2/Erk1/2, pStat3/Stat3, and pp90Rsk/pRsk1/2 in the livers of (**c**) control, Hamp-/- and (**f**) Hamp-/- mice maintained on an iron rich diet (IRD) (n = 3; 4;4 mice per group). M: Page Ruler Plus Prestained Protein Ladder (Thermo Scientific). Data were analyzed using GraphPad Prism software and results are shown as mean ± SEM (standard error of mean). For the statistical analysis, a nonparametric distribution and the unpaired Mann–Whitney U Test were used. Linear regression and Pearson correlation coefficients were computed for every data set with 95% confidence intervals. * p-values <0.05.

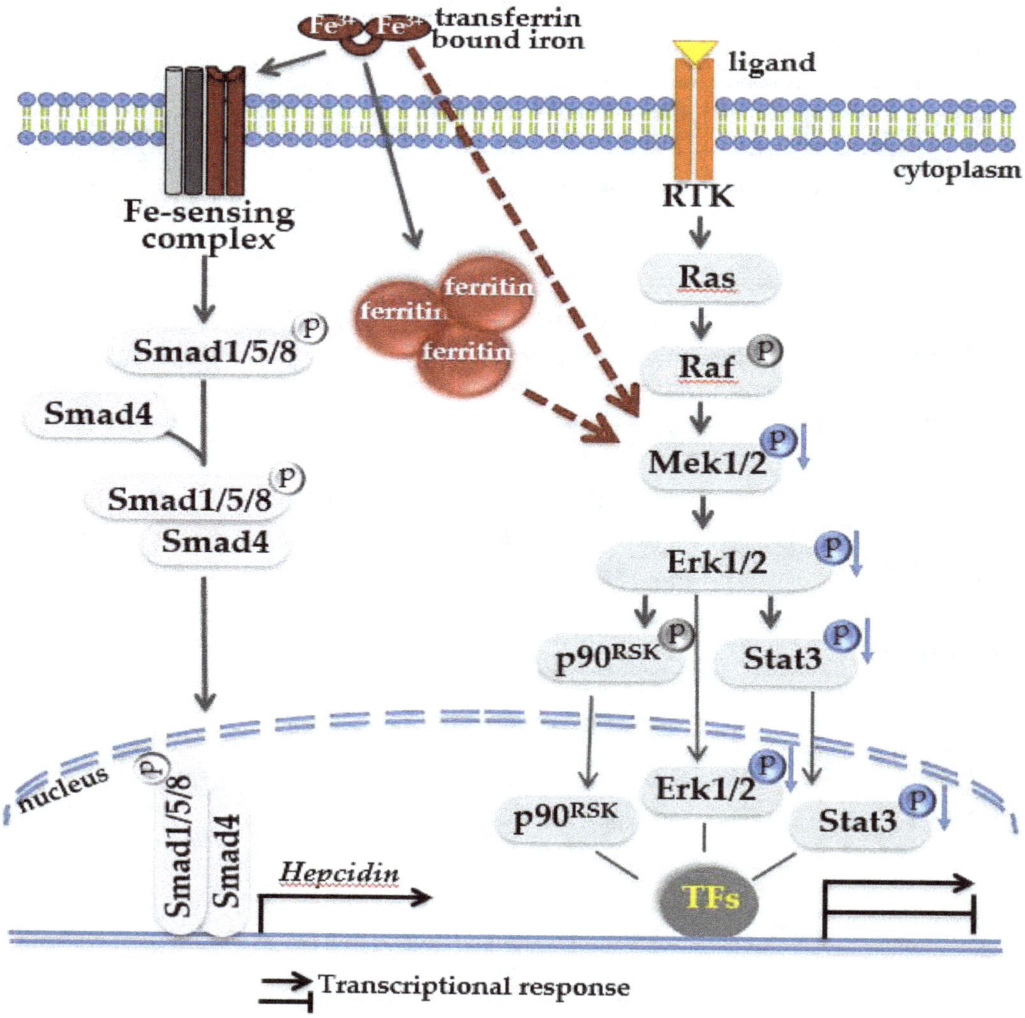

Figure 6. Proposed model of two signaling pathways operating in iron-loaded livers. Systemic iron overload results in heavy iron deposition in the liver, illustrated here in form of high ferritin. Under these conditions, high levels of circulating transferrin-bound iron is sensed by cell membrane multiprotein iron-sensing complex, resulting in the activation of intracellular Bmp-Smad signaling cascade and increased hepcidin transcription in the nucleus. Independent of Bmp-Smad-mediated hepcidin activation, through a yet unknown mechanism (proposed here by red arrows), a decrease in phosphorylation of Mek1/2-Erk1/2-Stat3 (indicated in blue) occurs which in turn may affect the property of pErk1/2 and pStat3 signaling molecules to regulate gene transcription, alone or in cooperation with other transcription factors (TFs). A decrease in the activity of Mek1/2-Erk1/2 signaling cascade can be considered as liver response to iron overload. We propose that a decrease in Mek1/2-Erk1/2 signaling activity may accelerate liver pathologies in addition to toxic effects of iron.

3. Materials and Methods

3.1. Mice and Treatments

Wild type *Hfe-/-* and *Hamp-/-* mutant mice, all males, were kept under a standard mouse diet containing 180 mg/kg iron (Ssniff, Soest, Germany). For the analysis livers were used from previously described wild-type mice undergoing intra peritoneal (i.p.) injection of iron-dextran solution [15,33] and from *Hamp-/-* and wild type mice fed with 3% carbonyl iron (Sigma, Germany) for 6 months [15,33]. Animal experiments were approved and performed in accordance to the Ulm University Animal Care

Committee and German Low for Welfare of laboratory animals in Baden-Württemberg, Germany (Project ID: 35/9185.81-3 / 972 / 1143).

3.2. Phosphoprotein Analysis in Liver Lysates

Protein lysates (10 μg in 50 μL) were prepared from liver tissues using Bio-Plex Cell Lysis Kit (BioRad Laboratories, Munich, Germany). The levels of intracellular phosphoproteins were measured using Bio-Plex Pro Cell Signaling MAPK Panel, 9-plex (BioRad Laboratories, Munich, Germany) according to the manufacturer's instructions. The data were analyzed using Bio-Plex Manager 6.1 Software Package.

3.3. Protein Isolation and Immunoblot Analysis

Protein extracts were prepared from flash-frozen tissue after homogenization in RIPA lysis buffer (Incomplete RIPA buffer, 7× protease inhibitor cocktail, 200mM sodium orthovandate, 1M sodium fluoride, 100mM PMSF) as previously described [15]. Total proteins (30–50 μg) were subjected to Western blot analysis with the following antibodies; anti-pMek1/2, anti-Mek1/2, anti-pErk1/2, anti-Erk1/2, anti-pp90Rsk, anti-pRsk1/2, anti-pStat3, and anti-Stat3 (all rabbit, Cell Signaling Technology, MA, USA; 1:1000 concentration). Mouse anti-vinculin (Santa Cruz, CA, USA; 1:2000) and mouse anti-β-actin (Sigma Aldrich, Missouri, USA; 1:10,000) were used as loading controls. Furthermore, membranes were washed and incubated with anti-rabbit or anti-mouse (Invitrogen, CA, USA; 1:5000) horseradish peroxidase-conjugated antibody. Western blot images were acquired using EMD Millipore Luminata HRP chemiluminescence substrate (Millipore, MA, USA) and signal acquired in Bio-Rad chemiluminescence detector (Bio-Rad Laboratories, CA, USA). The signals were semiquantified using image J (ImageJ; www://rsb.info.nih.gov/ij/).

3.4. Statistical Analysis

Data were analyzed using GraphPad Prism software and results are shown as mean ± standard error of mean. For the statistical analysis, a nonparametric distribution and the Mann–Whitney U test were used. Linear regression and Pearson correlation coefficients were computed for every data set with 95% confidence intervals. Statistically significant differences are indicated as $p < 05$ (*), $p < 01$ (**), and $p < 005$ (***).

Author Contributions: N.K.T. and N.B. performed the experiments; P.S. and I.C.C. provided resources and edited the manuscript; and M.V.S. designed the study, analyzed the data, and wrote the manuscript.

Acknowledgments: We thank the staff of the Animal Facility at the Ulm University.

References

1. Lesbordes-Brion, J.C.; Viatte, L.; Bennoun, M.; Lou, D.Q.; Ramey, G.; Houbron, C.; Hamard, G.; Kahn, A.; Vaulont, S. Targeted disruption of the hepcidin 1 gene results in severe hemochromatosis. *Blood* **2006**, *108*, 1402–1405. [CrossRef] [PubMed]
2. Deugnier, Y.; Turlin, B. Pathology of hepatic iron overload. *World J. Gastroenterol.* **2007**, *13*, 4755–4760. [CrossRef]
3. Kowdley, K.V. Iron Overload in Patients with Chronic Liver Disease. *Gastroenterol. Hepatol.* **2016**, *12*, 695–698.
4. Feder, J.N.; Gnirke, A.; Thomas, W.; Tsuchihashi, Z.; Ruddy, D.A.; Basava, A.; Dormishian, F.; Domingo, R., Jr.; Ellis, M.C.; Fullan, A.; et al. A novel MHC class I-like gene is mutated in patients with hereditary haemochromatosis. *Nat. Genet.* **1996**, *13*, 399–408. [CrossRef]

5. Levy, J.E.; Jin, O.; Fujiwara, Y.; Kuo, F.; Andrews, N.C. Transferrin receptor is necessary for development of erythrocytes and the nervous system. *Nat. Genet.* **1999**, *21*, 396–399. [CrossRef] [PubMed]
6. Vujic Spasic, M.; Kiss, J.; Herrmann, T.; Galy, B.; Martinache, S.; Stolte, J.; Grone, H.J.; Stremmel, W.; Hentze, M.W.; Muckenthaler, M.U. Hfe acts in hepatocytes to prevent hemochromatosis. *Cell Metab.* **2008**, *7*, 173–178. [CrossRef]
7. Wallace, D.F.; Summerville, L.; Subramaniam, V.N. Targeted disruption of the hepatic transferrin receptor 2 gene in mice leads to iron overload. *Gastroenterology* **2007**, *132*, 301–310. [CrossRef]
8. Wallace, D.F.; Summerville, L.; Crampton, E.M.; Frazer, D.M.; Anderson, G.J.; Subramaniam, V.N. Combined deletion of Hfe and transferrin receptor 2 in mice leads to marked dysregulation of hepcidin and iron overload. *Hepatology* **2009**, *50*, 1992–2000. [CrossRef]
9. Roetto, A.; Daraio, F.; Alberti, F.; Porporato, P.; Cali, A.; De Gobbi, M.; Camaschella, C. Hemochromatosis due to mutations in transferrin receptor 2. *Blood Cells Mol. Dis.* **2002**, *29*, 465–470. [CrossRef]
10. Niederkofler, V.; Salie, R.; Arber, S. Hemojuvelin is essential for dietary iron sensing, and its mutation leads to severe iron overload. *J. Clin. Investig.* **2005**, *115*, 2180–2186. [CrossRef] [PubMed]
11. Babitt, J.L.; Huang, F.W.; Wrighting, D.M.; Xia, Y.; Sidis, Y.; Samad, T.A.; Campagna, J.A.; Chung, R.T.; Schneyer, A.L.; Woolf, C.J.; et al. Bone morphogenetic protein signaling by hemojuvelin regulates hepcidin expression. *Nat. Genet.* **2006**, *38*, 531–539. [CrossRef] [PubMed]
12. Steinbicker, A.U.; Bartnikas, T.B.; Lohmeyer, L.K.; Leyton, P.; Mayeur, C.; Kao, S.M.; Pappas, A.E.; Peterson, R.T.; Bloch, D.B.; Yu, P.B.; et al. Perturbation of hepcidin expression by BMP type I receptor deletion induces iron overload in mice. *Blood* **2011**, *118*, 4224–4230. [CrossRef] [PubMed]
13. Ryan, J.D.; Ryan, E.; Fabre, A.; Lawless, M.W.; Crowe, J. Defective bone morphogenic protein signaling underlies hepcidin deficiency in HFE hereditary hemochromatosis. *Hepatology* **2010**, *52*, 1266–1273. [CrossRef]
14. Corradini, E.; Rozier, M.; Meynard, D.; Odhiambo, A.; Lin, H.Y.; Feng, Q.; Migas, M.C.; Britton, R.S.; Babitt, J.L.; Fleming, R.E. Iron regulation of hepcidin despite attenuated Smad1,5,8 signaling in mice without transferrin receptor 2 or Hfe. *Gastroenterology* **2011**, *141*, 1907–1914. [CrossRef] [PubMed]
15. Vujic Spasic, M.; Sparla, R.; Mleczko-Sanecka, K.; Migas, M.C.; Breitkopf-Heinlein, K.; Dooley, S.; Vaulont, S.; Fleming, R.E.; Muckenthaler, M.U. Smad6 and Smad7 are co-regulated with hepcidin in mouse models of iron overload. *Biochim. Biophys. Acta* **2013**, *1832*, 76–84. [CrossRef] [PubMed]
16. Calzolari, A.; Raggi, C.; Deaglio, S.; Sposi, N.M.; Stafsnes, M.; Fecchi, K.; Parolini, I.; Malavasi, F.; Peschle, C.; Sargiacomo, M.; et al. TfR2 localizes in lipid raft domains and is released in exosomes to activate signal transduction along the MAPK pathway. *J. Cell Sci.* **2006**, *119*, 4486–4498. [CrossRef] [PubMed]
17. Poli, M.; Luscieti, S.; Gandini, V.; Maccarinelli, F.; Finazzi, D.; Silvestri, L.; Roetto, A.; Arosio, P. Transferrin receptor 2 and HFE regulate furin expression via mitogen-activated protein kinase/extracellular signal-regulated kinase (MAPK/Erk) signaling. Implications for transferrin-dependent hepcidin regulation. *Haematologica* **2010**, *95*, 1832–1840. [CrossRef] [PubMed]
18. Ramey, G.; Deschemin, J.C.; Vaulont, S. Cross-talk between the mitogen activated protein kinase and bone morphogenetic protein/hemojuvelin pathways is required for the induction of hepcidin by holotransferrin in primary mouse hepatocytes. *Haematologica* **2009**, *94*, 765–772. [CrossRef]
19. Cargnello, M.; Roux, P.P. Activation and function of the MAPKs and their substrates, the MAPK-activated protein kinases. *Microbiol. Mol. Boil. Rev.* **2011**, *75*, 50–83. [CrossRef] [PubMed]
20. Lawan, A.; Bennett, A.M. Mitogen-Activated Protein Kinase Regulation in Hepatic Metabolism. *Trends Endocrinol. Metab.* **2017**, *28*, 868–878. [CrossRef] [PubMed]
21. Roskoski, R., Jr. ERK1/2 MAP kinases: Structure, function, and regulation. *Pharmacol. Res.* **2012**, *66*, 105–143. [CrossRef] [PubMed]
22. Sabio, G.; Davis, R.J. TNF and MAP kinase signalling pathways. *Semin. Immunol.* **2014**, *26*, 237–245. [CrossRef]
23. Gehart, H.; Kumpf, S.; Ittner, A.; Ricci, R. MAPK signalling in cellular metabolism: Stress or wellness? *EMBO Rep.* **2010**, *11*, 834–840. [CrossRef] [PubMed]
24. Sumara, G.; Formentini, I.; Collins, S.; Sumara, I.; Windak, R.; Bodenmiller, B.; Ramracheya, R.; Caille, D.; Jiang, H.; Platt, K.A.; et al. Regulation of PKD by the MAPK p38delta in insulin secretion and glucose homeostasis. *Cell* **2009**, *136*, 235–248. [CrossRef] [PubMed]
25. Barger, P.M.; Browning, A.C.; Garner, A.N.; Kelly, D.P. p38 mitogen-activated protein kinase activates peroxisome proliferator-activated receptor alpha: A potential role in the cardiac metabolic stress response.

J. Boil. Chem. **2001**, *276*, 44495–44501. [CrossRef]
26. Manieri, E.; Sabio, G. Stress kinases in the modulation of metabolism and energy balance. *J. Mol. Endocrinol.* **2015**, *55*, R11–R22. [CrossRef]
27. Bost, F.; Aouadi, M.; Caron, L.; Binetruy, B. The role of MAPKs in adipocyte differentiation and obesity. *Biochimie* **2005**, *87*, 51–56. [CrossRef] [PubMed]
28. Samuel, V.T.; Shulman, G.I. Nonalcoholic Fatty Liver Disease as a Nexus of Metabolic and Hepatic Diseases. *Cell Metab.* **2018**, *27*, 22–41. [CrossRef] [PubMed]
29. Khan, A.S.; Subramaniam, S.; Dramane, G.; Khelifi, D.; Khan, N.A. ERK1 and ERK2 activation modulates diet-induced obesity in mice. *Biochimie* **2017**, *137*, 78–87. [CrossRef]
30. Kujiraoka, T.; Satoh, Y.; Ayaori, M.; Shiraishi, Y.; Arai-Nakaya, Y.; Hakuno, D.; Yada, H.; Kuwada, N.; Endo, S.; Isoda, K.; et al. Hepatic extracellular signal-regulated kinase 2 suppresses endoplasmic reticulum stress and protects from oxidative stress and endothelial dysfunction. *J. Am. Heart Assoc.* **2013**, *2*, e000361. [CrossRef]
31. Yu, Y.; Richardson, D.R. Cellular iron depletion stimulates the JNK and p38 MAPK signaling transduction pathways, dissociation of ASK1-thioredoxin, and activation of ASK1. *J. Boil. Chem.* **2011**, *286*, 15413–15427. [CrossRef]
32. Chung, J.; Uchida, E.; Grammer, T.C.; Blenis, J. STAT3 serine phosphorylation by ERK-dependent and -independent pathways negatively modulates its tyrosine phosphorylation. *Mol. Cell. Boil.* **1997**, *17*, 6508–6516. [CrossRef]
33. Lunova, M.; Goehring, C.; Kuscuoglu, D.; Mueller, K.; Chen, Y.; Walther, P.; Deschemin, J.C.; Vaulont, S.; Haybaeck, J.; Lackner, C.; et al. Hepcidin knockout mice fed with iron-rich diet develop chronic liver injury and liver fibrosis due to lysosomal iron overload. *J. Hepatol.* **2014**, *61*, 633–641. [CrossRef] [PubMed]
34. Zerrad-Saadi, A.; Lambert-Blot, M.; Mitchell, C.; Bretes, H.; Collin de l'Hortet, A.; Baud, V.; Chereau, F.; Sotiropoulos, A.; Kopchick, J.J.; Liao, L.; et al. GH receptor plays a major role in liver regeneration through the control of EGFR and ERK1/2 activation. *Endocrinology* **2011**, *152*, 2731–2741. [CrossRef]
35. Poli, G.; Schaur, R.J. 4-Hydroxynonenal in the pathomechanisms of oxidative stress. *IUBMB Life* **2000**, *50*, 315–321. [CrossRef] [PubMed]
36. Tsukamoto, H.; Horne, W.; Kamimura, S.; Niemela, O.; Parkkila, S.; Yla-Herttuala, S.; Brittenham, G.M. Experimental liver cirrhosis induced by alcohol and iron. *J. Clin. Investig.* **1995**, *96*, 620–630. [CrossRef]
37. Jazirehi, A.R.; Vega, M.I.; Chatterjee, D.; Goodglick, L.; Bonavida, B. Inhibition of the Raf-MEK1/2-ERK1/2 signaling pathway, Bcl-xL down-regulation, and chemosensitization of non-Hodgkin's lymphoma B cells by Rituximab. *Cancer Res.* **2004**, *64*, 7117–7126. [CrossRef]
38. Rouault, T.A. Hepatic iron overload in alcoholic liver disease: Why does it occur and what is its role in pathogenesis? *Alcohol* **2003**, *30*, 103–106. [CrossRef]
39. Ioannou, G.N.; Dominitz, J.A.; Weiss, N.S.; Heagerty, P.J.; Kowdley, K.V. The effect of alcohol consumption on the prevalence of iron overload, iron deficiency, and iron deficiency anemia. *Gastroenterology* **2004**, *126*, 1293–1301. [CrossRef]
40. Harrison-Findik, D.D.; Klein, E.; Crist, C.; Evans, J.; Timchenko, N.; Gollan, J. Iron-mediated regulation of liver hepcidin expression in rats and mice is abolished by alcohol. *Hepatology* **2007**, *46*, 1979–1985. [CrossRef]
41. Aroor, A.R.; Shukla, S.D. MAP kinase signaling in diverse effects of ethanol. *Life Sci.* **2004**, *74*, 2339–2364. [CrossRef] [PubMed]
42. Sampey, B.P.; Stewart, B.J.; Petersen, D.R. Ethanol-induced modulation of hepatocellular extracellular signal-regulated kinase-1/2 activity via 4-hydroxynonenal. *J. Boil. Chem.* **2007**, *282*, 1925–1937. [CrossRef] [PubMed]
43. Chen, J.; Ishac, E.J.; Dent, P.; Kunos, G.; Gao, B. Effects of ethanol on mitogen-activated protein kinase and stress-activated protein kinase cascades in normal and regenerating liver. *Biochem. J.* **1998**, *334 Pt 3*, 669–676. [CrossRef]
44. Marmur, J.; Beshara, S.; Eggertsen, G.; Onelov, L.; Albiin, N.; Danielsson, O.; Hultcrantz, R.; Stal, P. Hepcidin levels correlate to liver iron content, but not steatohepatitis, in non-alcoholic fatty liver disease. *BMC Gastroenterol.* **2018**, *18*, 78. [CrossRef] [PubMed]
45. Datz, C.; Felder, T.K.; Niederseer, D.; Aigner, E. Iron homeostasis in the metabolic syndrome. *Eur. J. Clin. Investig.* **2013**, *43*, 215–224. [CrossRef]
46. Kowdley, K.V.; Belt, P.; Wilson, L.A.; Yeh, M.M.; Neuschwander-Tetri, B.A.; Chalasani, N.; Sanyal, A.J.; Nelson, J.E.; Network, N.C.R. Serum ferritin is an independent predictor of histologic severity and advanced fibrosis in patients with nonalcoholic fatty liver disease. *Hepatology* **2012**, *55*, 77–85. [CrossRef] [PubMed]

47. Nelson, J.E.; Klintworth, H.; Kowdley, K.V. Iron metabolism in Nonalcoholic Fatty Liver Disease. *Curr. Gastroenterol. Rep.* **2012**, *14*, 8–16. [CrossRef]
48. Younossi, Z.; Henry, L. Contribution of Alcoholic and Nonalcoholic Fatty Liver Disease to the Burden of Liver-Related Morbidity and Mortality. *Gastroenterology* **2016**, *150*, 1778–1785. [CrossRef]
49. Ma, C.; Zhang, Q.; Greten, T.F. Nonalcoholic fatty liver disease promotes hepatocellular carcinoma through direct and indirect effects on hepatocytes. *FEBS J.* **2018**, *285*, 752–762. [CrossRef]
50. Michelotti, G.A.; Machado, M.V.; Diehl, A.M. NAFLD, NASH and liver cancer. *Nat. Rev. Gastroenterol. Hepatol.* **2013**, *10*, 656–665. [CrossRef]
51. Fracanzani, A.L.; Valenti, L.; Bugianesi, E.; Vanni, E.; Grieco, A.; Miele, L.; Consonni, D.; Fatta, E.; Lombardi, R.; Marchesini, G.; et al. Risk of nonalcoholic steatohepatitis and fibrosis in patients with nonalcoholic fatty liver disease and low visceral adiposity. *J. Hepatol.* **2011**, *54*, 1244–1249. [CrossRef] [PubMed]
52. Manousou, P.; Kalambokis, G.; Grillo, F.; Watkins, J.; Xirouchakis, E.; Pleguezuelo, M.; Leandro, G.; Arvaniti, V.; Germani, G.; Patch, D.; et al. Serum ferritin is a discriminant marker for both fibrosis and inflammation in histologically proven non-alcoholic fatty liver disease patients. *Liver Int.* **2011**, *31*, 730–739. [CrossRef] [PubMed]
53. Fujita, N.; Sugimoto, R.; Takeo, M.; Urawa, N.; Mifuji, R.; Tanaka, H.; Kobayashi, Y.; Iwasa, M.; Watanabe, S.; Adachi, Y.; et al. Hepcidin expression in the liver: Relatively low level in patients with chronic hepatitis C. *Mol. Med.* **2007**, *13*, 97–104. [CrossRef] [PubMed]
54. Nishina, S.; Hino, K.; Korenaga, M.; Vecchi, C.; Pietrangelo, A.; Mizukami, Y.; Furutani, T.; Sakai, A.; Okuda, M.; Hidaka, I.; et al. Hepatitis C virus-induced reactive oxygen species raise hepatic iron level in mice by reducing hepcidin transcription. *Gastroenterology* **2008**, *134*, 226–238. [CrossRef]

Permissions

All chapters in this book were first published by MDPI; hereby published with permission under the Creative Commons Attribution License or equivalent. Every chapter published in this book has been scrutinized by our experts. Their significance has been extensively debated. The topics covered herein carry significant findings which will fuel the growth of the discipline. They may even be implemented as practical applications or may be referred to as a beginning point for another development.

The contributors of this book come from diverse backgrounds, making this book a truly international effort. This book will bring forth new frontiers with its revolutionizing research information and detailed analysis of the nascent developments around the world.

We would like to thank all the contributing authors for lending their expertise to make the book truly unique. They have played a crucial role in the development of this book. Without their invaluable contributions this book wouldn't have been possible. They have made vital efforts to compile up to date information on the varied aspects of this subject to make this book a valuable addition to the collection of many professionals and students.

This book was conceptualized with the vision of imparting up-to-date information and advanced data in this field. To ensure the same, a matchless editorial board was set up. Every individual on the board went through rigorous rounds of assessment to prove their worth. After which they invested a large part of their time researching and compiling the most relevant data for our readers.

The editorial board has been involved in producing this book since its inception. They have spent rigorous hours researching and exploring the diverse topics which have resulted in the successful publishing of this book. They have passed on their knowledge of decades through this book. To expedite this challenging task, the publisher supported the team at every step. A small team of assistant editors was also appointed to further simplify the editing procedure and attain best results for the readers.

Apart from the editorial board, the designing team has also invested a significant amount of their time in understanding the subject and creating the most relevant covers. They scrutinized every image to scout for the most suitable representation of the subject and create an appropriate cover for the book.

The publishing team has been an ardent support to the editorial, designing and production team. Their endless efforts to recruit the best for this project, has resulted in the accomplishment of this book. They are a veteran in the field of academics and their pool of knowledge is as vast as their experience in printing. Their expertise and guidance has proved useful at every step. Their uncompromising quality standards have made this book an exceptional effort. Their encouragement from time to time has been an inspiration for everyone.

The publisher and the editorial board hope that this book will prove to be a valuable piece of knowledge for researchers, students, practitioners and scholars across the globe.

List of Contributors

George J. Kontoghiorghes and Christina N. Kontoghiorghe
Postgraduate Research Institute of Science, Technology, Environment and Medicine, CY-3021 Limassol, Cyprus

Brian Chiou and James R. Connor
Department of Neurosurgery, Penn State College of Medicine, Hershey, PA 17033, USA

Fadi Bou-Abdallah and John J. Paliakkara
Department of Chemistry, State University of New York at Potsdam, Potsdam, NY 13676, USA

József Balla
HAS-UD Vascular Biology and Myocardial Pathophysiology Research Group, Hungarian Academy of Sciences, H-4032 Debrecen, Hungary
Division of Nephrology, Department of Medicine, Faculty of Medicine, University of Debrecen, H-4032 Debrecen, Hungary

György Balla
HAS-UD Vascular Biology and Myocardial Pathophysiology Research Group, Hungarian Academy of Sciences, H-4032 Debrecen, Hungary
Department of Pediatrics, Faculty of Medicine, University of Debrecen, H-4032 Debrecen, Hungary

Abolfazl Zarjou
Department of Medicine, University of Alabama at Birmingham, Birmingham, AL 35294, USA
Nephrology Research and Training Center, University of Alabama at Birmingham, Birmingham, AL 35294, USA

Laura E. Diepeveen, Coby M. Laarakkers, Antonius E. van Herwaarden and Rachel P.L. van Swelm
Department of Laboratory Medicine, Radboud University Medical Center, 6525 Nijmegen, The Netherlands

DorineW. Swinkels
Department of Laboratory Medicine, Radboud University Medical Center, 6525 Nijmegen, The Netherlands
Department of Laboratory Medicine, Translational Metabolic Laboratory, Radboud University Medical Center, 6500 HB Nijmegen, The Netherlands

Hanka Venselaar
Centre for Molecular and Biomolecular Informatics, Radboud Institute for Molecular Life Sciences, Radboud, University Medical Center, 6500 HB Nijmegen, The Netherlands

Edouard Bardou-Jacquet
Liver Diseases Department, French Reference Centre for Rare Iron Overload Diseases of Genetic Origin, University Hospital Pontchaillou, 35033 Rennes, France

Hans Groenewoud and Joanna IntHout
Department of Health Evidence, Radboud University Medical Center, 6525 Nijmegen, The Netherlands

Jack F. Wetzels
Department of Nephrology, Radboud University Medical Center, 6525 Nijmegen, The Netherlands

Robert R. Crichton
Faculty of Science, Universite catholique de Louvain, 1348 Louvain-la-Neuve, Belgium

Roberta J. Ward
Division of Brain Sciences, Imperial College, London W12 ONN, UK

Robert C. Hider
Institute of Pharmaceutical Science, King's College London, London SE1 9NH, UK

Xuejiao Sha, Hai Chen, Jingsheng Zhang and Guanghua Zhao
Beijing Advanced Innovation Center for Food Nutrition and Human Health, College of Food Science and Nutritional Engineering, Beijing Key Laboratory of Functional Food from Plant Resources, China Agricultural University, Beijing 100083, China

Olivier Loréal, Thibault Cavey, François Robin, Moussa Kenawi, Pascal Guggenbuhl and Pierre Brissot
INSERM, Univ Rennes, INRA, CHU Rennes, Institut NUMECAN (Nutrition Metabolisms and Cancer), F-35033 Rennes, France

David Alsina, Rosa Purroy, Joaquim Ros and Jordi Tamarit
Departament de Ciències Mèdiques Bàsiques, IRBLleida, Universitat de Lleida, 25198 Lleida, Spain

Roel Janssen
Department of Laboratory Medicine, Translational Metabolic Laboratory, Radboud University Medical Center, 6500 HB Nijmegen, The Netherlands

Hilde P.E. Peters
Department of Nephrology, Isala Hospital, 8025 Zwolle, The Netherlands

Houda Hamdi-Roze
Molecular Genetics Department, French Reference Centre for Rare Iron Overload Diseases of Genetic Origin, University Hospital Pontchaillou, 35033 Rennes, France

Hal Drakesmith
MRC Human Immunology Unit,Weatherall Institute of Molecular Medicine, University of Oxford, Oxford OX39DS, UK

Veronica Fiorito, Deborah Chiabrando and Emanuela Tolosano
Department of Molecular Biotechnology and Health Sciences, Molecular Biotechnology Center, University of Torino, 10126 Torino, Italy

Mayra Vera-Aviles, Eleni Vantana, Emmy Kardinasari, Ngat L. Koh and Gladys O. Latunde-Dada
King's College London, Department of Nutritional Sciences, Faculty of Life Sciences and Medicine, Franklin-Wilkins Building, 150 Stamford Street, London SE1 9NH, UK

Galina Melman and Artem Melman
Department of Chemistry & Biomolecular Science, Clarkson University, Potsdam, NY 13699, USA

Naveen Kumar Tangudu, Nils Buth, Ion C. Cirstea and Maja Vujić Spasić
Institute of Comparative Molecular Endocrinology, University of Ulm, Ulm 89081, Germany

Pavel Strnad
Department of Medicine III and IZKF, University Hospital Aachen, Aachen 52074, Germany

Index

A

Acute Kidney Injury, 76-77, 83-86, 216

Antioxidants, 1, 24, 26-27, 30, 33, 39, 41, 70, 74, 114, 125, 145, 153, 200, 209, 218

B

Basal Ganglia, 40, 53

Beta Globin, 4

Binding Ability, 116

Biomarker, 44, 52-54, 61, 95, 114, 208-209, 217

C

Cancer Cells, 2, 19, 25-27, 29, 44, 49, 55, 58-59

Cardiac Hypertrophy, 146-147, 153

Chaotropes, 62, 67-68, 73

Chelate Ligands, 64, 70, 73

Chelation, 1, 10-21, 24-26, 28-30, 34-35, 37, 40-43, 52, 66, 72-73, 78-79, 103-112, 114-115, 119, 125, 131, 147, 153-154, 179, 211

Chelators, 1-3, 8-23, 25-29, 31, 34-43, 64, 70-71, 74, 103-112, 117, 121, 131, 140, 147, 149-150, 212

Chronic Kidney Disease, 59, 76, 78, 83-84, 87, 102, 205-206, 212-217, 219

Cinnamic Acid Derivatives, 116-125

Cisplatin, 39, 68, 74, 79

Collagen Synthesis, 5

D

Diffusion Mechanism, 66, 68

Drug Delivery, 44, 48, 58

Drug Hydroxyurea, 22, 27

E

Electron Transfer, 6, 62-63, 67, 69-71, 74, 193

F

Ferritin, 3, 5, 7-9, 12-13, 16-21, 23, 29, 32-33, 36-38, 42, 44-77, 79-84, 86, 88, 105-108, 112-113, 116-125, 129, 132, 136, 138-139, 142-143, 146, 150, 155-159, 163, 165-168, 172, 174-176, 178, 183, 195, 206, 209, 214, 216-217, 230, 233

Ferritin Molecule, 50, 63, 116, 119

Ferrochelatase, 144, 151, 196

Ferroportin, 5, 7, 78-79, 81, 85, 90, 100-101, 126-127, 129, 131-134, 139, 146, 155-157, 159-160, 163-183, 195, 206-207, 215

Fibroblasts, 53, 60, 145-146, 151, 193, 202

Frataxin Deficiency, 140, 142, 144-149, 152-154, 196

Frataxin Deficient Yeast, 142, 145, 147

Frataxin-deficient Cells, 140, 144-145, 148

Friedreich's Ataxia, 17, 20-21, 24-25, 28-29, 36, 52-53, 110, 115, 140, 142, 149, 151-154, 195

G

Genetic Hemochromatosis, 126, 128-129, 131, 136-138

H

Heme Groups, 63, 144

Heme Metabolism, 184-185, 187, 191-194

Hemochromatosis, 1-2, 4, 7, 16, 29, 45, 51, 55, 78, 81, 86, 89, 96, 101, 103, 105, 113, 126, 128-139, 155-156, 175-181, 220, 231-232

Hemoglobin, 3-5, 8, 12-14, 17, 22, 31-32, 36-38, 40-42, 79, 85-86, 101, 126, 131-132, 139, 156, 158, 184, 187, 195, 197, 205, 207, 214-215

Hepcidin, 5, 7, 59, 78-79, 81, 85-87, 89-91, 93-98, 100-102, 126-129, 131-139, 155-157, 160-162, 164-177, 179-183, 206-207, 214-215, 220-221, 224, 227, 230-234

Hepcidin Deficiency, 126, 129, 132-133, 232

Hepcidin Protein, 90-91

Hippocampal Neurons, 53, 184

Horse Spleen Ferritin, 65-67, 69, 73

Hydroxide Core, 63-65, 68, 71

I

Intact Ferritin, 62, 64

Intracellular Concentration, 69, 210

Iron Accumulation, 14, 24-25, 35-36, 38, 40, 42, 53, 60, 72, 81, 103, 105-108, 113, 126, 128-129, 139, 145-149, 153, 155-156, 180

Iron Cations, 62-64, 66, 70-71, 76-78, 81

Iron Chelators, 12, 26-27, 31, 34, 36-37, 39-41, 74, 103-109, 111-112, 117, 121, 131, 140, 147, 149-150

Iron Deficiency Anemia, 7, 14, 16, 19, 28-29, 35, 43, 51, 55, 59, 61, 116, 173, 180, 182, 206, 214, 216, 233

Iron Delivery, 16, 20-21, 28, 44-46, 54, 57, 144, 151, 196

Iron Depletive Treatment, 126, 130-133

Iron Excretion, 11-14, 105, 132

Iron Homeostasis, 2, 7, 30, 32, 38, 40, 44, 52, 54-55, 59, 61, 72, 78, 83, 85-86, 90, 109-110, 127, 133, 135, 140, 142, 145-149, 152, 176, 181-182, 191, 195, 216-217, 233

Iron Metabolism, 1, 7-9, 14, 16-17, 20, 22-23, 26, 32-33, 37, 42, 55, 59-60, 76, 78, 80, 84-85, 87, 90, 96, 100, 102, 110, 114-115, 126, 132-136, 138-139, 142, 181-182, 197, 202, 207, 209, 219, 234

Iron Mobilization, 12, 17-20, 27, 37, 62, 64-66, 68-71, 112, 125, 131

Iron Overload, 1, 13-16, 19-21, 23, 25, 28-29, 31-37, 40-41, 45-46, 60, 70, 74, 77, 81, 88, 103, 105-106, 110-113, 126, 128-129, 131-132, 134-139, 146-147, 155-156, 158-159, 166-168, 202, 208-209, 211, 213-214, 217, 220-222, 224, 227-228, 230-233

Iron Proteins, 1, 3, 7, 22, 62

Iron Reductive Mobilization, 62, 64, 67, 69

Iron Release, 17, 20-21, 42, 47, 57, 63, 65-68, 70, 73-74, 116-119, 121-125, 127-128, 132, 173, 206

Iron Release Rates, 65, 67

Iron-sulfur Deficiency, 145, 148, 154

K

Kidney Injury, 76-80, 83-86, 101, 216

Kinetics, 62, 65, 67, 70, 73, 101, 112, 119, 125

L

Loss Of Function, 155, 160, 175, 179

Lysosomes, 56, 64, 79

M

Mitochondria, 4, 6, 20-21, 31-33, 44-45, 48, 57, 69, 77-78, 110, 115, 130, 142-143, 145, 147, 151-152, 184, 187-194, 198-203, 205, 208, 210, 217

N

Nanocage, 33, 44, 49, 58, 63, 72, 74

Nephrotoxicity, 55, 78-79, 85, 216

Neurodegeneration, 1, 14, 24-25, 27-29, 35, 42, 45, 53-55, 60-61, 114, 146-147, 149, 153, 184-185, 187-191, 193-195, 198, 200-203

Neurodegenerative Diseases, 12, 28, 38, 53, 55, 103-104, 110-111, 184, 187, 190-191, 193-195, 198-201

Neuroferritinopathy, 53, 60

Non Transferrin Bound Iron, 111, 126

O

Oxidative Stress, 1-2, 24, 29-31, 39-43, 52-54, 61, 78-79, 86, 106, 109, 115, 130, 136, 140, 142, 145, 147-148, 152-153, 184-185, 189-191, 197, 199, 205-211, 213, 216-219, 227, 233

P

Parkinson's Disease, 35, 40, 42, 53, 55, 60-61, 103, 107-108, 111, 113-114, 197-203

Pathophysiology, 38, 51, 60-61, 76, 87, 128-129, 140, 145-147, 174-175, 177, 195

Peritoneal Dialysis, 90-91, 100-102

Pituitary, 103-107, 113

Plasma Catalytic Iron Cation, 78

Protein Binding, 90-91, 95-96

Proximal Tubule, 79, 83-85

R

Reactive Oxygen Species, 2, 29, 44, 52, 129, 137, 145-146, 149, 188, 190, 198, 200, 203, 205, 234

Reduced Flavins, 64-67, 69, 71, 73

Reducing Agents, 12, 62, 64, 66, 69, 71

Ribonucleotide Reductase, 5-6, 12, 17, 22-23, 27, 32, 38

S

Sickle Cell Disease, 4, 30, 38, 103, 220

Soybean Seed Ferritin, 116-119, 123-124

Systemic Inflammation, 79, 130

T

Thalassemia Patients, 4, 13-14, 24, 28, 36, 38, 42, 105-106, 113

Transferrin Receptors, 17, 20, 23, 27, 32, 220

V

Vascular Calcification, 76-77, 80, 87-88, 205, 209, 217

www.ingramcontent.com/pod-product-compliance
Lightning Source LLC
LaVergne TN
LVHW060511210926
848485LV00005B/1062